Carol —
240-1986

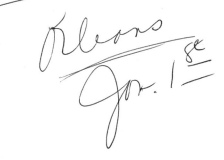
Kleans
Jan. 1st

294-1746 — Plymouth

FERMIN A. CARRANZA, Jr., Dr. Odont.

Professor and Chairman, Section of Periodontology
School of Dentistry, Center for the Health Sciences
Member, Dental Research Institute and
Clinical Research Center for Periodontal Disease
University of California, Los Angeles

DOROTHY A. PERRY, R.D.H., Ph.D.

Adjunct Assistant Professor, Section of Periodontology
School of Dentistry, Center for the Health Sciences
Member, Clinical Research Center for Periodontal Disease
University of California, Los Angeles

Clinical Periodontology for the Dental Hygienist

W. B. SAUNDERS COMPANY

Philadelphia   London   Toronto   Mexico City
Rio de Janeiro   Sydney   Tokyo   Hong Kong

W.B. SAUNDERS COMPANY
A Division of
Harcourt Brace & Company

The Curtis Center
Independence Square West
Philadelphia, Pennsylvania 19106

Library of Congress Cataloging-in-Publication Data
Carranza, Fermin A.
Clinical periodontology for the dental hygienist.
1. Periodontics.   2. Dental hygienists.   I. Perry, Dorothy A.   II. Title. [DNLM: 1. Dental Hygienists. 2. Periodontal Diseases. WU 240 C312c]
RK361.C37 1986   617.6'32   85-19625
ISBN 0-7216-1352-7

Listed here is the latest translated edition of this book together with the language of the translation and the publisher.

Spanish—*1st edition*—Nueva Editorial Interamericana, Mexico D.F., Mexico

Editor: Darlene Pedersen
Designer: Bill Donnelly
Production Manager: Laura Tarves
Manuscript Editor: Kate Mason
Page Layout Artist: Bill Donnelly
Indexer: Kate Mason

Clinical Periodontology for the Dental Hygienist   ISBN   0-7216-1352-7

Last digit is the print number.   9   8   7

Preface

The treatment of periodontal disease in the United States is in the hands of a team of professionals composed of general dentists, dental hygienists, and periodontists. The role of the dental hygienist is centered around instrumentation of root surfaces, maintenance care, and prevention; therefore a basic knowledge of clinical periodontology, including concepts of diagnosis and various therapeutic modalities, is essential to render high-quality care.

The last two editions of *Glickman's Clinical Periodontology* by Fermin A. Carranza, Jr. frequently have been adopted for dental hygiene courses. However, the author was repeatedly asked to prepare a shorter, more concise version that would contain the material of interest to the dental hygienist.

To produce this shorter version of the book, the senior author was fortunate to obtain the invaluable help of Dr. Dorothy A. Perry, a dental hygienist with a Ph.D. in education, whose greatest interest lies in the areas of teaching and clinical research.

This version was developed by rewriting material and omitting some topics that are not essential to the practice of dental hygiene. Great effort was made to retain all the clinically and conceptually relevant information.

A few words are in order with reference to the techniques of periodontal instrumentation. This area is of prime interest to the dental hygienist and would actually require an expansion of the information as it appears in *Glickman's Clinical Periodontology*. We chose to emphasize the conceptual aspects of periodontology and refer the students to other texts devoted entirely to the extensive and more technical subject of periodontal instrumentation.

The book covers two areas. The first deals with basic concepts of periodontal pathology and etiology, the second with clinical examination and therapeutic techniques. To perform a diagnosis, the dentist often relies on the hygienist for gathering relevant data and information; we attempted to emphasize this aspect of responsibility. Various modalities of periodontal surgery are briefly presented but retain the concepts and steps of interest to the hygienist as a surgical assistant and sometimes as the person in charge of postoperative care. This information is also valuable for an understanding of the benefits of surgical procedures in the continuum of care from Phase I therapy to maintenance care.

The authors are indebted to the contributors of the original book who generated information used for this version. In some cases their work was included with only minor changes because the subject matter required an in-depth presentation for the dental hygienist; other chapters were completely rewritten. We are glad to mention the following original collaborators whose efforts were essential for this book: Robert L. Merin (maintenance phase and results of treatment), Michael G. Newman (microbiology), Russell J. Nisengard (host response), Joan Ann Otomo (systemically compromised patients),

F. Reinaldo Saglie (normal gingiva and microbiology), Max O. Schmid (phase I therapy), Gerald Shklar (desquamative gingivitis), Thomas N. Sims (osseous surgery), William K. Solberg (occlusion), Vladimir W. Spolsky (epidemiology), and Henry H. Takei (flap surgery).

The authors also wish to acknowledge the excellent secretarial assistance of Marsha Hood and Angela Wong and the cooperation of many individuals in the W. B. Saunders Co., particularly Robert Reinhardt, Dental Editor. The W. B. Saunders Co. was extremely understanding and helpful in our effort to transcribe the "big" book onto computer disks and prepare this version directly on the text processor. Our task was eased by this electronic help.

Our families shared the load that preparing this book entailed, including not only the physical but the emotional strains involved. We wish to acknowledge the support of Rita Carranza and Bob Perry in our endeavors.

FERMIN A. CARRANZA, JR.

DOROTHY A. PERRY

Contents

Chapter 1

The Tissues of the Periodontium

The periodontium consists of the investing and supporting tissues of the tooth (gingiva, periodontal ligament, cementum and alveolar bone). The cementum is considered a part of the periodontium because, with the bone, it serves as the support for the fibers of the periodontal ligament. The periodontium is subject to morphologic and functional variations, as well as changes associated with age. This chapter deals with the normal features of the tissues of the periodontium, knowledge of which is necessary for an understanding of periodontal disease.

THE GINGIVA

The *oral mucosa* consists of three zones: the gingiva and the covering of the hard palate, termed the *masticatory mucosa*; the dorsum of the tongue, covered by *specialized mucosa*; and the *oral mucous membrane* lining the remainder of the oral cavity. *The gingiva is the part of the oral mucosa that covers the alveolar processes of the jaws and surrounds the necks of the teeth.*

Normal Clinical Features

The gingiva is divided anatomically into the marginal gingiva forming the gingival sulcus; the attached gingiva; and the interdental gingiva.

Marginal Gingiva (Unattached or Free Gingiva)

The marginal (unattached or free) gingiva is the terminal edge or border of the gingiva surrounding the teeth in a collar-like fashion (Figs. 1–1 and 1–2). In about 50 per cent of cases it is demarcated from the adjacent attached gingiva by a shallow linear depression, the *free gingival groove*. Usually about 1 mm wide, this groove forms the soft tissue wall of the *gingival sulcus*. The sulcus may be separated from the tooth surface with a periodontal probe.

Gingival Sulcus

The gingival sulcus is the shallow crevice or space around the tooth bounded by the surface of the tooth on one side and the epithelium lining

1

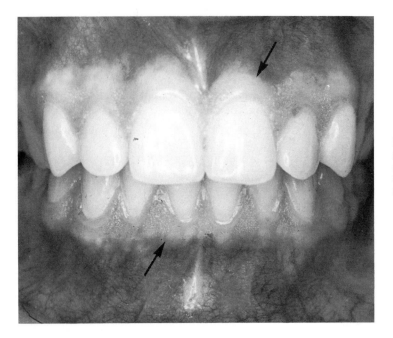

Figure 1–1. Normal gingiva in young adult. Note the demarcation (mucogingival line) *(arrows)* between the attached gingiva and darker alveolar mucosa.

the free margin of the gingiva on the other. It barely permits the entrance of a periodontal probe.

Sulcus depth is found in clinically healthy gingiva in man and animals. The depth of the gingival sulcus as determined in histologic sections has been reported as 1.5 to 1.8 mm, with variations from 0 to 6 mm.[35] Periodontal probes are used to determine the clinical depth of the sulcus. It should be clearly understood that the *histologic depth* of a sulcus need not be and is not exactly equal to the depth of penetration of the probe. The *probing depth* of the clinically normal gingival sulcus in man is 2 to 3 mm, because the probe will penetrate the epithelial lining of the sulcus.

Attached Gingiva

The *attached gingiva* is continuous with the marginal gingiva. It is firm, resilient, and tightly bound to the underlying periosteum of alveolar bone. The facial aspect of the attached gingiva extends to the relatively loose and movable alveolar mucosa, from which it is demarcated by the *mucogingival junction*.

The width of the attached gingiva is the distance between the mucogingival junction and the projection on the external surface of the bottom of the gingival sulcus or the periodontal pocket. It should not be confused with the width of the keratinized gingiva because the attached gingiva does not include the marginal (free) gingiva.

The width of the attached gingiva on the facial aspect differs in different areas of the mouth.[9] It is generally greatest in the incisor region (3.5 to 4.5 mm in the maxilla and 3.3 to 3.9 mm in the mandible) and less in the

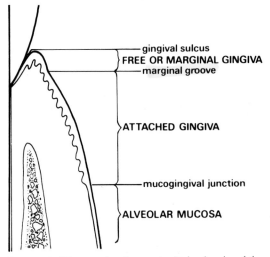

gingival sulcus
FREE OR MARGINAL GINGIVA
marginal groove

ATTACHED GINGIVA

mucogingival junction

ALVEOLAR MUCOSA

Figure 1–2. Diagram showing anatomic landmarks of the gingiva.

posterior segments, with the least width in the first premolar area (1.9 mm in the maxilla and 1.8 mm in the mandible).[3] The mucogingival junction remains stationary throughout adult life, and changes in the width of the attached gingiva are due to modifications in the position of its coronal end. In the absence of pathology, the width of the attached gingiva increases with age and in supraerupted teeth.[2] On the lingual aspect of the mandible, the attached gingiva terminates at the junction with the lingual alveolar mucosa, which is continuous with the mucous membrane lining the floor of the mouth. The palatal surface of the attached gingiva in the maxilla blends imperceptibly with the equally firm, resilient palatal mucosa.

Interdental Gingiva

The *interdental gingiva* occupies the gingival embrasure, which is the interproximal space beneath the area of tooth contact. It usually consists of two papillae, one facial and one lingual, and the *col*.[16] The col is a valley-like depression which connects the papillae and conforms to the shape of the interproximal contact area. When teeth are not in contact, the col is often absent. Even when teeth are in contact, the col may be absent in some individuals (Fig. 1–3). Each interdental papilla is pyramidal; the facial and lingual surfaces are tapered toward the interproximal contact area, and the mesial and distal surfaces are slightly concave. The lateral borders and tip of the interdental papillae are formed by a continuation of the marginal gingiva from the adjacent teeth. The intervening portion consists of attached gingiva.

In the absence of proximal tooth contact, the gingiva is firmly bound over the interdental bone and forms a smooth, rounded surface without interdental papillae.

Normal Microscopic Features

The gingiva consists of a central core of connective tissue covered by stratified squamous epithelium.

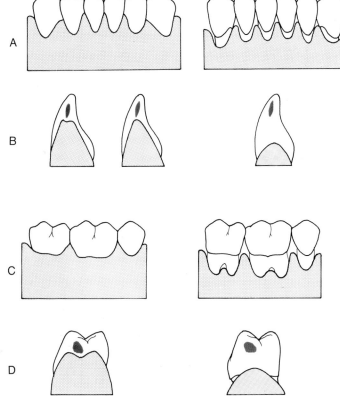

Figure 1–3. Diagram comparing anatomic variations of the interdental col in the normal gingiva *(left side)* and after gingival recession *(right side)*. A and B, Mandibular anterior segment, facial and buccolingual views, respectively. C and D, Mandibular posterior region, facial and buccolingual views, respectively. Tooth contact points are shown in *B* and *D*.

Gingival Epithelium

The gingival epithelium is made up of three areas: the oral or outer epithelium, the sulcular epithelium, and the junctional epithelium.

The *oral or outer epithelium* covers the crest and outer surface of the marginal gingiva and the surface of the attached gingiva. It consists of keratinized or parakeratinized stratified squamous epithelium.

The *sulcular epithelium* lines the gingival sulcus. It is a thin, nonkeratinized stratified squamous epithelium without rete pegs and

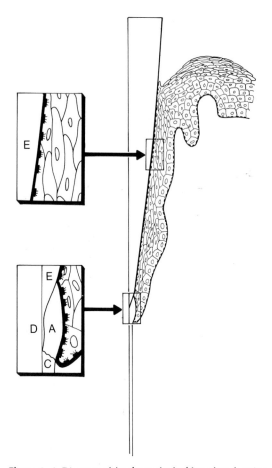

Figure 1–4. Diagram of the **dentogingival junction** showing the junctional epithelium adhering to the tooth surface. At upper left, an enlarged view of epithelial cells showing hemidesmosomes in those cells along the enamel (E) surface. Intervening between the epithelial cells and the enamel are the basal lamina and dental cuticle, respectively; both of these structures are represented by the single, thick line along the enamel. At lower left, an enlarged view of the cemento-enamel junction showing a small area of afibrillar cementum (A). C, cementum; D, dentin.

extends from the coronal limit of the junctional epithelium to the crest of the gingival margin. This epithelium is not normally keratinized. The sulcular epithelium is extremely important, because it may act as a semipermeable membrane through which injurious bacterial products pass into the gingiva and tissue fluid from the gingiva seeps into the sulcus.[45]

The *junctional epithelium* consists of a collarlike band of stratified squamous nonkeratinizing epithelium. It is three to four cell layers thick in early life, but the number of layers increases with age to 10 or even 20; its length ranges from 0.25 to 1.35 mm.

The attachment of the junctional epithelium to the tooth consists of a basal lamina (basement membrane)[29] that is comparable to that which attaches epithelium to connective tissue elsewhere in the body (Fig. 1–4). The basal lamina consists of a lamina densa (adjacent to the enamel) and a lamina lucida to which hemidesmosomes are attached.

The attachment of the junctional epithelium to the tooth is reinforced by the gingival fibers, which brace the marginal gingiva against the tooth surface. For this reason the junctional epithelium and the gingival fibers are a functional unit, referred to as the *dentogingival unit*.

Keratinization. Three types of surface differentiation can occur in gingival epithelium. (1) *Keratinization*, in which the surface cells form scales of keratin and lose their nuclei. Keratohyaline granules appear in the subsurface layer (granular layer or stratum granulosum). (2) *Parakeratinization*, in which the cells of the superficial layers retain their nuclei, albeit pyknotic, but show some signs of being keratinized; the granular layer is absent. (3) *Nonkeratinization*, in which the cells of the surface layers are nucleated and no signs of keratinization are present.

The epithelium covering the outer surface of the marginal gingiv~ and the attached gingiva is keratinized or parakeratinized or presents varied combinations of both conditions.[39] The most prevalent type of surface in this area is parakeratinization.[47] Keratinization is greatest on the palate followed by the gingiva, tongue, and cheek which is the least keratinized.

The gingival sulcular epithelium is normally nonkeratinized. However, it has the potential to keratinize if (1) it is reflected and exposed to the oral cavity[10, 12] or (2) the bacterial flora of the sulcus is eliminated. These findings suggest that the local irritation of the sulcus prevents sulcular keratinization.

Furthermore, research on free gingival grafts has shown that when connective tissue is transplanted from a keratinized area to a nonkeratinized area it becomes covered by keratinized epithelium.[25] This finding suggests a connective tissue–based genetic determination of the type of epithelial surface.

Renewal of Gingival Epithelium. The oral epithelium undergoes continuous *renewal*. Its thickness is maintained by a balance between new cell formation in the basal and spinous layers and the shedding of old cells at the surface. The mitotic rate is higher in nonkeratinized areas and is increased in gingivitis. The following turnover times have been reported for different areas of the oral epithelium in experimental animals: gingiva, 10 to 12 days; and junctional epithelium, 1 to 6 days.[43]

Gingival Fluid (Sulcular Fluid). Gingival or sulcular fluid seeps into the sulcus from the gingival connective tissue through the thin sulcular wall.[11, 15, 30] It is believed to (1) cleanse material from the sulcus, (2) contain plasma proteins which may improve adhesion of the epithelial attachment to the tooth, (3) possess antimicrobial properties, and (4) exert antibody activity in defense of the gingiva.

Gingival Connective Tissue

The connective tissue of the gingiva is known as the *lamina propria*. It is densely collagenous with few elastic fibers.

Gingival Fibers. The connective tissue of the marginal gingiva is densely collagenous, containing a prominent system of collagen fiber bundles called the *gingival fibers*. The gingival fibers have the following functions: (1) to brace the marginal gingiva firmly against the tooth, (2) to provide the rigidity necessary to withstand the forces of mastication without being deflected away from the tooth surface, and (3) to unite the free marginal gingiva with the cementum of the root and the adjacent attached gingiva. The gingival fibers are arranged in three groups: gingivodental, circular, and transseptal.[4, 28]

The *gingivodental group* of fibers are on the facial, lingual, and interproximal surfaces.

They are embedded in the cementum just beneath the epithelium at the base of the gingival sulcus and spread to the surface of the marginal gingiva and the periosteum of the facial and lingual alveolar bone and extend toward the crest of the interdental gingiva (Fig. 1–5).

The *circular group* of fibers course through the connective tissue of the marginal and interdental gingiva and encircle the tooth in ring-like fashion.

The *transseptal fibers* are located interproximally and form horizontal bundles that extend between the cementum of approximating teeth into which they are embedded.

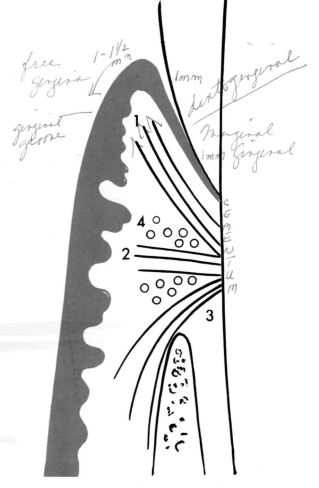

Figure 1–5. Diagrammatic illustration of the **gingivodental fibers** extending from the cementum (1) to the crest of the gingiva, (2) to the outer surface, and (3) external to the periosteum of the labial plate. Circular fibers (4) are shown in cross section.

Connective Tissue Cellular Elements. The preponderant cellular element in the gingival connective tissue is the *fibroblast*. Numerous fibroblasts are found between the fiber bundles. As in connective tissue elsewhere in the body, fibroblasts synthesize and secrete the collagen fibers, as well as elastin, the noncollagenous proteins, glycoproteins, and glycosaminoglycans. Mast cells, which are distributed throughout the body, are numerous in the connective tissue of the oral mucosa and the gingiva.[13]

In clinically normal gingiva, small foci of *plasma cells* and *lymphocytes* are found in the connective tissue near the base of the sulcus. *Neutrophils* can be seen in relatively high numbers in both the gingival connective tissue and the sulcus. Their presence is believed to be related to the penetration of antigenic substances from the oral cavity via the sulcular and junctional epithelia. However, *in spite of the frequency of their occurrence, the inflammatory infiltrate cells are not a normal component of the gingival tissue.*

Blood Supply, Lymphatics, and Nerves. There are three sources of blood supply to the gingiva: (1) *Supraperiosteal arterioles* along the facial and lingual surfaces of the alveolar bone (Fig. 1–6), from which capillaries extend along the sulcular epithelium and between the rete pegs of the external gingival surface.[26] (2) *Vessels of the periodontal ligament*, which extend into the gingiva and anastomose with capillaries in the sulcus area. (3) *Arterioles, which emerge from the crest of the interdental septa*[18] and extend parallel to the crest of the bone to anastomose with vessels of the periodontal ligament, with capillaries in the gingival crevicular areas, and with vessels which run over the alveolar crest.

The *lymphatic drainage* of the gingiva begins in the lymphatics of the connective tissue papillae. It progresses into the collecting network external to the periosteum of the alveolar process and then to the regional lymph nodes.[44] In addition, lymphatics just beneath the junctional epithelium extend into the

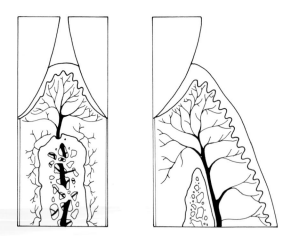

Figure 1–6. Diagrammatic representation of arteriole penetrating the interdental alveolar bone to supply the interdental tissues *(left)*, and a supraperiosteal arteriole overlying the facial alveolar bone, sending branches to the surrounding tissue *(right)*.

periodontal ligament and accompany the blood vessels.

Gingival innervation is derived from fibers arising from nerves in the periodontal ligament and from the labial, buccal, and palatal nerves.[7]

Correlation of Normal Clinical and Microscopic Features

To understand the normal clinical features of the gingiva, one must be able to interpret them in terms of the microscopic structures they represent.

Color

The color of the attached and marginal gingivae is generally described as *coral pink* and is produced by the vascular supply, the thickness and degree of keratinization of the epithelium, and the presence of pigment-containing cells. The color varies in different persons and appears to be correlated with

Figure 1–7. *Top,* Clinically normal gingiva in young adult. *Bottom,* Heavily pigmented (melanotic) gingiva in middle-aged adult. (From Glickman, I., and Smulow, J. B.: Periodontal Disease: Clinical, Radiographic, and Histopathologic Features. Philadelphia, W. B. Saunders Company, 1974.)

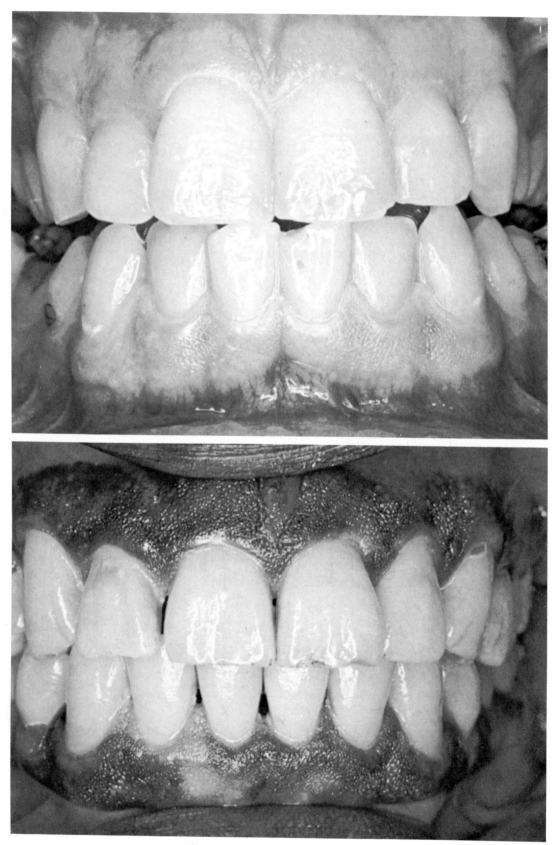

Figure 1–7. *See legend on opposite page.*

the cutaneous pigmentation. It is lighter in blond individuals with a fair complexion than in swarthy brunettes.

The attached gingiva is demarcated from the adjacent alveolar mucosa on the buccal aspect by a clearly defined mucogingival line. The alveolar mucosa is red, smooth, and shiny rather than pink and stippled. Microscopically, the epithelium of the alveolar mucosa is thinner, nonkeratinized, and contains no rete pegs. Also, the connective tissue of the alveolar mucosa is loosely arranged, and the blood vessels are more numerous, accounting for the difference in appearance.

Physiologic Pigmentation (Melanin). Melanin, a non–hemoglobin-derived brown pigment, is responsible for the normal pigmentation of the skin, gingiva, and remainder of the oral mucous membrane (Fig. 1–7). It is present in all normal individuals, often not in sufficient quantities to be detected clinically, but is absent or severely diminished in albinos. Melanin pigmentation in the oral cavity is prominent in blacks.

Contour

The contour or shape of the gingiva varies considerably and depends upon the shape of the teeth, their alignment in the arch, the location and size of the area of proximal contact, and the dimensions of the facial and lingual gingival embrasures. The marginal gingiva envelops the teeth in collarlike fashion and follows a scalloped outline on the facial and lingual surfaces. It forms a straight line along teeth with relatively flat surfaces. On teeth with pronounced mesiodistal convexity (e.g., maxillary canines) or teeth in labial version, the normal arcuate contour is accentuated and the gingiva is located farther apically. On teeth in lingual version the gingiva is horizontal and thickened (Fig. 1–8).

The *shape of the interdental gingiva* is governed by the contour of the proximal tooth surfaces and the location and shape of gingival embrasures. When the proximal surfaces of the crowns are relatively flat faciolingually and the roots are close together, the interdental bone is thin mesiodistally, and the gingival embrasures and interdental gingiva are narrow. Conversely, with proximal surfaces that flare away from the area of contact, the mesiodistal diameter of the interdental gingiva is broad (Fig. 1–9). The

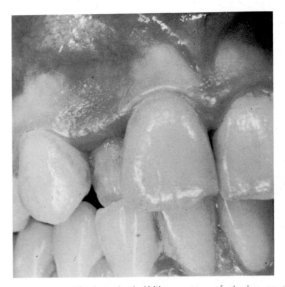

Figure 1–8. Thickened, shelf-like contour of gingiva on tooth in lingual version aggravated by local irritation caused by plaque accumulation.

height of the interdental gingiva varies with the location of the proximal contact.

Consistency

Healthy gingiva is *firm and resilient* and, with the exception of the movable free mar-

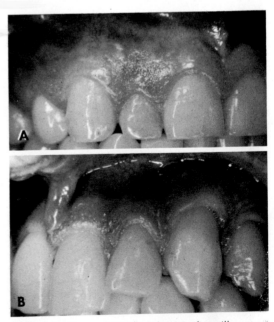

Figure 1–9. Shape of interdental gingival papillae correlated with shape of teeth and embrasures. *A*, Broad interdental papillae; *B*, narrow interdental papillae.

gin, *tightly bound to the underlying bone.* This is due to the collagenous nature of the lamina propria and its contiguity with the mucoperiosteum of the alveolar bone. The gingival fibers also contribute to the firmness of the gingival margin.

Surface Texture

Gingiva presents a textured surface like an orange peel and is referred to as being *stippled*. Stippling is best viewed by drying the gingiva (Fig. 1–10). *The attached gingiva is stippled; the marginal gingiva is not.* The central portion of the interdental papillae is usually stippled, but the marginal borders are smooth. The pattern and extent of stippling vary from person to person and in different areas of the same mouth.[22, 37] It is less prominent on lingual than on facial surfaces and may be absent in some persons.

Microscopically, stippling is produced by alternate rounded protuberances and depressions in the gingival surface. The papillary layer of the connective tissue projects into the elevations, and both the elevated and the depressed areas are covered by stratified squamous epithelium.

Stippling is a form of adaptive specialization or reinforcement for function. It is a feature of healthy gingiva, and reduction or loss of stippling is a common sign of gingival disease. When the gingiva is restored to health following treatment, the stippled appearance returns.

Position

The position of the gingiva refers to the level at which the *gingival margin is attached to the tooth.* When the tooth erupts into the oral cavity, the margin and sulcus are at the tip of the crown; as eruption progresses, they are seen closer to the root. During this eruption process the junctional epithelium and oral epithelium undergo extensive alterations and remodeling, while at the same time maintaining the shallow physiologic depth of the sulcus. Exposure of the root by the apical migration of the gingiva is called *gingival recession* or *atrophy.*

PERIODONTAL LIGAMENT

The periodontal ligament is the connective tissue structure that surrounds the root and connects it with the bone. It is continuous with the connective tissue of the gingiva and communicates with the marrow spaces through vascular channels in the bone.

Normal Microscopic Features

Principal Fibers

The most important elements of the periodontal ligament are the principal fibers, which are collagenous, arranged in bundles, and follow a wavy course when viewed in longitudinal section (Fig. 1–11). The principal fibers are arranged in the following groups: transseptal, alveolar crest, horizontal, oblique, and apical (Fig. 1–12). Terminal portions of the principal fibers that insert into cementum and bone are termed *Sharpey's fibers.*

Transseptal Group. These fibers extend interproximally over the alveolar crest and are embedded in the cementum of adjacent teeth (Fig. 1–13). The transseptal fibers are a remarkably constant finding. They are reconstructed even after destruction of the alveolar bone has occurred in periodontal disease.

Alveolar Crest Group. These fibers extend obliquely from the cementum just beneath

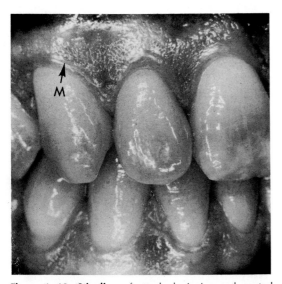

Figure 1–10. Stippling of attached gingiva and central portions of interdental papillae. The gingival margin (M) is smooth.

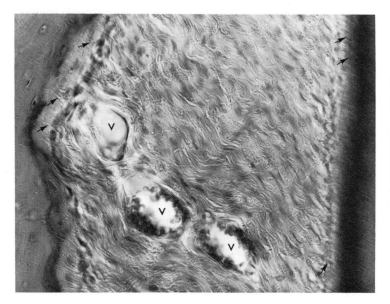

Figure 1–11. Principal fibers of the periodontal ligament follow a wavy course when sectioned longitudinally. The formative function of the periodontal ligament is illustrated by the newly formed osteoid and osteoblasts along a previously resorbed bone surface *(left)* and the cementoid and cementoblasts *(right)*. Note the fibers embedded in the forming calcified tissues *(arrows)*. V, vascular channels.

the junctional epithelium to the alveolar crest. Their function is to counterbalance the coronal thrust of the more apical fibers, thus helping to retain the tooth within its socket[14] and resist lateral tooth movements.

Horizontal Group. These fibers extend at right angles to the long axis of the tooth from the cementum to the alveolar bone. Their function is similar to that of the alveolar crest fibers.

Oblique Group. These fibers, the largest group in the periodontal ligament, extend

from the cementum in a coronal direction obliquely to the bone. They deflect the vertical masticatory stresses and transform them into tension on the alveolar bone.

Apical Group. The apical fibers radiate from the cementum to the bone at the fundus of the socket. They do not occur on incompletely formed roots.

Other Fibers

Other well-formed fiber bundles interdigitate at right angles or splay around and between regularly arranged fiber bundles.

Cellular Elements

The cellular elements of the periodontal ligament are fibroblasts, endothelial cells, cementoblasts, osteoblasts, osteoclasts, tissue macrophages, and strands of epithelial cells termed the "epithelial rests of Malassez" or "resting epithelial cells."[46]

The *epithelial rests* form a latticework in the periodontal ligament and appear as either isolated clusters of cells or interlacing strands. They are sometimes considered to be remnants of the Hertwig root sheath, and participate in the formation of periapical cysts and lateral root cysts.

The periodontal ligament may also contain calcified masses called cementicles that may be adherent to, or detached from, the root surfaces.

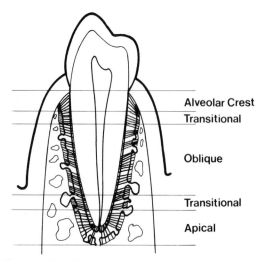

Alveolar Crest
Transitional

Oblique

Transitional

Apical

Figure 1–12. Diagram showing arrangement of **principal fiber bundles.**

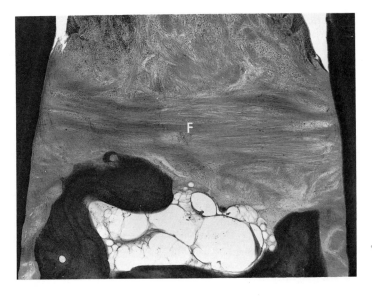

Figure 1–13. Transseptal fibers (F) at the crest of the interdental bone.

Vascular Supply and Innervation

The blood supply is derived from the *inferior and superior alveolar arteries* and reaches the periodontal ligament from three sources: *apical vessels, penetrating vessels from the alveolar bone, and anastomosing vessels from the gingiva.*[17]

Lymphatics supplement the venous drainage system. Those draining the region just beneath the junctional epithelium pass into the periodontal ligament and accompany the blood vessels into the periapical region. From there they pass through the alveolar bone to the inferior dental canal in the mandible, or the infraorbital canal in the maxilla, and to the submaxillary group of lymph nodes.

The periodontal ligament is abundantly supplied with sensory nerve fibers capable of transmitting *tactile, pressure*, and *pain sensations* by the trigeminal pathways.[5, 7] Nerve bundles pass into the periodontal ligament from the periapical area and through channels from the alveolar bone. The nerve bundles follow the course of the blood vessels and terminate as either free nerve endings or elongate spindle-like structures. The latter are *proprioceptive receptors* that account for the sense of localization when a tooth is touched.

Functions

The functions of the periodontal ligament are *physical, formative, nutritional*, and *sensory*.

Physical Function

The physical functions of the periodontal ligament entail the following: transmission of occlusal forces to the bone (Fig. 1–14), attachment of the teeth to the bone, maintenance of the gingival tissues in their proper relationship to the teeth, resistance to the impact of occlusal forces (shock absorption), and provision of a "soft tissue casing" to protect the vessels and nerves from injury by mechanical forces.

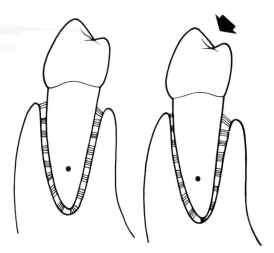

Figure 1–14. *Right,* **Distribution of faciolingual forces** *(arrow)* **around the axis of rotation** *(black circle on root)* in a mandibular premolar. The periodontal ligament fibers are compressed in areas of pressure and tension. *Left,* The same tooth in a resting state.

Formative Function

The periodontal ligament serves as the periosteum for cementum and bone. Cells of the periodontal ligament participate in the formation and resorption of these tissues, which occur during physiologic tooth movement, the accommodation of the periodontium to occlusal forces, and the repair of injuries.

Nutritional and Sensory Functions

The periodontal ligament supplies nutrients to the cementum, bone, and gingiva by way of the blood vessels and provides lymphatic drainage. The innervation of the periodontal ligament provides *proprioceptive and tactile sensitivity.*

CEMENTUM

Cementum is the calcified mesenchymal tissue that forms the outer covering of the

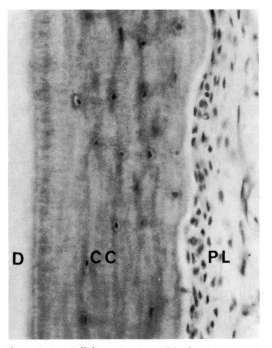

Figure 1–16. Cellular cementum (CC) showing cementocytes lying within lacunae. Cellular cementum is thicker than acellular cementum (cf. Fig. 1–15). There is also evidence of incremental lines, but they are less distinct than in acellular cementum. The cells adjacent to the surface of the cementum in the periodontal ligament (PL) space are cementoblasts. D, dentin. × 300.

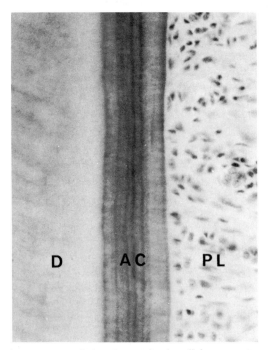

Figure 1–15. A light micrograph of **acellular cementum** (AC) showing incremental lines running parallel to the long axis of the tooth. These lines represent the appositional growth of cementum. Note the thin light lines running into the cementum perpendicular to the surface; these represent Sharpey's fibers of the periodontal ligament (PL). D, dentin. × 300.

anatomic root. It may exert a far more critical role in the development of periodontal disease than has thus far been demonstrated.

Normal Microscopic Features

There are two main forms of root cementum: *acellular (primary) and cellular (secondary)*. Both consist of a calcified interfibrillar matrix and collagen fibrils. Both acellular and cellular cementum are arranged in *lamellae* separated by incremental lines parallel to the long axis of the root (Figs. 1–15 and 1–16). These lines represent rest periods in cementum formation and are more mineralized than the adjacent cementum. Sharpey's fibers make up most of the structure of *acellular cementum,* and have a principal role in supporting the tooth. Most of the fibers are inserted at approximately right angles into the root surface and penetrate deep into the cementum, but others enter from several different directions.

The distribution of acellular and cellular

cementum varies. The coronal half of the root is usually covered by the acellular type, and cellular cementum is more common in the apical half. With age, the greatest increase in cementum is of the cellular type in the apical half of the root and in the furcation areas.

The Cemento-enamel Junction

The *cemento-enamel junction* is the area where the anatomic crown terminates at the root surface. The cementum at and immediately apical to the cemento-enamel junction is of particular clinical importance in root scaling procedures. Three relationships involving the cementum, dentin, and enamel may exist at the cemento-enamel junction.[32] Cementum *overlaps the enamel* in about 60 to 65 per cent of the cases (Fig. 1–17); in approximately 30 per cent of the cases there is an *edge-to-edge butt joint*; and in 5 to 10 per cent the *cementum and enamel fail to meet.* When gingival recession occurs in the last group, it may be accompanied by an accentuated sensitivity where the dentin is exposed.

Thickness of Cementum

The *thickness of cementum* on the coronal half of the root varies from 16 to 60 microns, or about the thickness of a hair. It attains its greatest thickness, up to 150 to 200 microns, in the apical third, and also in the bifurcation and trifurcation areas.[33] Between the ages of 11 and 70 the average thickness of the cementum increases threefold, with the greatest increase in the apical region.[49]

Cementogenesis

Cementum formation starts, as does formation of bone and dentin, with the deposition of a meshwork of irregularly arranged collagen fibrils sparsely distributed in an interfibrillar ground substance or matrix called *precementum* or *cementoid*.[40] It increases in thickness by apposition of the matrix by cementoblasts.

Cementum deposition continues after the teeth have erupted into contact with their functional antagonists and throughout life. Cementum formation is most rapid in the apical regions where it compensates for tooth eruption and attrition.

Hypercementosis

Hypercementosis (cementum hyperplasia) is a prominent thickening of the cementum. It may be localized to one tooth or may affect the entire dentition. Hypercementosis occurs as a generalized thickening of the cementum, with nodular enlargement of the apical third of the root. It also appears in the form of spike-like excrescences (cemental spikes) created by either the coalescence of cementicles that adhere to the root[21] or the calcification of periodontal fibers at the sites of insertion into the cementum. The etiology of hypercementosis is not completely understood.

Cementicles

Cementicles are globular masses of cementum arranged in concentric lamellae that lie free in the periodontal ligament or adhere to

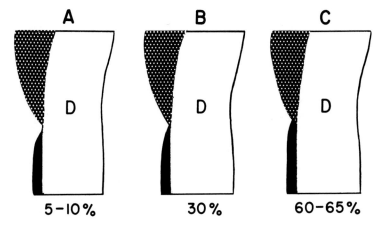

Figure 1–17. Statistical representation of normal variations in tooth morphology at the **cemento-enamel junction.** *A,* Space between enamel and cementum with dentin (D) exposed. *B,* End-to-end relationship of enamel and cementum. *C,* Cementum overlapping the enamel. (After Hopewell-Smith.)

the root surface. Cementicles may develop from calcified epithelial rests, around small spicules of cementum or alveolar bone traumatically displaced into the periodontal ligament, from calcified Sharpey's fibers, or from calcified thrombosed vessels within the periodontal ligament.[31]

Cementum Resorption and Repair

The cementum of erupted as well as of unerupted teeth is subject to resorption. The resorptive changes may be of microscopic proportion or sufficiently extensive to present a radiographically detectable alteration in the root contour. Cementum resorption is extremely common. In a microscopic study of 261 teeth it occurred in 236 (90.5 per cent).[23]

Cementum resorption may be due to local or systemic causes or may be idiopathic. Among the local conditions in which it occurs are trauma from occlusion,[34] orthodontic movement,[38] pressure from malaligned erupting teeth, cysts and tumors,[27] teeth without functional antagonists, embedded teeth, replanted and transplanted teeth,[1] periapical disease, and periodontal disease.

Fusion of the cementum and alveolar bone with obliteration of the periodontal ligament is termed *ankylosis*. This occurs in teeth with cemental resorption, which suggests that it may represent a form of abnormal repair. Ankylosis may also develop following chronic periapical inflammation, tooth replantation, and occlusal trauma and around embedded teeth.

ALVEOLAR BONE

The *alveolar process* is the bone that forms and supports the tooth sockets (alveoli). It consists of the inner socket wall of thin compact bone called the *alveolar bone proper (cribriform plate)*, the *supporting alveolar bone* which consists of cancellous trabeculae, and the facial and lingual plates of compact bone, called the the cortical plates. The interdental septum consists of cancellous supporting bone enclosed within a compact border (Fig. 1–18).

Normal Microscopic Features

Cells and Intercellular Matrix

Alveolar bone consists of a calcified matrix with *osteocytes* enclosed within spaces termed lacunae. The osteocytes extend processes into radiating canaliculi. The canaliculi form an anastomosing system through the intercellular matrix of the bone, which brings oxygen and nutrients via the blood to the osteocytes and removes metabolic waste products. Blood vessels branch extensively and travel through the periosteum. Bone growth occurs by apposition of an organic matrix that is deposited by osteoblasts.

Although the alveolar bone tissue is constantly changing in its internal organization, it retains approximately the same form from childhood through adult life. Bone deposition by osteoblasts is balanced by resorption by osteoclasts during the processes of tissue remodeling and renewal.

The bone matrix that is laid down by osteoblasts is not mineralized and is referred to as *osteoid*. While new osteoid is being deposited, the older osteoid located below the surface becomes mineralized.

The *osteoclasts* are large, multinucleated cells that are often seen on the surface of bone within eroded bony depressions referred to as *Howship's lacunae*. The main function of these cells is considered to be resorption of bone.

The Socket Wall

The periodontal ligament fibers that anchor the tooth in the socket are embedded for a considerable distance into the alveolar bone, where they are referred to as *Sharpey's fibers*. Some Sharpey's fibers are completely calcified, but most contain an uncalcified central core within a calcified outer layer.[41] The socket wall consists of dense lamellated bone, some of which is arranged in haversian systems, and *bundle bone*. Bundle bone is the term describing the bone adjacent to the periodontal ligament that contains Sharpey's fibers. It is arranged in layers with intervening appositional lines, parallel to the root. Bundle bone is gradually resorbed on the side of the marrow spaces and replaced by lamellated bone.

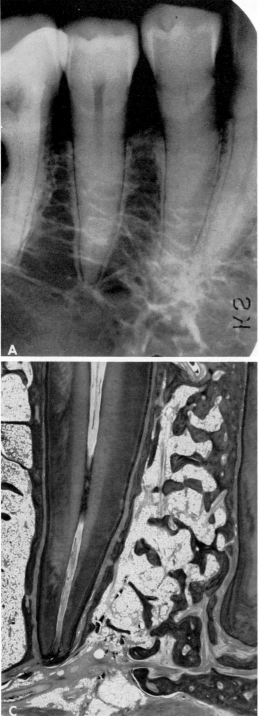

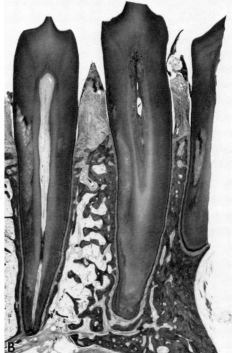

Figure 1–18. Interdental septa. *A*, Mandibular premolar area. Note the prominent lamina dura. *B*, Interdental septa between the canine *(right)* and premolars. The central cancellous portion is bordered by the dense bony cribriform plates of the socket. (This forms the lamina dura around the teeth in the radiograph). *C*, Interdental septum between the premolars, showing central cancellous bone and dense cribriform plate around the roots.

The *cancellous portion of the alveolar bone* consists of trabeculae that enclose irregularly shaped marrow spaces lined with a layer of thin, flattened endosteal cells. There is wide variation in the trabecular pattern of the cancellous bone,[36] which is affected by occlusal forces. The matrix of the cancellous trabeculae consists of irregularly arranged lamellae separated by marked incremental and resorption lines indicative of previous bone activity, with an occasional haversian system.

Vascular Supply, Lymphatics, and Nerves

The cribriform plate of the tooth socket appears radiographically as a thin, radiopaque line, termed the *lamina dura*. However, it is perforated by numerous channels, containing blood, lymph vessels, and nerves, which link the periodontal ligament with the cancellous portion of the alveolar bone.

The Interdental Septum

The interdental septum consists of cancellous bone bordered by the socket walls of approximating teeth and the facial and lingual cortical plates (Fig. 1–18).

The average distance between the crest of the alveolar bone and the cemento-enamel junction in the mandibular anterior region of young adults varies between 0.96 mm and 1.22 mm.[24] With age, the distance between the bone and the cemento-enamel junction increases throughout the mouth (1.88 mm to 2.81 mm.[20] However, this phenomenon may not be as much a function of age as of periodontal disease.

External Contour of Alveolar Bone

The *bone contour normally conforms to the prominence of the roots, with intervening vertical depressions which taper toward the margin* (Fig. 1–19). Alveolar bone anatomy varies from patient to patient and has important clinical implications. *The height and thickness of the facial and lingual bony plates are affected by the alignment of the teeth, angulation of the root to the bone, and occlusal forces.* On teeth in labial version, the margin of the labial bone is located farther apically than on teeth in

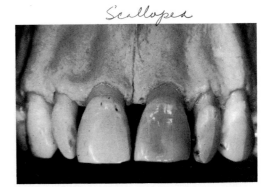

Figure 1–19. Normal bone contour conforms to the prominence of the roots.

proper alignment. The bone margin is thinned to a knife edge and presents an accentuated arc in the direction of the apex. On teeth in lingual version, the facial bony plate is thicker than normal. The margin is blunt and rounded, and horizontal rather than arcuate.

Fenestrations and Dehiscences

Isolated areas in which the root is denuded of bone and the root surfaces are covered only by periosteum and overlying gingiva are termed *fenestrations*. In this instance the marginal bone is intact. When the denuded areas extend through the marginal bone, the defect is called a *dehiscence* (Fig. 1–20). Such defects occur on approximately 20 per cent of the teeth; they occur more often on the facial bone than on the lingual, more com-

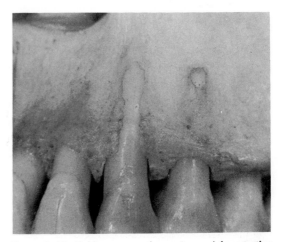

Figure 1–20. Dehiscence on the canine and **fenestration** of the first premolar.

monly on anterior teeth than on posterior teeth, and are frequently bilateral.

Lability of Alveolar Bone – *changing & remodeling*

In contrast to its apparent rigidity, alveolar bone is the least stable of the periodontal tissues; its structure is in a constant state of flux. The physiologic lability of alveolar bone is maintained by a sensitive balance between bone formation and bone resorption, regulated by local and systemic influences. Bone is resorbed in areas of pressure and formed in areas of tension.

Physiologic Migration of Teeth and Reconstruction of Alveolar Bone

With time and wear the proximal contact areas of the teeth are flattened and the teeth tend to move mesially. This is a gradual process with intermittent periods of activity, rest, and repair. *Alveolar bone is reconstructed in compliance with the physiologic mesial migration of the teeth.* Bone resorption is increased in areas of pressure along the mesial surfaces of the teeth, and new layers of bundle bone are formed in areas of tension on the distal surfaces.

Occlusal Forces and Alveolar Bone

There are two aspects to the relationship between occlusal forces and alveolar bone. *The bone exists for the purpose of supporting teeth during function* and, in common with the remainder of the skeletal system, *depends upon the stimulation it receives from function for the preservation of its structure.* There is therefore a constant and sensitive balance between occlusal forces and the structure of alveolar bone.

Alveolar bone undergoes constant physiologic remodeling in response to occlusal forces. Osteoclasts and osteoblasts redistribute bone substance to meet new functional demands very efficiently. Bone is removed from where it is no longer needed and added where new needs arise.

AGING AND THE PERIODONTIUM

Disease of the periodontium occurs in childhood, adolescence, and early adult-

hood, but the prevalence of periodontal disease and the tissue destruction and tooth loss it causes increases with age. Many tissue changes occur with aging, some of which may affect the disease experience of the periodontium. *It is difficult to draw a sharp line between physiologic aging and the cumulative effects of disease.*

Attrition

The most obvious change in the teeth with age is a loss of tooth substance caused by attrition. Occlusal wear reduces cusp height and inclination, with a resultant increase in the food table area and loss of sluiceways. The degree of attrition is influenced by the musculature, consistency of food, tooth hardness, occupational factors, and habits such as bruxism and clenching. The rate of attrition may be coordinated with other age changes such as continuous tooth eruption and gingival recession (Fig. 1–21).

Reduction in bone height that occurs with aging is not necessarily related to occlusal wear.[6] In those cases in which bone support is reduced, the clinical crown tends to become disproportionately long and creates excessive leverage upon the bone. Attrition appears to preserve the balance between the teeth and their bony support by reducing the clinical crowns.

Mesial Migration

Wear of teeth also occurs on the proximal surfaces, accompanied by mesial migration of the teeth. Proximal wear reduces the anteroposterior length of the dental arch by approximately 0.5 cm by age 40.[8, 48] Anteroposterior narrowing from proximal wear is greater in teeth that taper toward the cervical, such as the incisors. Progressive attrition and proximal wear result in a reduced maxillary-mandibular overjet in molar areas and anterior edge-to-edge bites.

Masticatory Efficiency

Loss of masticatory efficiency in aged individuals is a common finding. Slight atrophy of the buccal musculature has been de-

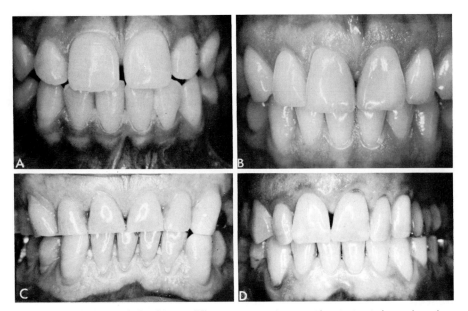

Figure 1–21. Tooth-periodontium relationships at different ages. *A,* Age 12. The gingiva is located on the enamel, and the clinical crown is shorter than the anatomic crown. *B,* Age 25. The gingiva is attached close to the cemento-enamel junction. *C,* Age 50. Slight occlusal wear and slight recession. *D,* Age 72. Moderate attrition and slight to moderate recession. These variations may be due not to an aging process but to the cumulative effect of injurious factors.

scribed as a physiologic feature of aging,[19] however, reduction in masticatory efficiency is more likely to be caused by unreplaced missing teeth, loose teeth, poorly fitting dentures, or an unwillingness to wear dentures. Reduced masticatory efficiency leads to poor chewing habits, a preponderance of soft foods in the diet, and the possibility of associated digestive disturbances.

Causative Factors

With time, chronic disease can produce many oral changes, and it is difficult to determine how much physiologic aging contributes to the total picture. Some contend that gingival recession, attrition, and reduction in bone height in the aged result more from disease and factors in the oral environment than from physiologic aging. Although gingival recession, attrition, and bone loss commonly occur with age, they are not present in everyone and vary considerably in the same age group. Marked attrition may be present in older individuals with relatively little alveolar bone loss and may also be produced in young and middle-aged adults by bruxing and clenching habits. Increased

alveolar bone loss in the aged has been related to less efficient oral hygiene,[42] bone loss, pathologic migration of the teeth, and a possible decrease in the cellular immune response to bacterial plaque. The associated loss of vertical dimension in the aged may be the result of periodontal disease and failure to replace missing teeth.

References

1. Agnew, R. G., and Fong, C. C.: Histologic studies on experimental transplantation of teeth. Oral Surg., 9:18, 1956.
2. Ainamo, A., and Ainamo, J.: The width of attached gingiva on supraerupted teeth. J. Periodont. Res., 13:194, 1978.
3. Ainamo, J., and Löe, H.: Anatomical characteristics of gingiva. A clinical and microscopic study of the free and attached gingiva. J. Periodontol., 37:5, 1966.
4. Arnim, S. S., and Hagerman, D. A.: The connective tissue fibers of the marginal gingiva. J. Am. Dent. Assoc., 47:271, 1953.
5. Avery, J. K., and Rapp, R.: Pain conduction in human dental tissues. Dent. Clin. North Am., July 1959.
6. Baer, P. N., et al.: Alveolar bone loss and occlusal wear. Periodontics, 1:45, 1963.
7. Bernick, S.: Innervation of the teeth and periodontium. Dent. Clin. North Am., July 1959, p. 503.
8. Black, C. V.: Pathology of the Hard Tissues of the

Teeth. Oral Diagnosis. 8th ed. Woodstock, Ill., MedicoDental Publishing Company, 1948, p. 389.

9. Bowers, G. M.: A study of the width of the attached gingiva. J. Periodontol., 34:210, 1963.
10. Bral, M. M., and Stahl, S. S.: Keratinizing potential of human crevicular epithelium. J. Periodontol., 48:381, 1977.
11. Brill, N., and Björn, H.: Passage of tissue fluid into human gingival pockets. Acta Odontol. Scand., 17:11, 1959.
12. Caffesse, R. G., Karring, T., and Nasjleti, C. E.: Keratinizing potential of sulcular epithelium. J. Periodontol., 48:140, 1977.
13. Carranza, F. A., Jr., and Cabrini, R. L.: Mast cells in human gingiva. Oral Surg., 8:1093, 1955.
14. Carranza, F. A., Sr., and Carranza, F. A., Jr.: The management of the alveolar bone in the treatment of the periodontal pocket. J. Periodontol., 27:29, 1956.
15. Cimasoni, G.: The crevicular fluid. Monographs in Oral Science. Vol. 3. Basel, S. Karger, 1974.
16. Cohen, B.: Morphological factors in the pathogenesis of periodontal disease. Br. Dent. J., 107:31, 1959.
17. Cohen, L.: Further studies into the vascular architecture of the mandible. J. Dent. Res., 39:936, 1960.
18. Folke, L. E. A., and Stallard, R. E.: Periodontal microcirculation as revealed by plastic microspheres. J. Periodont. Res., 2:53, 1967.
19. Freeman, J.T.: The basic factors of nutrition in old age. Geriatrics, 2:41, 1947.
20. Gargiulo, A. W., Wentz, F. M., and Orban, B.: Dimensions and relations of the dentogingival junction in humans. J. Periodontol., 32:216, 1961.
21. Gottlieb, B., and Orban, B.: Biology and Pathology of the Tooth and Its Supporting Mechanism. Trans. by M. Diamond. New York, The Macmillan Company, 1938, p. 70.
22. Greene, A. H.: A study of the characteristics of stippling and its relation to gingival health. J. Periodontol., 33:176, 1962.
23. Henry, J. L., and Weinmann, J. P.: The pattern of resorption and repair of human cementum. J. Am. Dent. Assoc., 42:271, 1951.
24. Herulf, G.: On det marginala alveolarbenet hos ungdom i studiealdernenrontgenstudie. Svensk TandklakareTidsskrift., 43:42, 1950.
25. Karring, T., Lang, N. P., and Löe, H.: The role of gingival connective tissue in determining epithelial differentiation. J. Periodont. Res., 10:1, 1975.
26. Kindlova, M.: The blood supply of the marginal periodontium in Macaccus Rhesus. Arch. Oral Biol., 10:869, 1965.
27. Kronfeld, R.: Biology of the cementum. J. Am. Dent. Assoc., 25:1451, 1938.
28. Kronfeld, R.: Histopathology of the Teeth and Their Surrounding Structures. Philadelphia, Lea & Febiger, 1939.
29. Listgarten, M. A.: Electron microscopic study of the gingivodental junction of man. Am. J. Anat., 119:147, 1966.
30. Mandel, J. I., and Weinstein, E.: The fluid of the gingival sulcus. Periodontics, 2:147, 1964.
31. Mikola, O. J., and Bauer, W. H.: Cementicles and fragments of cementum in the periodontal membrane. Oral Surg., 2:1063, 1949.
32. Noyes, F. B., Schour, I., and Noyes, H. J.: A Textbook of Dental Histology and Embryology, 5th ed. Philadelphia, Lea & Febiger, 1938, p. 113.
33. Orban, B.: Oral Histology and Embryology, 2nd ed. St. Louis, C. V. Mosby Company, 1944, p. 161.
34. Orban, B.: Tissue changes in traumatic occlusion. J. Am. Dent. Assoc., 15:2090, 1928.
35. Orban, B., and Kohler, J.: The physiologic gingival sulcus. Z. Stomatol., 22:353, 1924.
36. Parfitt, G. J.: An investigation of the normal variations in alveolar bone trabeculation. Oral Surg., 15:1453, 1962.
37. Rosenberg, H., and Massler, M. J.: Gingival stippling in young adult males. J. Periodontol., 38:473, 1967.
38. Rudolph, C. E.: An evaluation of root resorption occurring during orthodontic therapy. J. Dent. Res., 19:367, 1940.
39. Schilli, W.: The most superficial zone of the stratum corneum of the gingiva. Oral Surg., 25:896, 1968.
40. Selvig, K. A.: An ultrastructural study of cementum formation. Odontol. Scand., 22:105, 1964.
41. Selvig, K. A.: The fine structure of human cementum. Acta Odontol. Scand., 23:423, 1965.
42. Shklar, G.: The effects of aging upon oral mucosa. J. Invest. Dermatol., 47:115, 1966.
43. Skougaard, M. R., and Beagrie, G. S.: The renewal of gingival epithelium in marmosets (*Callithrix jacchus*) as determined through autoradiography with thymidine-H₃. Acta Odontol. Scand., 20:467, 1962.
44. Stillman, P. R., and McCall, J. O.: Textbook of Clinical Periodontics. New York, Macmillan, 1922.
45. Thilander, H.: Permeability of the gingival pocket epithelium. Int. Dent. J., 14:416, 1964.
46. Valderhaug, J. P., and Nylen, M. U.: Function of epithelial rests as suggested by their ultrastructure. J. Periodont. Res., 1:69, 1966.
47. Weinmann, J. P., and Meyer, J.: Types of keratinization in the human gingiva. J. Invest. Dermatol., 32:87, 1959.
48. Wood, H. E.: Causal factors in shortening tooth series with age. J. Dent. Res., 17:1, 1938.
49. Zander, H. A., and Hurzeler, B.: Continuous cementum apposition. J. Dent. Res., 37:1035, 1958.

Chapter 2

Gingival Diseases

THE ROLE OF INFLAMMATION IN GINGIVAL DISEASE

Gingivitis, inflammation of the gingiva, is the most common form of gingival disease. It is present in all forms of gingival disease because bacterial plaque, which causes inflammation, and irritational factors, which favor plaque accumulation, are very often present in the gingival environment. The inflammation caused by dental plaque gives rise to associated degenerative, necrotic, and proliferative changes in the gingival tissues. There is a tendency to designate all forms of gingival disease as gingivitis, as if inflammation were the only disease process involved. However, pathologic processes not caused by local irritation, such as atrophy, hyperplasia, and neoplasia, also occur in the gingiva. Differentiation between inflammation and other pathologic processes is necessary when evaluating gingival pathology.

The role of *inflammation* in individual cases of gingivitis varies as follows:

1. Inflammation may be the *primary* and *only* pathologic change. This is by far the most prevalent type of gingival disease.

2. Inflammation may be a *secondary* feature, superimposed upon systemically caused gingival disease. For example, inflammation commonly complicates gingival hyperplasia caused by the systemic administration of phenytoin.

3. Inflammation may be the precipitating factor responsible for clinical changes in patients with systemic conditions that alone would not produce clinically detectable gingival disease. Gingivitis during pregnancy is one example.

TYPES OF GINGIVAL DISEASE

The most common type of gingival disease is the simple inflammatory involvement caused by bacterial plaque attached to the tooth surface. This type of gingivitis, sometimes called chronic marginal gingivitis or simple gingivitis, may remain stationary for indefinite periods of time or may proceed to destruction of the supporting structures (periodontitis). The causes of progression are not clearly understood.

In addition, the gingiva can present symptoms of other diseases, sometimes but not always related to the usual periodontal problems. Several of these conditions are listed:

1. Acute necrotizing ulcerative gingivitis.

2. Acute herpetic gingivostomatitis and other viral diseases.

3. Allergic gingivitis, caused by various allergies.

4. Several dermatoses that attack the gingival tissues induce characteristic types of gingival disease, such as that seen in lichen planus, pemphigus, erythema multiforme, and others.

5. Gingivitis may be initiated by bacterial plaque, but the tissue response may be conditioned by systemic factors. This is the case in pregnancy, puberty gingivitis, and vitamin C deficiency.

6. The gingival response to a variety of pathogenic agents may include an increase in volume; this is termed gingival enlargement.

7. Different benign and malignant tumors may appear in the gingiva, either as primary or metastatic tumors.

COURSE AND DURATION OF GINGIVITIS

Acute gingivitis is a painful condition that comes on suddenly and is of short duration.

Subacute gingivitis is a less severe phase of the acute condition.

Recurrent gingivitis is the disease that reappears after having been eliminated by treatment or that disappears spontaneously and reappears.

Chronic gingivitis is the type most commonly encountered. This disease comes on slowly, is of long duration, and is painless unless complicated by acute or subacute exacerbations (Fig. 2–1). Patients seldom recollect having had any acute symptoms. Chronic gingivitis is a fluctuating disease in which inflamed areas persist or become normal and normal areas become inflamed.[29]

DISTRIBUTION OF GINGIVITIS

The distribution of gingivitis is characterized by location.

Localized gingivitis is confined to the gingiva of a single tooth or group of teeth.

Generalized gingivitis involves the entire mouth.

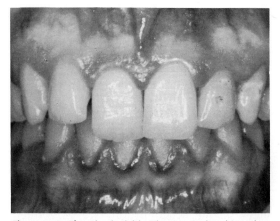

Figure 2–1. Chronic gingivitis. The marginal and interdental gingivae are smooth, edematous, and discolored.

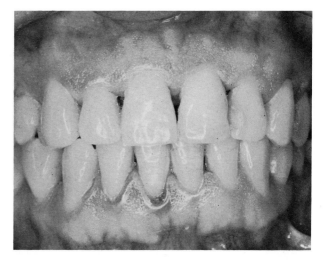

Figure 2–2. Localized marginal gingivitis in the mandibular anterior region.

Marginal gingivitis involves the gingival margin but may include a portion of the contiguous attached gingiva (Fig. 2–2).

Papillary gingivitis involves the interdental papillae and often extends into the adjacent portion of the gingival margin. The earliest signs of gingivitis most often occur in the papillae, which are therefore more frequently involved than is the gingival margin.

Diffuse gingivitis involves the gingival margin, attached gingiva, and interdental papillae (Fig. 2–3).

Disease in individual cases may also be described by combining the following terms:

Localized marginal gingivitis is confined to one or more areas of the marginal gingiva.

Localized diffuse gingivitis extends from the margin to the mucobuccal fold, but is limited in area.

Localized papillary gingivitis is confined to one or more interdental spaces in a limited area (Fig. 2–4).

Generalized marginal gingivitis is involvement of the gingival margin in relation to all the teeth. Usually, the interdental papillae are also involved (Fig. 2–5).

Generalized diffuse gingivitis involves the entire gingiva. Usually, the alveolar mucosa is also affected; therefore the demarcation between it and the attached gingiva is obliterated (Fig. 2–6). Systemic conditions are involved in the etiology of generalized diffuse gingivitis except in cases caused by acute infection or generalized chemical irritation.

PATHOLOGY OF GINGIVITIS

Gingivitis is associated with the presence of oral microorganisms in the gingival sulcus. These organisms are capable of synthesizing potentially harmful products that cause damage to intercellular constituents such as collagen, ground substance, glycocalyx (cell coat) as well as to epithelial and connective tissue cells. The resulting widening of the intercellular spaces between the junctional epithelial cells during early gingivitis may permit injurious agents derived from bacteria, or bacteria themselves, to gain access to the connective tissue.

Vascular changes are the first response to

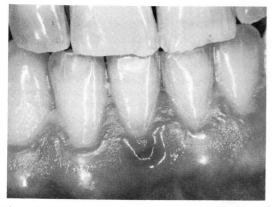

Figure 2–3. Localized diffuse gingivitis. Both the marginal and attached gingiva are involved.

that bleeding upon probing appears earlier than changes in color or other visual signs of inflammation;[36, 43] moreover, bleeding is a more objective sign than color change in the diagnosis of early gingival inflammation. Gingival bleeding varies in severity, duration, and the ease with which it is provoked.

Chronic and Recurrent Bleeding

The most common cause of abnormal recurrent gingival bleeding is chronic inflammation.[44] The bleeding is provoked by mechanical trauma such as that from toothbrushing, toothpicks, or food impaction; by biting into solid foods such as apples; or by grinding the teeth (bruxism).

In the chronically inflamed state the capillaries are engorged and closer to the surface; also, the thinned, degenerated epithelium is less protective, so that ordinarily innocuous stimuli cause rupture of the capillaries, which is seen clinically as gingival bleeding (Fig. 2–8). The severity of the bleeding and the ease with which it is provoked depend upon the intensity of the inflammation.

Acute Bleeding

Acute episodes of gingival bleeding are caused by injury or may occur spontaneously in acute gingival disease. Laceration of the gingiva by aggressive toothbrushing or sharp pieces of food causes gingival bleeding even in the absence of gingival disease. Gingival burns from hot foods or chemicals also increase the ease of gingival bleeding. Spontaneous bleeding or bleeding upon slight provocation occurs in *acute necrotizing ulcerative gingivitis*. In this condition, engorged blood vessels in the inflamed connective tissue are exposed by desquamation of necrotic surface epithelium.

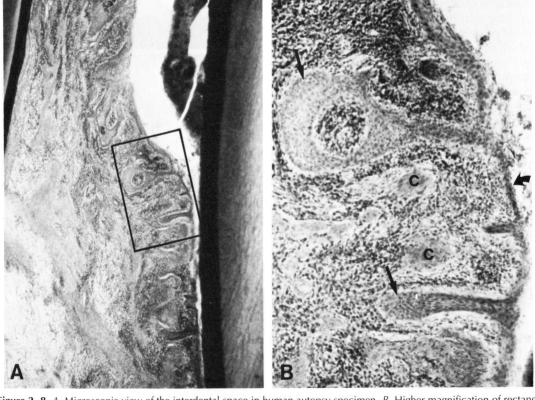

Figure 2–8. *A,* Microscopic view of the interdental space in human autopsy specimen. *B,* Higher magnification of rectangle in *A.* Note the dense inflammatory infiltrate, the thinned epithelium *(curved arrow),* the extension of rete pegs *(straight arrows),* and the remnants of collagen fibers *(C).*

Gingival Bleeding Associated with Systemic Disturbances

There are systemic disorders in which gingival hemorrhage, unprovoked by mechanical irritation, occurs spontaneously, or in which gingival bleeding following irritation is excessive and difficult to control. These are called *hemorrhagic diseases* and represent a wide variety of conditions that vary in etiology and clinical manifestations. Such conditions have one feature in common: namely, abnormal bleeding in the skin, internal organs, and other tissues besides the oral mucous membrane. The reader is directed to books on clinical hematology that analyze this point in greater detail.

Color Changes in the Gingiva

Color Changes in Chronic Gingivitis

Change in color is a very important clinical sign of gingival disease. The normal gingival color is "coral pink," owing to the tissue vascularity, modified by the overlying epithelial layers. For this reason, the gingiva will become redder when (1) there is an increase in vascularization or (2) the degree of epithelial keratinization becomes reduced or disappears. The color will become paler when (1) vascularization is reduced (associated with fibrosis of the corium) or (2) epithelial keratinization increases. Therefore, chronic inflammation will intensify the red or bluish-red color owing to vascular proliferation and to reduction of keratinization due to epithelial compression by the inflamed tissue. Venous stasis will add a bluish hue. Starting as slightly reddened, the color changes through varying shades of red, reddish blue, and deep blue with increasing chronicity of the inflammatory process. The changes start in the interdental papillae and gingival margin and spread to the attached gingiva (see Fig. 2–1). Proper diagnosis and treatment require an understanding of the tissue changes which alter the color of the gingiva at the clinical level.

Color Changes in Acute Gingivitis

Color changes in acute gingival inflammation differ in nature and distribution from those in chronic gingivitis. The color changes may be marginal, diffuse, or patchlike, depending upon the acute condition. In *acute necrotizing ulcerative gingivitis* the involvement is marginal, in *herpetic gingivostomatitis* it is diffuse, and in *acute reactions to chemical irritation* it is usually patchlike.

Color changes vary with the intensity of the inflammation. In all instances there is an initial bright red erythema. If the condition does not worsen, this is the only color change until the gingiva reverts to normal. In severe acute inflammation, the red color changes to a shiny slate gray, which gradually becomes a dull whitish gray. The gray discoloration produced by tissue necrosis is demarcated from the adjacent gingiva by a thin, sharply defined erythematous zone.

Metallic Pigmentation

Heavy metals absorbed systemically from therapeutic use or the environment may discolor the gingiva and other areas of the oral mucosa.[40] This is different from tattooing produced by the accidental embedding of amalgam[6] or other metal fragments. *Bismuth, arsenic, and mercury* produce a black line in the gingiva that follows the contour of the margin. The pigmentation may also appear as isolated black blotches involving the marginal, interdental, and attached gingivae. *Lead* results in a bluish-red or deep blue linear pigmentation of the gingival margin (burtonian line)[14] and *silver* (argyria) in a violet marginal line, often accompanied by a diffuse bluish-gray discoloration throughout the oral mucosa.[49]

Gingival pigmentation from systemically absorbed metals results from perivascular precipitation of metallic sulfides in the subepithelial connective tissue. Gingival pigmentation is not an effect of systemic toxicity. It occurs only in areas of inflammation, where the increased permeability of irritated blood vessels permits seepage of the metal into the surrounding tissue. In addition to inflamed gingiva, mucosal areas irritated by biting or abnormal chewing habits, such as the inner surface of the lips, the cheek at the level of the occlusal line, and the lateral border of the tongue, are common pigmentation sites.

Gingival or mucosal pigmentation is eliminated by *removing the local irritating factors and restoring tissue health,* without necessarily discontinuing the metal-containing drugs required for therapeutic purposes. *Temporary correction* is obtained by topical application of concentrated peroxide or by insufflating the gingiva with oxygen to oxidize the dark metallic sulfides. The discoloration reappears unless the procedures are repeated.

Color Changes Associated with Systemic Factors

Some systemic diseases may cause color changes in the oral mucosa, including the gingiva.[15] In general, these abnormal pigmentations are nonspecific in nature and should stimulate further diagnostic efforts or referral to the proper specialist.[56] Endogenous oral pigmentations can be due to melanin, bilirubin, or iron.[49]

Melanin oral pigmentations can be normal physiologic pigmentations that are commonly found in individuals of darker races (see Chapter 1), including Caucasian brunettes. Diseases that increase melanin pigmentation include the following: *Addison's disease*, which is caused by adrenal dysfunction and produces isolated patches of discoloration varying from bluish black to brown; *Peutz-Jeghers syndrome*, which produces intestinal polyposis and melanin pigmentation in the oral mucosa and lips; and *Albright's syndrome* (polyostotic fibrous dysplasia) and *von Recklinghausen's disease* (neurofibromatosis),

both of which produce areas of oral melanin pigmentation.

Skin and mucous membranes can also be stained by bile pigments. *Jaundice* is best detected by examination of the sclera, but the oral mucosa may also acquire a yellowish color. The deposition of iron in *hemochromatosis* may produce a blue-gray pigmentation of the oral mucosa. Several endocrine and metabolic disturbances may produce color changes: these include diabetes and pregnancy. Blood dyscrasias such as anemia, polycythemia, and leukemia may also induce color changes.

Exogenous factors capable of producing color changes in the gingiva include atmospheric irritants, such as coal and metal dust, and coloring agents in food or lozenges. Tobacco causes a gray hyperkeratosis of the gingiva. Localized bluish-black areas of pigment are commonly due to amalgam implanted in the mucosa.

Changes in the Consistency of the Gingiva

Both chronic and acute inflammations produce changes in the normal firm resilient consistency of the gingiva. Chronic gingivitis is a conflict between destructive and reparative changes, and the consistency of the gingiva deter-

TABLE 2–1. CLINICAL AND HISTOPATHOLOGIC CHANGES IN GINGIVAL CONSISTENCY

Chronic Gingivitis	
Clinical Changes	*Underlying Microscopic Features*
1. Soggy puffiness that pits on pressure	1. Infiltration by fluid and cells of the inflammatory exudate
2. Marked softness and friability, with ready fragmentation upon exploration with a probe and pinpoint surface areas of redness and desquamation	2. Degeneration of connective tissue and epithelium associated with injurious substances which provoke the inflammation and the inflammatory exudate. Change in the connective tissue–epithelium relationship, with the inflamed, engorged connective tissue expanding to within a few epithelial cells of the surface. Thinning of the epithelium and degeneration associated with edema and leukocytic invasion, separated by areas in which the rete pegs are elongated into the connective tissue.
3. Firm, leathery consistency	3. Fibrosis and epithelial proliferation associated with longstanding chronic inflammation
Acute Gingivitis	
Clinical Changes	*Underlying Microscopic Features*
1. Diffuse puffiness and softening	1. Diffuse edema of acute inflammatory origin; fatty infiltration in xanthomatosis
2. Sloughing with grayish flake-like particles of debris adhering to the eroded surface.	2. Necrosis with the formation of a pseudomembrane composed of bacteria, polymorphonuclear leukocytes and degenerated epithelial cells in a fibrinous meshwork
3. Vesicle formation	3. Inter- and intracellular edema with degeneration of the nucleus and cytoplasm and rupture of the cell wall

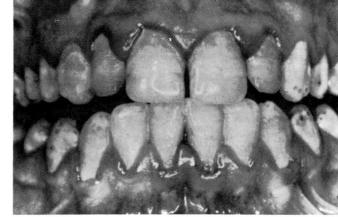

Figure 2–9. Chronic gingivitis. Note the swelling and discoloration produced when inflammatory exudate and tissue degeneration are the predominant microscopic changes. The gingiva is soft, friable, and bleeds easily. Note also the mottled teeth.

soft, smooth, shiny

mined by the relative balance between the two. Table 2–1 is a summary of clinical and microscopic changes associated with gingival consistency.

Changes in the Surface Texture of the Gingiva

Loss of surface stippling is an early sign of gingivitis. In chronic inflammation the surface is either smooth and shiny or firm and nodular, depending upon whether the dominant changes are exudative or fibrotic (Figs. 2–9 and 2–10).

Changes in Gingival Contour

Changes in gingival contour are for the most part associated with gingival enlarge-ment, but changes may also occur in other conditions.

Stillman's clefts are apostrophe-shaped indentations extending from and into the gingival margin for varying distances. The clefts generally occur on the facial surface (Fig. 2–11). The clefts may repair spontaneously or persist as surface lesions of deep periodontal pockets that penetrate into the supporting tissues. Their association with trauma from occlusion has not been substantiated. The length of the clefts varies from a slight break in the gingival margin to a depth of 5 to 6 mm or more.

McCall's festoons are life saver–shaped enlargements of the marginal gingiva (Fig. 2–12) that occur most frequently in the canine and premolar areas on the facial surface. In the early stages, the color and consistency of the gingiva are normal. Accumulation of food debris leads to secondary inflammatory

firm, fibrotic

Figure 2–10. Chronic gingivitis. Note the firm gingiva with minutely nodular surface produced when fibrosis predominates in the inflammatory process.

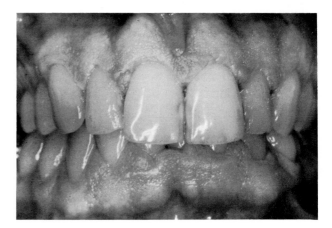

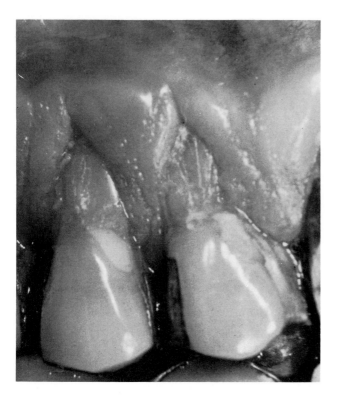

Figure 2–11. **Stillman's clefts** in the gingiva.

changes. Trauma from occlusion and mechanical stimulation are suggested etiologic factors; however, festoons occur on teeth without occlusal antagonists.

GINGIVAL RECESSION

Recession is the *exposure of the root surface by an apical shift in the position of the gingiva.* A distinction between the "actual" and "apparent" positions of the gingiva must be made. The *actual position* is the level of the epithelial attachment on the tooth, whereas the *apparent position* is the level of the crest of the gingival margin. *It is the actual position of the gingiva, not the apparent position, which determines the severity of recession.* This determines two types of recession: *visible,* which is clinically observable; and *hidden,* which is covered by gingiva and can only be measured by inserting a probe to the level of epithelial

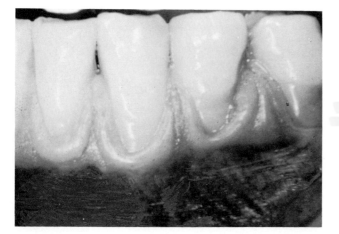

Life Saver –

Figure 2–12. **McCall's festoons.** Note the characteristic rim-like enlargement of the gingival margin.

Canines/ PM - facial

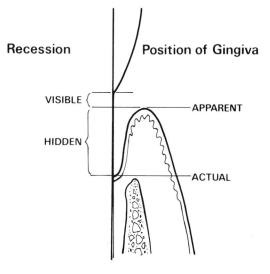

Recession | Position of Gingiva

VISIBLE {

HIDDEN {

APPARENT

ACTUAL

Figure 2–13. Diagram illustrating **apparent and actual position of the gingiva** and **visible and hidden recession.**

attachment (Fig. 2–13). The total amount of recession is the sum of the two. *Recession refers to the location of the gingiva, not its condition* (Fig. 2–14). Receded gingiva is often inflamed but may be normal except for its position (Fig. 2–15). Recession may be localized to a tooth or group of teeth or generalized throughout the mouth (Fig. 2–16).

Etiology of Recession

Gingival recession increases with age; the incidence varies from 8 per cent in children to 100 per cent after the age of 50.[60] This has led some authors to assume that recession may be a physiologic process related to aging. However, convincing evidence for a physiologic shift of the gingival attachment has never been presented.[39] The gradual apical shift is most probably the result of the cumulative effect of minor pathologic involvement and/or repeated minor direct trauma to the gingiva. *The following factors have been implicated in the etiology of gingival recession: faulty toothbrushing (gingival abrasion), tooth malposition, gingival inflammation, and high frenum attachment.* Trauma from occlusion has also been suggested, but its mechanism of action has never been demonstrated.

Although toothbrushing is important for gingival health, *faulty toothbrushing may cause gingival recession.* Recession tends to be more frequent and severe in patients with comparatively healthy gingiva, little bacterial plaque, and good oral hygiene.[27, 47]

Susceptibility to recession is influenced by the position of teeth in the arch,[58] the angle of the root in the bone, and the mesiodistal curvature of the tooth surface.[45]

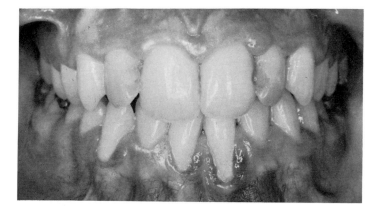

Figure 2–14. Recession around malposed anterior teeth. The gingiva is markedly inflamed.

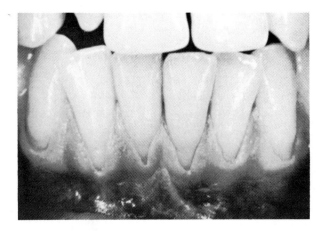

Figure 2–15. Recession associated with malposed teeth. Note excellent condition of the gingiva.

Several aspects of gingival recession make it clinically significant. Exposed root surfaces are susceptible to caries. Wearing away of exposed cementum leaves an underlying dentinal surface that may be extremely sensitive, particularly to touch. Interproximal recession creates spaces in which plaque, food, and bacteria accumulate and are difficult to clean.

GINGIVAL ENLARGEMENT

Gingival enlargement (increase in size) is a common feature of gingival disease. There are many types of gingival enlargement, which vary according to the etiologic factors and pathologic processes that produce them.[21] The lesions may by localized, generalized, marginal, papillary, diffuse, or discrete. Gingival enlargements are classified as inflammatory, noninflammatory, combined, conditioned, neoplastic and developmental.

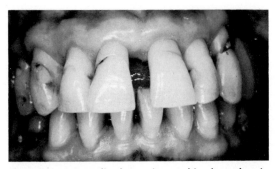

Figure 2–16. Generalized recession resulting from chronic periodontal disease.

Inflammatory Enlargement

Gingival enlargement may result from chronic or acute inflammatory changes. Enlargements induced by chronic changes are by far the more common.

Chronic Inflammatory Enlargement

Chronic inflammatory gingival enlargement originates as a slight ballooning of the interdental papilla, marginal gingiva, or both. In the early stages it produces a life saver–like bulge around the involved teeth. This bulge increases in size until it covers part of the crowns. The enlargement is generally papillary or marginal and *may be localized or generalized* (Figs. 2–17 and 2–18). It progresses slowly and painlessly unless it is complicated by acute infection or trauma (Fig. 2–19).

Occasionally, chronic inflammatory gingival enlargement *occurs as a discrete sessile or pedunculated mass resembling a tumor.* It may be interproximal or on the marginal or attached gingiva. The lesions are slow-growing and usually painless. They may undergo spontaneous reduction in size, followed by reappearance and continued enlargement. Painful ulceration in the fold between the mass and the adjacent gingiva sometimes occurs.

Chronic inflammatory gingival enlargement is *caused by prolonged local irritation.*

Gingival Changes Associated with Mouth Breathing. Gingivitis and gingival enlargement are often seen in mouth breathers,

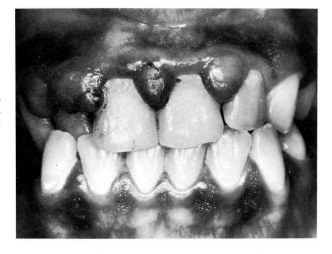

Figure 2–17. Chronic inflammatory gingival enlargement. In this patient the enlargement is localized to the anterior region and is associated with irregularity of teeth.

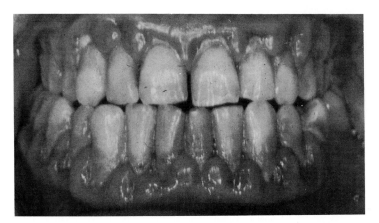

Figure 2–18. Generalized chronic inflammatory gingival enlargement.

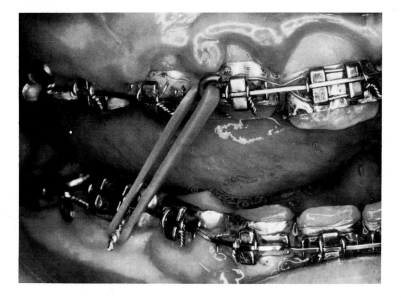

Figure 2–19. Chronic inflammatory gingival enlargement. The enlargement in this case is associated with plaque accumulation around an orthodontic appliance.

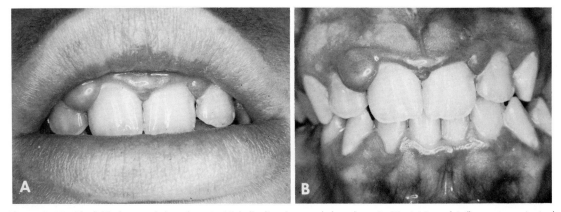

Figure 2–20. Gingivitis in mouth breather. A, High lip line in mouth breather. B, Gingivitis and inflammatory gingival enlargement in exposed area of gingiva.

usually in the maxillary anterior area[38] (Fig. 2–20). The gingiva appears red and edematous, with a diffuse surface shininess of the exposed area. In many cases the altered gingiva is clearly demarcated from the adjacent unexposed normal gingiva. The exact manner in which mouth breathing causes gingival changes has not been demonstrated. Its harmful effect is generally attributed to irritation from surface dehydration; however, comparable changes could not be produced by "air drying" the gingiva of experimental animals.[33]

Acute Inflammatory Enlargement

A *gingival abscess* is a localized, painful, rapidly expanding lesion that is usually of sudden onset. It is generally limited to the marginal gingiva or interdental papilla. In its early stages it appears as a red swelling with a smooth, shiny surface. Within 24 to 48 hours, the lesion is usually fluctuant and pointed, with a surface orifice from which a purulent exudate may be expressed. The adjacent teeth are often sensitive to percussion. If permitted to progress, the lesion generally ruptures spontaneously.

The *gingival abscess* consists of a purulent focus in the connective tissue surrounded by a diffuse infiltration of polymorphonuclear leukocytes, edematous tissue, and vascular engorgement. The surface epithelium presents varying degrees of intracellular and extracellular edema, invasion by leukocytes, and ulceration.

Acute inflammatory gingival enlargement

is a response to irritation from foreign substances such as a toothbrush bristle, a piece of apple skin or a popcorn hull forcefully embedded into the gingiva. The lesion is confined to the gingiva and should not be confused with periodontal or lateral abscesses.

Noninflammatory Hyperplastic Enlargement (Gingival Hyperplasia)

The term hyperplasia refers to an increase in the size of tissue or an organ produced by an increase in the number of its component cells. Noninflammatory gingival hyperplasia is produced by factors other than local irritation. It is not common and occurs most often in association with phenytoin therapy.

Gingival Hyperplasia Associated with Phenytoin Therapy ✓ 8/80% of users get

Enlargement of the gingiva caused by phenytoin (commonly known in the United States by its trade name, Dilantin; in other countries, Epanutin), an anticonvulsant used in the treatment of epilepsy, occurs in some patients receiving the drug. Its reported incidence varies from 3 to 84.5 per cent.[2, 22, 28]

The primary or basic lesion starts as a painless, beadlike enlargement of the facial and lingual gingival margin and interdental papillae. As the condition progresses, the marginal and papillary enlargements unite, and may develop into a massive tissue fold covering a considerable portion of the crowns, which can interfere with occlusion (Fig. 2–21). When uncomplicated by inflammation, the lesion is mulberry-shaped, firm, pale pink, and resilient, with a minutely lobulated surface and without a tendency to bleed. *Phenytoin-induced hyperplasia may occur in mouths devoid of local irritants and may be absent in mouths in which local irritants are profuse.* The enlargement is chronic and slowly increases in size until it interferes with occlusion or becomes so unsightly that the patient seeks help. When surgically removed, it recurs. Spontaneous disappearance occurs within a few months after the drug is discontinued.

Local irritants (e.g., materia alba, calculus, overhanging margins of restorations, and food impaction) favor plaque accumulation, thereby causing inflammation that often complicates gingival hyperplasia caused by the drug. *It is important to distinguish between the increase in size caused by the phenytoin-induced hyperplasia and the complicating inflammation caused by local irritation.* Secondary inflammatory changes add to the size of the lesion caused by phenytoin, produce red or bluish-red discoloration, obliterate the lobulated surface demarcations, and create an increased tendency toward bleeding.

The enlargement is basically a hyperplastic reaction initiated by the drug, with inflammation a secondary complicating factor. Some feel that inflammation is a prerequisite for development of the hyperplasia and that it can be prevented by the removal of local irritants and fastidious oral hygiene.[34, 46] Others find that oral hygiene by means of toothbrushing[16] or the use of a chlorhexidine toothpaste[52] reduces the inflammation but does not lessen the hyperplasia or prevent it.[16]

Familial, Hereditary, or Idiopathic Hyperplastic Enlargement

This is a rare condition of undetermined etiology that affects the attached gingiva, the marginal gingiva, and the interdental papillae. This is in contrast to phenytoin-induced hyperplasia, which is often limited to the gingival margin and interdental papillae. The enlarged gingiva is pink, firm, almost leathery in consistency, and presents a characteristic minutely "pebbled" surface. The hyperplasia is appropriately designated as *idiopathic*, although some cases have been explained on a hereditary basis.[17, 61]

Combined Enlargement

This condition results when gingival hyperplasia is complicated by secondary inflammatory changes. Gingival hyperplasia creates conditions favoring plaque accumulation by accentuating the depth of the gingival sulcus, interfering with effective hygiene measures, and allowing deflection from the normal excursive pathways of food. These secondary inflammatory changes increase the size of

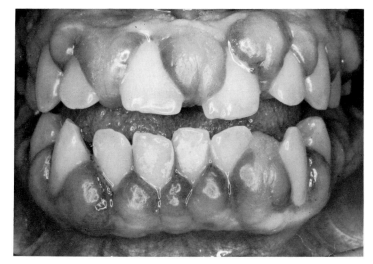

Figure 2–21. Gingival enlargement associated with phenytoin therapy. Note the prominent papillary lesions. The gingiva is firm and nodular. There is marginal inflammation along the crevices deepened by the gingival overgrowth.

the pre-existing gingival hyperplasia and produce combined gingival enlargement. Often, secondary inflammation obscures the features of the pre-existent noninflammatory hyperplasia so that the entire lesion appears to be inflammatory.

Conditioned Enlargement

This type of enlargement occurs when the systemic condition of individuals exaggerates or distorts the usual gingival response to local irritation and produces a corresponding modification of the clinical features of chronic gingivitis. The specific clinical picture depends upon the nature of the modifying systemic influence; the most common being the hormone induced changes in pregnancy and puberty. Individuals with leukemias or vitamin C deficiencies can also present conditioned gingival enlargement. *Local irritation is necessary for the initiation of this type of enlargement.*

Enlargement in Pregnancy *P. Intermedia*

In *pregnancy*, gingival enlargement may be marginal and generalized or occur as single or multiple "tumors." The prevalence of marginal gingival enlargement in pregnancy has been reported as 10 per cent[7] and 70 per cent.[61] The gingival enlargement does not occur without clinical evidence of local irritation. *Pregnancy does not cause the condition; the altered tissue metabolism in pregnancy accentuates the response to local irritants.*[30]

The clinical picture varies considerably. Enlargement is usually generalized and tends to be more prominent interproximally than on the facial and lingual surfaces. The gingiva is bright red or magenta, soft, friable and has a smooth, shiny surface. Bleeding occurs spontaneously or upon slight provocation (Fig. 2–22).

The so-called pregnancy tumor is not a neoplasm; it is an inflammatory response to local irritation. It usually appears after the third month of pregnancy, but may occur earlier,[35] and has a reported incidence of 1.8 to 5 per cent.[42] The lesion appears as a discrete, mushroom-like, flattened spherical mass protruding from the gingival margin or, more frequently, from the interproximal space, attached by a sessile or pedunculated base.

Most gingival disease during pregnancy can be prevented by the removal of local irritants and the institution of fastidious oral hygiene at the outset. Treatment during pregnancy that is limited to the removal of tissue, without complete elimination of local irritants, is followed by recurrence. Commonly, gingival enlargement is reduced following parturition but the complete elimination of the residual inflammatory lesion requires the removal of all local irritants.

Enlargement in Puberty

Enlargement of the gingiva is frequently seen during *puberty*. It occurs in both males and females and appears in areas of local irritation. The size of the gingival enlargement is far in excess of that usually seen associated with comparable amounts of local irritants. This enlargement is marginal, and is frequently characterized by prominent bulbous interproximal papillae. Often the lin-

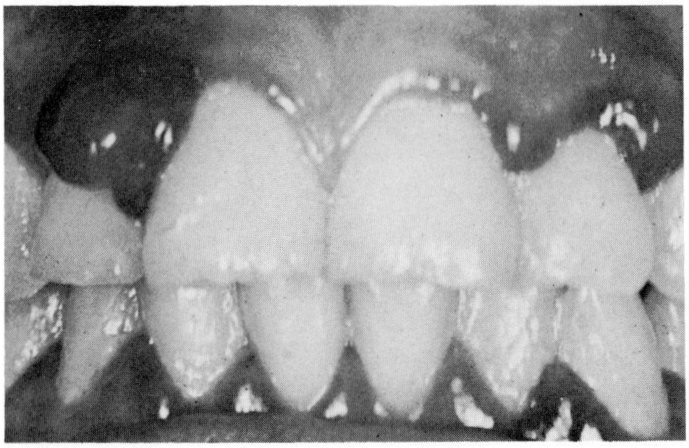

Figure 2–22. Generalized marginal gingivitis in a pregnant woman. Note the localized gingival enlargement (pregnancy tumor) between teeth #7 and #8.

gual surfaces are relatively unaltered because the mechanical action of the tongue and the excursion of food prevent much accumulation of local irritants in this area.

All of the clinical features generally associated with chronic inflammatory gingival disease are present in this condition. *It is the degree of enlargement and the tendency toward massive recurrence in the presence of relatively little local irritation that distinguish the gingival enlargement of puberty from uncomplicated chronic inflammatory gingival enlargement.* After puberty, the enlargement undergoes spontaneous reduction, but it does not disappear until local irritants are removed.

Nonspecific Conditioned Enlargement (Granuloma Pyogenicum)

Granuloma pyogenicum is a nonspecific, tumor-like gingival enlargement considered to be an exaggerated conditioned response to minor trauma. The exact nature of the systemic conditioning factor has not been identified.[32]

Neoplastic Enlargement (Gingival Tumors)

Benign Tumors of the Gingiva

Epulis. *Epulis* is a generic term used clinically to designate all tumors and tumor-like lesions of the gingiva. Most lesions referred to as epulis are inflammatory rather than neoplastic. In fact, neoplasms account for a very small proportion of gingival enlargements.

Fibroma. *Fibromas* of the gingiva arise from the gingival connective tissue or from the periodontal ligament. They are slow-growing, spherical tumors that tend to be firm, nodular, and pedunculated but may appear soft and vascular.

Nevus. The *nevus* may be pigmented or nonpigmented. It commonly occurs on the skin, but a few cases of gingival nevi have been reported. The lesion is benign and slow-growing, varying in color from pale gray to dark brown. It may be flat or raised slightly above the gingival surface, sessile or nodular.[5]

Hemangioma. *Hemangiomas* are benign blood vessel tumors occasionally occurring on the gingiva. These tumors are soft, pain-less, and may be pedunculated. The color varies from deep red to purple, and the tumor blanches on the application of pressure.

Papilloma. *Papilloma* of the gingiva appears as a hard, wart-like protuberance from the gingival surface. It may be small and discrete or appear as a broad, hard elevation of the gingiva with a minutely irregular surface.

Peripheral Giant Cell Reparative Granuloma. *Giant cell lesions* of the gingiva arise interdentally or from the gingival margin, occur most frequently on the labial surface, and may be sessile or pedunculated. They vary in appearance from a smooth, regularly outlined mass to an irregularly shaped, multi-lobulated protuberance with surface indentations. There are no pathognomonic clinical features that differentiate these lesions from other forms of gingival enlargement. Microscopic examination is required for definitive diagnosis.

Malignant Tumors of the Gingiva

Carcinoma. The gingiva is not a frequent site of oral malignancy. *Squamous cell carcinoma is the most common malignant tumor of the gingiva.* Only 1.9[19] to 5.4 per cent[1] of oral carcinomas occur on the gingiva, with the mandible, usually the molar area, being the most common site. Leukoplakia is often associated with the tumor.

Malignant Melanoma. *Malignant melanoma* is a rare oral tumor that tends to occur in the gingiva of the anterior maxilla.[4] The malignant melanoma is usually darkly pigmented and is often preceded by the occurrence of localized pigmentation.[8] It may be flat or nodular and is characterized by rapid growth and early metastasis.

Sarcoma. *Fibrosarcoma, lymphosarcoma, and reticulum cell sarcoma* of the gingiva are rare; only isolated cases have been described in the literature.[10, 25, 58]

Developmental Enlargement

Developmental enlargement appears as a bulbous distortion of the labial and marginal contours of the gingiva of teeth during eruption. It is caused by superimposition of the bulk of the gingiva upon the normal prominence of the enamel in the gingival half of the crown. The enlargement often persists until the junctional epithelium has migrated from the enamel to the cemento-enamel junction.

In a strict sense, developmental gingival enlargement is physiologic, and it ordinarily presents no problem. However, when complicated by marginal inflammation, the composite picture gives the impression of extensive gingival enlargement. Treatment to alleviate the marginal inflammation, rather than resection of the enlargement, is indicated.

ACUTE NECROTIZING ULCERATIVE GINGIVITIS

Acute necrotizing ulcerative gingivitis (ANUG) is an inflammatory destructive disease of the gingiva that presents characteristic signs and symptoms. Other terms by which this condition is commonly known are Vincent's infection and trench mouth.

Bacellus Vincentii
Borrelia Vincentii
Clinical Features *Prevotella Intermedia*

Necrotizing ulcerative gingivitis most often occurs as an *acute* disease. Its relatively mild and more persistent form is referred to as *subacute*. *Recurrent* disease is marked by periods of remission and exacerbation. Sometimes diagnoses of *chronic* necrotizing ulcerative gingivitis are made. However, it is difficult to justify this separate designation because comparable microscopic and clinical features are present in most periodontal pockets with ulceration and destruction of gingival tissue.

Acute necrotizing ulcerative gingivitis is characterized by *sudden onset,* frequently following an episode of debilitating disease or acute respiratory infection. Change in living habits, protracted work without adequate rest, and stress are frequent features of the patients' histories.

Characteristic lesions are punched-out, crater-like depressions at the crest of the gingiva that involve the interdental papillae, and often the marginal gingiva (Fig. 2–23). The surface of the gingival craters is covered by a gray, pseudomembranous slough demarcated from the remainder of the gingival mucosa by a pronounced linear erythema (Fig. 2–23).

The lesions progressively destroy the gingiva and underlying periodontal tissues (Fig. 2–23B). A fetid odor, increased salivation, and spontaneous gingival hemorrhage or pronounced bleeding upon slight stimulation are characteristic clinical signs (Fig. 2–23C).

Acute necrotizing ulcerative gingivitis can occur in otherwise disease-free mouths or superimposed upon chronic gingivitis (Fig. 2–23D) *or periodontal pockets.* Involvement may be limited to a single tooth or group of teeth or may be widespread throughout the mouth.

The lesions are extremely sensitive to the touch, and the patient complains of a constant radiating, gnawing pain that is intensified by spicy or hot foods and mastication. There is a metallic foul taste, and the patient is conscious of an excessive amount of "pasty" saliva.

Individuals with this disease are usually ambulatory, with a minimum of systemic complications. *Local lymphadenopathy and a slight elevation in temperature* are common features of the mild and moderate stages of the disease. In severe cases there are marked systemic complications such as high fever, increased pulse rate, leukocytosis, loss of appetite, and general lassitude. Systemic reactions are more severe in children. *Insomnia, constipation, gastrointestinal disorders, headache, and mental depression sometimes accompany the condition.*

The clinical course is indefinite. If untreated, acute necrotizing ulcerative gingivitis may result in progressive destruction of the periodontium and denudation of the roots, accompanied by an increase in the severity of toxic systemic complications. Often the disease undergoes a diminution in severity, leading to a subacute stage with varying degrees of clinical symptomatology. *The disease may subside spontaneously without treatment.* Such patients generally present a history of repeated remissions and exacerbations. Recurrence of the condition in previously treated patients is frequent.

Microscopically, the lesions appear as a nonspecific acute necrotizing inflammation at the gingival margin, involving both the stratified squamous epithelium and the underlying connective tissue. The surface epithelium is destroyed and replaced by a meshwork of fibrin, necrotic epithelial cells, polymorphonuclear leukocytes, and various types of microorganisms, seen clinically as the pseudo-

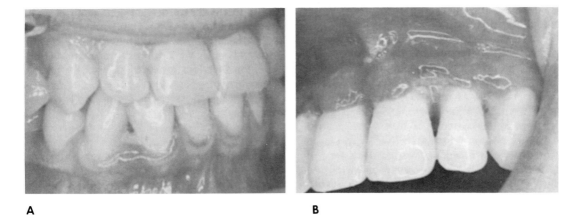

A   B

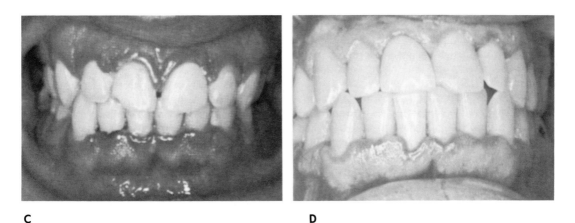

C   D

Figure 2–23. Acute necrotizing ulcerative gingivitis. *A,* Typical punched out interdental papilla between mandibular canine and lateral incisor. *B,* Typical lesions with progressive tissue destruction. *C,* Typical lesions with spontaneous hemorrhage. *D,* Typical lesions have produced irregular gingival contour in a patient with chronic gingivitis.

membrane. The underlying connective tissue is markedly hyperemic, with numerous engorged capillaries and a dense infiltration of polymorphonuclear leukocytes and appears clinically as linear erythema. Spirochetes have been shown to penetrate the living tissue to a depth of about 300 microns.[37]

Smears taken of the lesions present scattered bacteria (predominantly spirochetes and fusiform bacilli), desquamated epithelial cells, and occasional polymorphonuclear leukocytes. The spirochetal organisms form a light-staining, conspicuous, interlacing network throughout the microscopic field.

Diagnosis is based upon clinical findings. A bacterial smear may be used to corroborate the clinical diagnosis, but it is not necessary or definitive because the bacterial picture is not appreciably different from that in marginal gingivitis, periodontal pockets, pericoronitis, or herpetic gingivostomatitis.[51]

Etiology

Plaut in 1894[48] and Vincent in 1896[59] introduced the concept that acute necrotizing ulcerative gingivitis is caused by specific bacteria, namely a fusiform bacillus and a spirochetal organism. The current opinion is that it is caused by a *complex of bacterial organisms* but requires underlying tissue changes to facilitate the pathogenic activity of the bacteria.[24] In addition to *fusiform bacilli* and *spirochetes, vibrios* and *streptococci* are invariably included in the complex of bacteria isolated from lesions of acute necrotizing ulcerative gingivitis.

Preexisting gingivitis, injury to the gingiva, and smoking are important *predisposing factors*. Although necrotizing ulcerative gingivitis may appear in otherwise disease-free mouths, the disease most often occurs *superimposed upon preexisting chronic gingival disease and periodontal pockets*.

Acute necrotizing ulcerative gingivitis is often superimposed upon gingiva altered by severe systemic disease such as nutritional deficiency or other debilitating diseases.

Psychologic factors appear to be important and common in the etiology of acute necrotizing ulcerative gingivitis. The disease often occurs under stressful situations such as induction into the army and school examinations.[18, 20] The mechanisms whereby psychological factors create or predispose to gingival disease have not been established.

Epidemiology and Prevalence

Acute necrotizing ulcerative gingivitis often occurs in epidemic patterns. At one time it was considered contagious, but this has not been substantiated.[54] The disease can occur at any age, with the highest prevalence reported between ages 15 and 30.[11, 57] It is not common in children in the United States, Canada, and Europe, but it has been reported in children from low socioeconomic groups in underdeveloped countries.[31]

Communicability

Acute necrotizing ulcerative gingivitis is not a communicable disease. The distinction must be made between communicability and transmissibility when referring to disease characteristics. The term *transmissible* denotes a capacity for the maintenance of an infectious agent in successive passage through a susceptible animal host.[50] The term *communicable* signifies a capacity for the maintenance of infection by natural modes of spread such as direct contact through drinking water, food, and eating utensils; via the airborne route; or by means of arthropod vectors. Communicable diseases may be described as contagious. It has been demonstrated that disease associated with the fusospirochetal bacterial complex is transmissible; the occurrence of

the disease in epidemic-like outbreaks does not necessarily mean that it is contagious. The affected groups may be afflicted by the disease because of common predisposing factors rather than because of its spread from person to person. In all likelihood both a predisposed host and appropriate bacteria are necessary for the production of this disease.

ACUTE HERPETIC GINGIVOSTOMATITIS

Acute herpetic gingivostomatitis is an infection of the oral cavity caused by the herpes simplex virus.[12, 41, 55] Secondary bacterial infection frequently complicates the clinical picture. Acute herpetic gingivostomatitis occurs most frequently in infants and children below the age of 6 years,[55] but it is also seen in adolescents and adults. It occurs with equal frequency in males and females.

Clinical Features

The condition appears as a diffuse, erythematous, shiny involvement of the gingiva and the adjacent oral mucosa, with varying degrees of edema and gingival bleeding (Fig. 2–24). Initially, discrete spherical gray vesicles appear that coalesce and rupture, forming painful small ulcers. The ulcers, seen clinically more often than vesicles, have red, elevated, halo-like margins and depressed yellowish or grayish-white central portions.

The course of the disease is limited to 7 to 10 days. The diffuse gingival erythema and edema that appear early in the disease persist for several days after the ulcerative lesions have healed. Scarring does not occur.

Acute herpetic gingivostomatitis may appear in a *localized* form following dental procedures in the oral cavity. The affected areas are surfaces of the oral mucosa traumatized by cotton rolls, areas of vigorously applied digital pressure, or intraoral injection sites. The condition appears 1 or 2 days after the trauma, and the involvement presents a diffuse, shiny erythema with numerous pinpoint vesicles confined to an area that can be clearly demarcated from the adjacent uninvolved mucosa.

Herpetic gingivostomatitis is accompanied

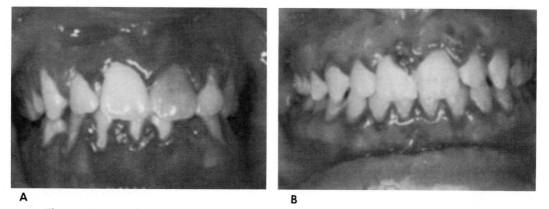

Figure 2–24. Acute herpetic gingivostomatitis. *A,* Typical diffuse erythema. *B,* Vesicles on the gingiva.

by generalized "soreness" of the oral cavity, which interferes with eating and drinking. The ruptured vesicles are the focal sites of pain and are particularly sensitive to touch, thermal changes, condiments, fruit juices, and the excursive action of coarse foods. Infants with the disease may be irritable and refuse to take food.

The diagnosis is usually established from the patient's history and the clinical findings. Material may be obtained from the lesions and submitted to the laboratory for confirmatory tests.

Acute herpetic gingivostomatitis should be differentiated from *aphthous stomatitis (canker sore).* This is a condition characterized by the appearance of discrete spherical vesicles that rupture after 1 or 2 days and form depressed spherical ulcers. The ulcers consist of a saucer-like red or grayish-red central portion and an elevated rim-like periphery. The lesions may occur anywhere in the oral cavity; the mucobuccal fold and the floor of the mouth are common sites. Aphthous stomatitis is painful. It may occur as a single lesion or as lesions scattered throughout the mouth. The duration of each lesion is 7 to 10 days. As a rule, the lesions are larger than those seen in acute herpetic gingivostomatitis. Aphthous stomatitis is a different clinical entity than acute herpetic gingivostomatitis.[13] The ulcerations may look the same in the two conditions, but diffuse erythematous involvement of the gingiva and acute toxic systemic symptoms do not occur in aphthous stomatitis.

Communicability

Acute herpetic gingivostomatitis is contagious[9] and is usually seen in infants and children. Most adults have developed immunity to herpes simplex virus as the result of subclinical infection during childhood.

PERICORONITIS

The term *pericoronitis* refers to inflammation of the gingiva in relation to the crown of an incompletely erupted tooth. It occurs most frequently in the mandibular third molar area.[51, 53] Pericoronitis may be acute, subacute, or chronic.

The partially erupted or impacted mandibular third molar is the most common site of pericoronitis. The space between the crown of the tooth and the overlying gingival flap is an ideal area for the accumulation of food debris and bacterial growth. Even in patients with no clinical signs or symptoms, the gingival flap is often chronically inflamed and presents varying degrees of ulceration along its inner surface (Fig. 2–25). Acute inflammatory involvement is episodic.

Acute pericoronitis is identified by varying degrees of involvement of the pericoronal flap and adjacent structures, as well as systemic complications. Inflammatory response results in an increase in the bulk of the flap, which interferes with complete closure of the jaws. The flap is traumatized by contact with the opposing teeth and the inflammatory

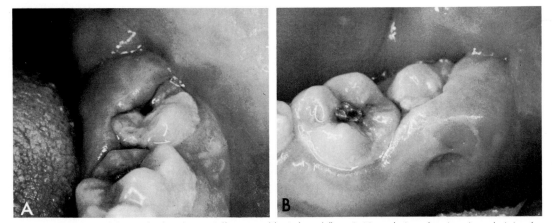

Figure 2–25. Pericoronitis. *A,* Third molar partially covered by infected flap. *B,* Lingual view showing sinus draining from infected flap.

involvement is aggravated. *The clinical picture is that of a markedly red, swollen, suppurating lesion that is exquisitely tender, with radiating pains to the ear, throat, and floor of the mouth.* There is usually a foul taste and an inability to close the teeth together. Swelling of the cheek in the region of the angle of the jaw and lymphadenitis are common findings. There may also be toxic systemic complications such as fever, leukocytosis, and malaise.

DESQUAMATIVE GINGIVITIS

Desquamative gingivitis is not a specific disease entity but rather a nonspecific gingival manifestation of a variety of systemic disturbances, some of which are better understood at present than others. The large majority of cases of so-called chronic desquamative gingivitis represent either lichen planus or mucous membrane pemphigoid. *Since mucous membrane pemphigoid is a relatively rare disease, the majority of cases of so-called desquamative gingivitis are probably lichen planus.*

Careful examination of the mouth may reveal other manifestations of lichen planus, such as reticulate lesions of the buccal mucosa, but some cases of lichen planus start with gingival involvement, and other lesions appear as the disease progresses. In mucous membrane pemphigoid, there may be conjunctival lesions as well as involvement of other mucous membrane sites, such as the

nasal mucosa, vagina, rectum, and urethra. In this case also, early involvement may be confined to the gingiva, and other oral lesions may follow. Diagnosis is possible by histologic studies which differentiate between bullous lesions, resembling the histopathologic features of mucous membrane pemphigoid, and lichenoid lesions, with features similar to those of lichen planus.

Clinical Features

The clinical features of mild, moderate, and severe forms of so-called desquamative gingivitis have been described.[23] Lingual surfaces are usually less severely involved than labial because the tongue and friction from food reduce the amount of local irritants, therefore limiting inflammation.

Mild Form. The mild form occurs most frequently in females between 17 and 23 years of age. Painless, diffuse erythema of the marginal, interdental, and attached gingivae is present and the condition usually comes to the attention of the patient or dentist because of the overall discoloration.

Moderate Form. This condition is seen most frequently in persons between 30 and 40 years of age. Patients complain of burning sensations and sensitivity to thermal changes. Inhalation of air is painful. These individuals cannot tolerate condiments, and toothbrushing causes painful denudation of the gingival surface. Clinical features include the patchy distribution of bright red and gray

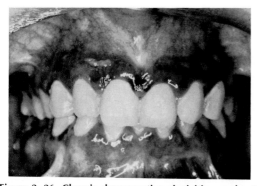

Figure 2–26. Chronic desquamative gingivitis—moderate form. There is generalized edema and erythema associated with inflammation and exposure of underlying connective tissue.

areas involving the marginal and attached gingivae. The surface is smooth and shiny, and the normally resilient gingiva becomes soft (Fig. 2–26). There is slight pitting upon pressure, and the epithelium is not firmly adherent to the underlying tissues. Massaging the gingiva with the finger results in peeling of the epithelium and exposure of the underlying bleeding connective tissue surface. The oral mucosa in the remainder of the mouth is extremely smooth and shiny.

Severe Form. This occurs as scattered, irregularly shaped areas in which the gingiva is denuded and strikingly red in appearance. Since the gingiva separating the red areas is grayish-blue, in overall appearance the gingiva seems speckled. The surface epithelium

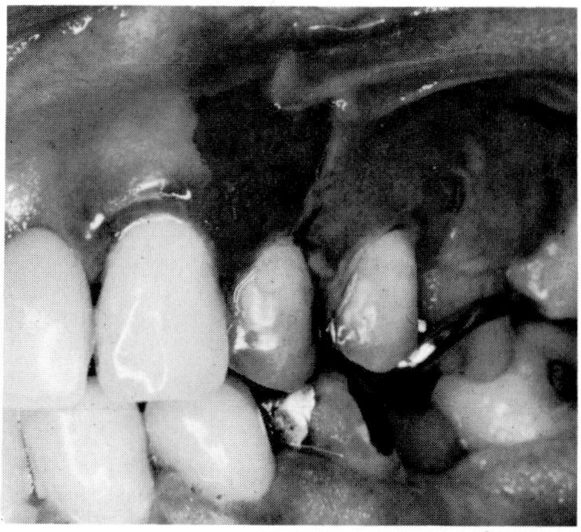

Figure 2–27. Chronic desquamative gingivitis—severe form. There is complete denudation of the epithelium with exposure of underlying erythematous inflamed connective tissue.

appears shredded and friable (Fig. 2–27) and can be peeled off in small patches.

Occasionally surface vessels rupture, release a serous fluid, and expose an underlying surface that is red and raw. A blast of air directed at the gingiva may cause elevation of the epithelium and the consequent formation of a bubble. The areas of involvement seem to shift to different locations on the gingiva. The mucosa is smooth and shiny and may present fissuring in the cheeks adjacent to lines of occlusion.

The condition is extremely painful. Affected individuals cannot tolerate coarse foods, condiments, or temperature changes. There is a constant dry, burning sensation throughout the oral cavity.

Microscopic Features

Microscopically, desquamative gingivitis appears as one of two types: (1) bullous lesions resembling the features of mucous membrane pemphigoid or (2) lichenoid lesions with features similar to those of lichen planus.

Therapy

The therapy for so-called desquamative gingivitis must be based, if possible, on an understanding of the basic disease process causing the gingival reaction.

Careful oral examinations must be carried out so that other lesions may be discovered leading to an accurate differential diagnosis. In lichen planus the gingivae are rarely affected without other oral mucosal lesions being present.

Carefully taken histories will uncover possible coexistent extraoral disease.

Biopsy studies often point to the diagnosis of lichen planus or mucous membrane pemphigoid. They will also reveal unusual cases in which a desquamative gingivitis is a chronic bacterial infection such as tuberculosis, or a mycotic infection such as candidiasis.

Palliative local treatment is essential for all forms of desquamative gingivitis. The patient must be carefully instructed in plaque control using a soft toothbrush, since the gingival surface is easily abraded by toothbrushing. Oxidizing mouthwashes (hydrogen peroxide

USP 3 per cent diluted to one third peroxide and two thirds warm water) should be used twice daily. The reduction of marginal gingivitis results in some reduction of the inflammation and desquamation of the attached gingiva. Treatment with topical corticosteroid ointments[26] and creams may be attempted, but their success has been limited.

Systemic therapy is sometimes used in cases of severe gingival involvement. Consultation with the patient's physician is required prior to the use of any systemic corticosteroid therapy. It is also important to note that systemic therapy for lichen planus is rarely helpful.

In many cases of desquamative gingivitis it may not be possible to determine the basic etiology. However, applied local therapy together with diligence and patience will eventually improve the condition, and the etiologic background may be discovered upon the eventual appearance of other lesions or symptoms. Particular care and patience are required in the atrophic gingivitis of aging, since there is no systemic therapy that has been found useful, other than nutritional supplements if the patient's nutritional status is deficient. Nutritional supplements[52] are of no value unless the patient suffers from a true nutritional deficiency.

References

1. Ackerman, L. V., and del Regato, J. A.: Cancer: Diagnosis, Treatment and Prognosis. St. Louis, C. V. Mosby Company, 1947.
2. Angelopoulos, A. P., and Goaz, P. W.: Incidence of diphenylhydantoin gingival hyperplasia. Oral Surg., 34:898, 1972.
3. Attstrom, R., and Egelberg, J.: Emigration of blood neutrophils and monocytes into the gingival crevices. J. Periodont. Res., 5:48, 1970.
4. Baxter, H. A., Brown, J. B., and Byars, L. T.: Malignant melanomas. Am. J. Orthod., 27:90, 1941.
5. Bernier, J. L., and Tiecke, R. W.: Nevus of the gingiva. J. Oral Surg., 8:165, 1950.
6. Buchner, A., and Hansen, L. A.: Amalgam pigmentation (amalgam tattoo) of the oral mucosa. A clinicopathologic study of 268 cases. Oral Surg., 49:139, 1980.
7. Burket, L. W.: Oral Medicine. Philadelphia, J. B. Lippincott Company, 1946, p. 295.
8. Chaudry, A. P., Hampel, A., and Gorlin, R. J.: Primary malignant melanoma of the oral cavity: a review of 105 cases. Cancer, 11:923, 1958.
9. Chilton, N. W.: Herpetic stomatitis. Am. J. Orthod. Oral Surg., 30:335, 1944.
10. Cook, H. P.: Oral lymphomas. Oral Surg., 4:690, 1961.
11. Dean, H. T., and Singleton, J. E., Jr.: Vincent's infection—a wartime disease. Am. J. Public Health, 35:433, 1945.
12. Dodd, K., Johnston, L. M., and Buddingh, G. J.: Herpetic stomatitis. J. Pediatr., 12:95, 1938.
13. Dodd, R., and Ruchman, J.: Herpes simplex virus not the etiologic agent of recurrent stomatitis. Pediatrics, 5:833, 1950.
14. Dummett, C. O.: Abnormal color changes in gingivae. Oral Surg., 2:649, 1949.
15. Dummett, C. O.: Oral tissue color changes. Ala. J. Med. Sci., 6:274, 1979.
16. Elzay, R. P., and Swenson, H. M.: Effect of an electric toothbrush on dilantin sodium induced gingival hyperplasia. N.Y. J. Dent., 34:13, 1964.
17. Emerson, T. G.: Hereditary gingival hyperplasia. A family pedigree of four generations. Oral Surg., 19:1, 1965.
18. Emslie, R. D.: Cancrum oris. Dent. Pract., 13:481, 1963.
19. Gardner, A. F., Schwartz, F. L., and Pallen, H. S.: Carcinoma of the oral regions. Ann. Dent., 21:80, 1962.
20. Giddon, D. B., Zackin, S. J., and Goldhaber, P.: Acute necrotizing gingivitis in college students. J. Am. Dent. Assoc., 68:381, 1964.
21. Glickman, I.: A basic classification of gingival enlargement. J. Periodontol., 21:131, 1950.
22. Glickman, I., and Lewitus, M.: Hyperplasia of the gingiva associated with dilantin (sodium diphenyl hydantoinate) therapy. J. Am. Dent. Assoc., 28:199, 1941.
23. Glickman, I., and Smulow, J. B.: Chronic desquamative gingivitis: its nature and treatment. J. Periodontol., 35:397, 1964.
24. Goldhaber, P., and Giddon, D. B.: Present concepts concerning the etiology and treatment of acute necrotizing ulcerative gingivitis. Int. Dent. J., 14:468, 1964.
25. Goldman, H. M.: Sarcoma. Am. J. Orthod., 30:311, 1944.
26. Goldman, H. M., and Ruben, M. P.: Desquamative gingivitis and its response to topical triamcinolone therapy. Oral Surg., 21:579, 1966.
27. Gorman, N. J.: Prevalence and etiology of gingival recession. J. Periodontol., 38:316, 1967.
28. Hall, W. B.: Dilantin hyperplasia: a preventable lesion. J. Periodont. Res., 4(Suppl.):36, 1969.
29. Hoover, D. R., and Lefkowitz, W.: Fluctuation in marginal gingivitis. J. Periodontol., 36:310, 1965.
30. Hugoson, A.: Gingival inflammation and female sex hormones. A clinical investigation of pregnant women and experimental studies in dogs. J. Periodont. Res., 5(Suppl.):1, 1970.
31. Jimenez, M., and Baer, P. N.: Necrotizing ulcerative gingivitis in children: a 9 year clinical study. J. Periodontol., 46:715, 1975.
32. Kerr, D. A.: Granuloma pyogenicum. Oral Surg., 4:155, 1951.
33. Klingsberg, J., Cancellaro, L. A., and Butcher, E. O.: Effects of air drying in rodent oral mucous membrane. A histologic study of simulated mouth breathing. J. Periodontol., 32:38, 1961.
34. Larmas, L. A., Mäkinen, K. K., and Paunio, K. U.: A histochemical study of amylaminopeptidase in hydantoin induced hyperplastic, healthy and inflamed human gingiva. J. Periodont. Res., 8:21, 1973.

35. Lee, K. W.: The fibrous epulis and related lesions. Granuloma pyogenicum, "pregnancy tumor," fibroepithelial polyp and calcifying fibroblastic granuloma. A clinicopathological study. Periodontics, 6:277, 1968.

36. Lenox, J. A., and Kopczyk, R. A.: A clinical system for scoring a patient's oral hygiene performance. J. Am. Dent. Assoc., 86:849, 1973.

37. Listgarten, M. A.: Electron microscopic observations on the bacterial flora of acute necrotizing ulcerative gingivitis. J. Periodontol., 36:328, 1965.

38. Lite, T., et al.: Gingival patterns in mouth breathers. A clinical and histopathologic study and a method of treatment. Oral Surg., 8:382, 1955.

39. Löe, H.: The structure and physiology of the dentogingival junction. In Miles, A. E. (ed.): Structural and Chemical Organization of Teeth. Vol. 2. New York, Academic Press, 1967.

40. McCarthy, F. P., and Dexter, S. O., Jr.: Oral manifestations of bismuth. N. Engl. J. Med., 213:345, 1935.

41. McNair, S. T.: Herpetic stomatitis. J. Dent. Res., 29:647, 1950.

42. Maier, A. W., and Orban, B.: Gingivitis in pregnancy. Oral Surg., 2:334, 1949.

43. Meitner, S. W., et al.: Identification of inflamed gingival surfaces. J. Clin. Periodontol., 6:93, 1979.

44. Milne, A. M.: Gingival bleeding in 848 army recruits. An assessment. Br. Dent. J., 122:111, 1967.

45. Morris, M. L.: The position of the margin of the gingiva. Oral Surg., 11:969, 1958.

46. Nuki, K., and Cooper, S. H.: The role of inflammation in the pathogenesis of gingival enlargement during the administration of diphenylhydantoin sodium in cats. J. Periodont. Res., 7:91, 1972.

47. O'Leary, T. J., Drake, R. V., Crump, P., and Allen, N. F.: The incidence of recession in young males—a further study. J. Periodontol., 42:264, 1971.

48. Plaut, H. C.: Studien zur bakteriellen Diagnostik der Diphtherie und der Anginen. Dtsch. Med. Wochnschr., 20:920, 1894.

49. Prinz, H.: Pigmentations of oral mucous membrane. Dent. Cosmos, 74:554, 1932.

50. Rosebury, T.: Is Vincent's infection a communicable disease? J. Am. Dent. Assoc., 29:823, 1942.

51. Rosebury, T., MacDonald, J. B., and Clark, A.: A bacteriologic survey of gingival scrapings from periodontal infections by direct examination, guinea pig inoculation and anaerobic cultivation. J. Dent. Res., 29:718, 1950.

52. Roth, H., and Ross, I. F.: The treatment of desquamative gingivitis. Oral Surg., 9:391, 1956.

53. Salman, I.: Pericoronal infection. Dent. Outlook, 26:460, 1939.

54. Schluger, S.: Necrotizing ulcerative gingivitis in the army. Incidence, communicability, and treatment. J. Am. Dent. Assoc., 38:174, 1949.

55. Scott, T. F. M., Steigman, A. S., and Convey, J. H.: Acute infectious gingivostomatitis: etiology, epidemiology, and clinical picture of common disorders caused by virus of herpes simplex. J.A.M.A., 117:999, 1941.

56. Shklar, G., and McCarthy, P. L.: The Oral Manifestations of Systemic Disease. Boston, Butterworth, 1976.

57. Stammers, A. F.: Vincent's infection. Br. Dent. J., 76:171, 1944.

58. Thoma, K. H., Holland, D. J., Woodbury, H. W., Burrow, J. G., and Sleeper, E. I.: Malignant lymphoma of the gingiva. Oral Surg., 1:57, 1948.

59. Vincent, H.: Sur l'aétiologie et sur les lésions anatomopathologiques, de la poutriture d'hôpital. Ann. de l'Inst. Pasteur, 10:448, 1896.

60. Woofter, C.: The prevalence and etiology of gingival recession. Periodont. Abstracts, 17:45, 1969.

61. Zackin, S. J., and Weisberger, D.: Hereditary gingival fibromatosis. Oral Surg., 14:828, 1961.

Chapter 3

Marginal Periodontitis

Periodontal disease is a generic term for all types of pathologic involvement of the periodontal tissues. These include neoplastic and degenerative diseases as well as inflammatory diseases. Inflammatory diseases of the periodontium include "gingival and periodontal diseases" that are the major cause of tooth loss in adults. Gingival disease is described in Chapter 2.

Chronic destructive periodontitis can be classified as follows:

1. *Periodontitis* is characterized by pocket formation and bone loss.
   A. *Simple adult, or marginal periodontitis* is characterized by pocket formation and bone loss and may be present in slowly progressive or rapidly progressive forms.
   B. *Compound periodontitis* consists of marginal periodontitis with added changes caused by trauma from occlusion.
   C. *Juvenile forms of periodontitis* may be present in generalized or localized forms.
2. *Trauma from occlusion* is injury to the periodontium induced by excessive forces.
3. *Periodontal atrophy* is the reduction in height of the alveolar bone accompanied by *gingival recession;* it is due to the cumulative effects of repeated injuries to the periodontium.

A. *Presenile atrophy* is reduction in bone height that is uniform throughout the mouth and without apparent local cause.
B. *Disuse atrophy* results from lack of functional stimulation to the periodontium.

Both trauma from occlusion and periodontal atrophy are, in their pure forms, accommodation phenomena to changes in the oral environment. They are included under "periodontal diseases" for the sake of completeness and convenience for the clinician. This chapter will cover the pathology of simple periodontitis.

THE PERIODONTAL POCKET

The periodontal pocket is defined as a pathologically deepened gingival sulcus. It is one of the important clinical features of periodontal disease that leads to destruction of the supporting periodontal tissues and tooth loss.

Periodontal pockets are generally painless but may give rise to the following symptoms: localized pain or a sensation of pressure after eating, which gradually diminishes; a foul taste in localized areas; radiating pain "deep in the bone"; and toothache in the absence

47

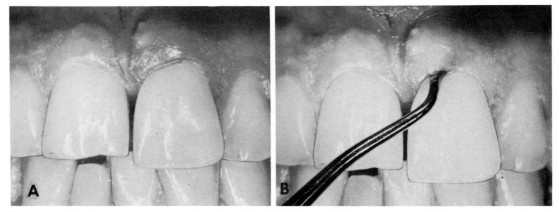

Figure 3–1. Periodontal pockets. *A,* Extrusion of maxillary left incisor and diastema associated with periodontal pocket. *B,* Entire length of periodontal probe inserted to the base of periodontal pocket on central incisor.

of caries. However, *the only reliable method for locating periodontal pockets and determining their extent is careful probing of the gingival margin along each tooth surface* (Fig. 3–1).

Several clinical signs suggest the presence of periodontal pockets. These are:

1. Enlarged, bluish-red marginal gingiva with a "rolled" edge separated from the tooth surface.

2. A reddish-blue vertical zone extending from the gingival margin to the attached gingiva and sometimes into the alveolar mucosa.

3. A break in the facio-lingual continuity of the interdental gingiva.

4. Shiny, discolored, and puffy gingiva associated with exposed root surfaces.

5. Gingival bleeding.

6. Purulent exudate of the gingival margin or its appearance in response to digital pressure on the lateral aspect of the margin.

7. Looseness, extrusion, and migration of teeth.

8. The development of diastemata where none had existed.

Classification

Periodontal pockets are classified as gingival pockets or periodontal pockets according

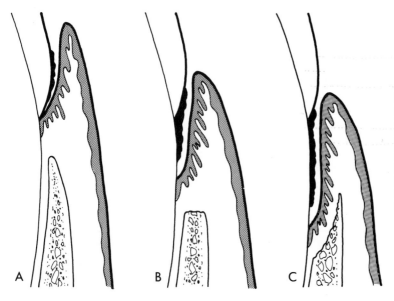

Figure 3–2. Different types of periodontal pockets. *A,* Gingival pocket. There is no destruction of the supporting periodontal tissues. *B,* Suprabony pocket. The base of the pocket is coronal to the level of the underlying bone. Bone loss is horizontal. *C,* Infrabony pocket. The base of the pocket is apical to the level of the adjacent bone. Bone loss is vertical.

to morphology and their relationship to adjacent structures (Fig. 3–2).

The *gingival pocket* is formed by gingival enlargement without destruction of the underlying periodontal tissues. The sulcus is deepened because of the increased bulk of the gingiva. Gingival pockets are described in Chapter 2.

Periodontal pockets occur when the supporting periodontal tissues are destroyed and can be of two types: (1) *suprabony* (supracrestal, supra-alveolar), in which the bottom of the pocket is coronal to the underlying alveolar bone; and (2) *infrabony* (intrabony, subcrestal, or intra-alveolar), in which the bottom of the pocket is apical to the level of the adjacent alveolar bone. In this type the lateral pocket wall lies between the tooth surface and the alveolar bone.

Pockets of different depths and types may occur on different surfaces of the same tooth and on approximating surfaces of the same interdental space. Pockets are also classified as *simple*, involving one root surface; *compound*, involving two or more root surfaces; and *complex*, a spiraling pocket around two or more root surfaces.

Pathogenesis

Periodontal pockets are caused by microorganisms and their products, which produce pathologic tissue changes leading to deepening of the gingival sulcus. This deepening may occur by (1) movement of the gingival margin in the direction of the crown producing a gingival pocket, (2) apical migration of the junctional epithelium and separation from the root surface, or (3) more commonly, a combination of both processes (Fig. 3–3).

Changes involving the transition from normal gingival sulci to pathologic periodontal pockets are associated with different proportions of bacterial cells in dental plaque. Healthy gingiva is associated with few microorganisms, mostly coccoid cells and straight rods. Diseased gingiva is associated with increased percentages of spirochetes and motile rods.[19, 20]

Pocket formation starts as an inflammatory change in the connective tissue wall of the gingival sulcus caused by bacterial plaque. The cellular and fluid inflammatory exudate causes degeneration of

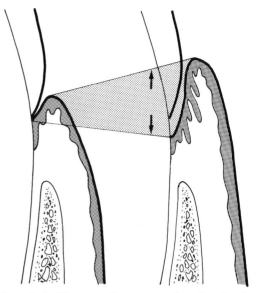

Figure 3–3. Diagrammatic representation of pocket formation. There is expansion in two directions *(arrows)* from the normal gingival sulcus *(left)* to the periodontal pocket *(right).*

the surrounding connective tissue, including the gingival fibers.

Two zones have been described in the process of destruction of connective tissue attachment.[9, 34] Just apical to the junctional epithelium is an area of destroyed collagen fibers, which becomes occupied by inflammatory cells and edema. Immediately apical to this is a zone of partial destruction, then an area of normal attachment.

Along with collagen destruction, the junctional epithelium proliferates along the root in the form of finger-like projections two or three cells in thickness. The coronal portion detaches from the root as it migrates apically, as a result of increased invasion of polymorphonuclear leukocytes. Thus, the sulcus bottom shifts apically, and the oral sulcular epithelium occupies a gradually increasing portion of the sulcular lining.[35]

With continued inflammation, the gingiva increases in bulk, and the crest of the gingival margin extends toward the crown. The junctional epithelium continues to migrate along the root and separate from it. The epithelium of the lateral wall of the pocket proliferates to form cordlike extensions into the inflamed connective tissue. Leukocytes and edema from the inflamed connective tissue infiltrate the epithelium lining the pocket, resulting in varying degrees of degeneration and necrosis (Fig. 3–4)

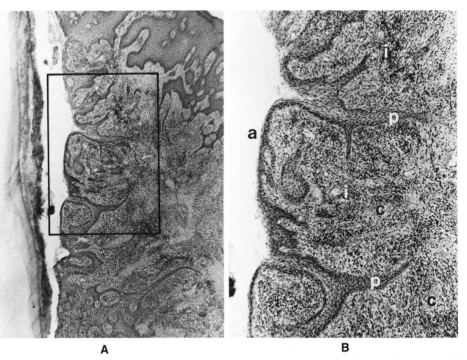

A   **B**

Figure 3–4. *A,* **Low-power view of the lateral wall of a periodontal pocket.** Note the dense inflammatory infiltrate and the proliferating epithelium. *B,* High-power view of rectangle in Figure 3–4*A.* Note the areas of atrophic epithelium (a) and areas of epithelial proliferation (p). The connective tissue is densely infiltrated (i); some remnants of collagen fibers (c) can be seen.

The transformation of a gingival sulcus into a periodontal pocket creates an area where plaque removal becomes impossible, therefore causing more gingival inflammation, which enhances pocket formation and allows more plaque accumulation. *The rationale for pocket reduction is based on the need to eliminate areas of plaque accumulation.*

Periodontal Disease Activity

For many years the loss of attachment produced by periodontal disease was thought to be a slow but continuously progressive phenomenon. In recent years and as a consequence of studies on the specificity of plaque bacteria, this concept of disease activity has changed.

Periodontal pockets are now thought to go through periods of quiescence and exacerbation. *Periods of quiescence* are characterized by a reduced inflammatory response and little or no loss of bone and connective tissue attachment. A build-up of unattached plaque, with its gram-negative, motile, and anaerobic bacteria, starts a *period of exacerbation* in which bone and connective tissue

attachments are lost and the pockets deepen. Destructive periods may last for days, weeks, or longer and are eventually followed by periods of remission or quiescence, in which a more stable condition characterized by a gram-positive flora is established.

These periods of quiescence and exacerbation are also known as *periods of activity and inactivity.* Clinically, active periods show increased bleeding and greater amounts of gingival exudate. Histologically, thinned or ulcerated pocket epithelium and an inflammatory infiltrate are present. The infiltrate is composed predominantly of plasma cells[8] and/or polymorphonuclear leukocytes.[30] Bacterial samples from the pocket lumen, analyzed with darkfield microscopy, show higher proportions of motile organisms and spirochetes.[20] Over a period of time, bone loss can be detected radiographically.

Histopathology

The Soft Tissue Wall

The connective tissue is edematous and densely infiltrated with plasma cells, lymphocytes, and a scattering of polymorpho-nuclear leukocytes. The blood vessels are increased in number, dilated, and engorged. The connective tissue presents varying degrees of degeneration. Single or multiple necrotic foci are occasionally present.[29] In addition to exudative and degenerative changes, the connective tissue presents proliferation of the endothelial cells, with newly formed capillaries, fibroblasts, and collagen fibers. The junctional epithelium at the base of the pocket is shorter than usual but never disappears.

The most severe degenerative changes in the periodontal pocket occur along the lateral wall (Fig. 3–4). Epithelial buds or interlacing cords of epithelial cells project from the lateral wall into the adjacent inflamed connective tissue. These epithelial projections, as well as the remainder of the lateral epithelium, are densely infiltrated by leukocytes and edema from the inflamed connective tissue. Progressive degeneration and necrosis of the epithelium lead to ulceration of the lateral wall, exposure of the underlying markedly inflamed connective tissue, and suppuration. In some cases acute inflammation is superimposed upon the underlying chronic changes.

Bacterial invasion of the apical and lateral areas of the pocket wall may occur in human chronic periodontitis. Filaments, rods, and coccoid organisms with predominant gram-negative cell walls appear in intercellular spaces of the epithelium,[10] and accumulate on the basement lamina.[33] Bacteria can also traverse the basement lamina and invade the subepithelial connective tissue.[33]

The severity of the degenerative changes is not necessarily related to pocket depth. Ulceration of the lateral wall may occur in shallow pockets, and deep pockets are occasionally observed which present only slight degeneration.

Periodontal pockets are chronic inflammatory lesions constantly undergoing repair. Complete healing does not occur because of the persistence of local irritants which continue to stimulate fluid and cellular exudate, causing degeneration of newly formed tissue elements.

The balance between exudative and constructive changes determines the color, consistency, and surface texture of the pocket wall. If the inflammatory fluid and cellular exudate predominate, the pocket wall is bluish-red, soft, spongy, and friable, with a smooth, shiny surface. If there is a relative predominance of newly formed connective tissue cells and fibers, the pocket wall is firm and pink. Clinically, the former appears as an edematous pocket, the latter as a fibrotic pocket. Edematous and fibrotic pockets represent opposite extremes of the same pathologic process rather than different disease entities. They are subject to constant modification, depending upon the predominant changes occurring.

The outer appearance of a periodontal pocket may be misleading because it is not necessarily a true indication of what is taking place throughout the pocket wall. The most severe changes in periodontal pockets occur along the inner aspect. In some cases inflammation and ulceration on the inside of the pocket are walled off, resulting in the outward appear-

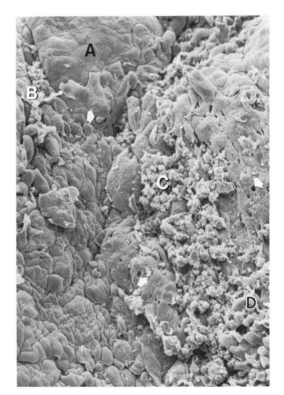

Figure 3–5. Scanning electron microscopic frontal view of periodontal pocket wall. Different areas can be seen in the pocket wall surface. A, area of quiescence; B, bacterial accumulation; C, bacterial-leukocyte interaction; D, intense cellular desquamation. Arrows point to emerging leukocytes and holes left by them in the pocket wall. × 800.

ance of pink and fibrotic gingiva despite the degeneration taking place within.

Microtopography of the Gingival Wall of the Pocket

Scanning electron microscopy has permitted the description of the soft tissue wall of the pocket where different types of activity take place.[32] Areas of different activity are irregularly oval or elongated, adjacent to one another, and measure about 50 to 200 microns. This suggests that the pocket wall is constantly changing as a result of the interaction between the host and the bacteria (Fig. 3–5). The following areas have been described:

1. *Areas of relative quiescence* show a relatively flat surface with minor depressions and mounds and occasional shedding of cells.

2. *Areas of bacterial accumulation* appear as depressions on the epithelial surface, with abundant debris and bacterial clumps penetrating into the enlarged intercellular spaces. These bacteria are mainly cocci, rods, and filaments, with a few spirochetes.

3. *Areas of emergence of leukocytes* are seen passing through the pocket wall from holes located in the intercellular spaces.

4. *Areas of leukocyte-bacterial interaction* appear, showing numerous leukocytes covered with bacteria in the apparent process of phagocytosis. Bacterial plaque associated with the epithelium is seen either as an organized matrix covered by a fibrin-like material in contact with the surface of cells or as bacteria penetrating into the intercellular spaces.

5. *Areas of intense epithelial desquamation* are seen consisting of semi-attached and folded epithelial squames, sometimes partially covered with bacteria.

6. *Areas of ulceration* show exposed connective tissue (Fig. 3–6).

7. *Areas of hemorrhage* are characterized by numerous erythrocytes (see Fig. 3–6).

The transition from one area to another is proposed to occur as bacteria accumulate in previously quiescent areas, triggering the emergence of leukocytes and the leukocyte-bacterial interaction. This would lead to intense epithelial desquamation and, finally, to ulceration and hemorrhage.

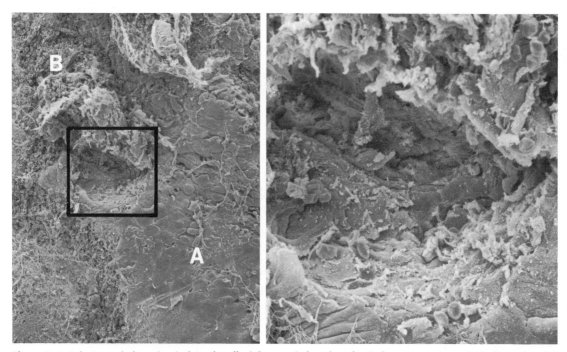

Figure 3–6. *Left,* **Area of ulceration in lateral wall of deep periodontal pocket in human specimen.** A, Surface of pocket epithelium in a quiescent state; B, area of hemorrhage. × 800. *Right,* Higher magnification of square in figure at left. Connective tissue fibers and cells can be seen in bottom of ulcer. Scanning electron microscopy. × 3000.

Pocket Contents

Periodontal pockets contain debris consisting of microorganisms and their products (enzymes, endotoxins, and other metabolic products), dental plaque, gingival fluid, food remnants, salivary mucin, desquamated epithelial cells, and leukocytes. Plaque-covered calculus usually projects from the tooth surface. If a purulent exudate is present, it consists of living, degenerated, and necrotic leukocytes (predominantly polymorphonuclear), living and dead bacteria, serum, and a scant amount of fibrin.[23] The contents of periodontal pockets filtered free of organisms and debris have been demonstrated to be toxic when injected subcutaneously into experimental animals.[14]

The presence of pus or the ease with which it can be expressed from the pocket merely reflects the nature of the inflammatory changes in the pocket wall. It is no indication of the depth of the pocket or the severity of the destruction of the supporting tissues. *Pus is a common feature of periodontal disease, but it is only a secondary sign.* Extensive pus formation may occur in shallow pockets, whereas deep pockets may present little or no pus.

The Root Surface Wall

The root surface walls of periodontal pockets often undergo changes that are significant because they may *perpetuate the periodontal infection, cause pain, and complicate periodontal treatment.* Changes in cementum can be classified according to structural, chemical, and cytotoxic features.

Structural changes include the following:

1. *Presence of pathologic granules,*[4, 5] which may represent areas of collagen degeneration or where collagen fibrils had not been fully mineralized.

2. *Areas of increased mineralization,*[36] which are probably due to the exchange of minerals and organic components at the cementum-saliva interface upon exposure to the oral cavity.

3. *Areas of demineralization,* which are probably related to *root caries* (Fig. 3–7). Exposure to oral fluid and bacterial plaque results in

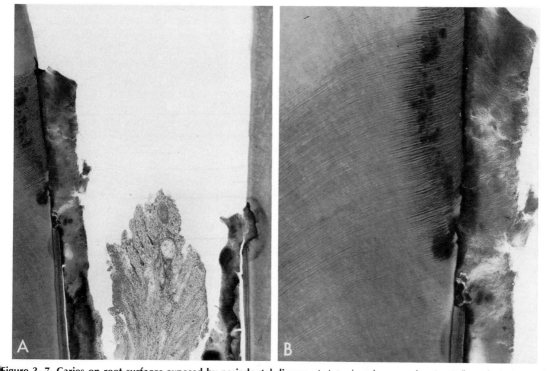

Figure 3–7. Caries on root surfaces exposed by periodontal disease. *A,* Interdental space, showing inflamed gingiva and caries on proximal tooth surfaces. *B,* Caries of cementum and dentin, showing bacterial invasion of dentinal tubules. Note the filamentous structure of the dental plaque and darker staining of calculus adherent to the root.

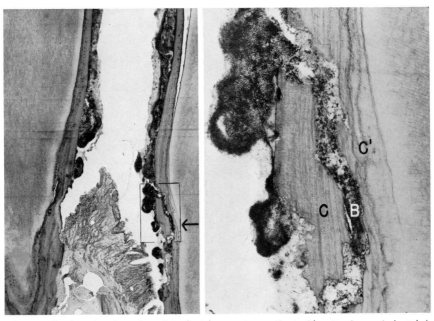

Figure 3–8. *Left,* Mesiodistal section through an interdental space in a patient with extensive periodontal destruction. An area of **cementum necrosis** is enclosed within the rectangle designated by the arrow. *Right,* Detailed section of area enclosed in the rectangle showing **necrotic fragment of cementum** (C) separated from lamellated cementum (C') by clumps of bacteria (B).

proteolysis of the embedded remnants of Sharpey's fibers; the cementum may be softened and undergo fragmentation and cavitation (Fig. 3–8).[16]

Involvement of the cementum is followed by bacterial penetration of the dentinal tubules, resulting in destruction of the dentin. In severe cases, large sections of necrotic cementum become detached from the tooth and separated from it by masses of bacteria. The undisturbed tooth may not be painful, but penetration of the defective cementum with a probe may cause pain. A prevalence rate study of root caries in individuals 20 to 64 years old revealed that 42 per cent had one or more root caries lesions and that the number of lesions tends to increase with age.[17]

Caries of the root may lead to *pulpitis,* sensitivity to sweets and thermal changes, or severe pain. Pathologic exposure of the pulp occurs in severe cases. Root caries may cause toothaches in patients with periodontal disease and without evidence of coronal decay. *Caries of the cementum requires special attention when the pocket is treated.* The necrotic cementum must be removed by scaling and root planing until firm tooth surface is reached, even if this entails extension into the dentin.

Cemental Resorption. Areas of cellular resorption of cementum and dentin are common in roots uninvolved with periodontal disease.[37] These are of no particular significance as long as the roots are covered by periodontal ligament, and they are apt to undergo repair. However, if the roots are exposed by progressive pocket formation before repair occurs, they appear as isolated cavitations that penetrate into the dentin. These areas can be differentiated from caries of the cementum by their clear-cut outline and hard surface. Once exposed to the oral cavity, they may be sources of considerable pain and require restoration.

Cytotoxic Changes. Bacterial penetration into the cementum can be found as deep as the cemento-dentinal junction.[7, 40] In addition, bacterial products such as endotoxins[3] have also been detected in the cementum wall of periodontal pockets. When root fragments from teeth with periodontal disease are placed in tissue culture, they induce irreversible morphologic changes in the cells of the culture. Such changes are not produced by normal roots.[15] Diseased root fragments also prevent the in vitro attachment of human gingival fibroblasts, whereas nor-

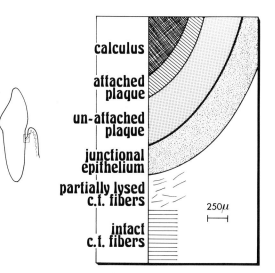

Figure 3–9. Diagrammatic representation of the area of the bottom of a pocket.

calculus

attached plaque

un-attached plaque

junctional epithelium

partially lysed c.t. fibers

250μ

intact c.t. fibers

mal root surfaces allow the cells to attach freely.[2, 3] When reimplanted in the oral mucosa of the patient, diseased root fragments induce an inflammatory response even if autoclaved.[22]

The following areas are found on the cemental walls of periodontal pockets (Fig. 3–9):

1. Cementum covered by calculus, where all previously described changes can be found.

2. Attached plaque, which covers calculus and extends apically to a variable degree, probably to 500 microns.

3. Areas of unattached bacterial plaque.

4. Junctional epithelium attached to the cementum, approximately 50 to 200 microns in length.

5. Areas of partially destroyed connective tissue fibers.

6. Areas of intact connective tissue fibers. All these areas are of particular interest since they are the sites where pocket instrumentation occurs.

Pulp Changes Associated with Periodontal Pockets

The spread of infection from periodontal pockets may cause pathologic changes in the pulp that give rise to painful symptoms or adversely affect the response of the pulp to restorative procedures. Involvement of the pulp in periodontal disease occurs through either the apical foramen or the lateral canals in the root after infection

spreads from the pocket through the periodontal ligament.

Gingival Recession, Pocket Depth, and Bone Loss

Pocket formation causes recession of the gingiva and denudation of the root surface. The severity of recession is generally, but not always, correlated with the depth of the pocket. This is because the *degree of recession depends upon the location of the base of the pocket on the root surface, whereas the depth is the distance between the base of the pocket and the crest of the gingiva.* Pockets of the same depth may be associated with different degrees of recession, and pockets of different depths may be associated with the same amount of recession (Figs. 3–10 and 3–11). Exposure of the roots after pockets are eliminated depends upon the amount of recession before treatment is instituted. A realistic appraisal of the existing recession associated with periodontal pockets will prevent the erroneous impression that it is caused by the treatment.

Severity of bone loss is generally correlated with pocket depth. But extensive bone loss may be associated with shallow pockets and slight loss with deep pockets. Destruction of alveolar bone may also occur in the absence of periodontal pockets, associated with trauma from occlusion or marked recession. Normally, the distance between the junctional epithelium and the alveolar bone is relatively constant, about 0.5 to 2 mm.[38]

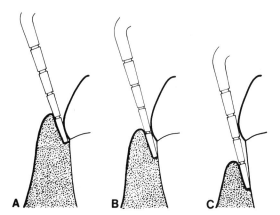

Figure 3–10. Same pocket depth—different amounts of recession. *A,* Gingival pocket—no recession. *B,* Periodontal pocket of similar depth as *A,* but with some degree of recession. *C,* Pocket depth same as in *A* and *B* but with still more recession.

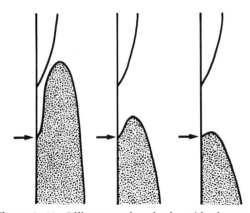

Figure 3–11. Different pocket depths with the same amount of recession. Arrows point to bottom of pocket. Distance between arrow and cemento-enamel junctions remains the same in spite of different pocket depths.

Suprabony and Infrabony Pockets

The principal differences between infrabony and suprabony pockets are the relationship of the soft tissue wall of the pocket to the alveolar bone, the pattern of bone destruction, and the direction of the transseptal fibers of the periodontal ligament.[6] These features are summarized in Table 3–1.

In the *infrabony pocket*, the base is apical to the level of the alveolar bone, and the pocket wall lies between the tooth and bone. These most often occur interproximally but may be located on the facial and lingual surfaces. Often the pockets spread from the original surfaces to one or more contiguous surfaces. The *suprabony pocket* has its base coronal to the crest of the bone. *The inflammatory, proliferative, and degenerative changes in infrabony and suprabony pockets are the same, and both* lead to destruction of the supporting periodontal tissues.

Infrabony pockets are caused by the same local irritants as those causing suprabony pockets. Trauma from occlusion may add to the effect of inflammation by altering the alignment of the transseptal periodontal fibers, diverting the inflammation directly into the periodontal ligament space rather than into the interdental septum, or by injuring the periodontal ligament fibers, aggravating the destruction produced by inflammation.[11, 12]

EXTENSION OF INFLAMMATION TO THE SUPPORTING PERIODONTAL TISSUES

The extension of inflammation from the marginal gingiva into the supporting periodontal tissues marks the transition from *gingivitis* to *periodontitis. Periodontitis is always preceded by gingivitis, but not all gingivitis proceeds to periodontitis.* Some cases never transform to periodontitis, and others progress very quickly. The factors responsible for the extension of inflammation to the supporting structures, converting gingivitis to periodontitis, are not known. However, *the transition is associated with changes in the composition of bacterial plaque and in the composition of the cellular infiltrate.* In advanced stages of disease the number of motile organisms and spirochetes increases, whereas the number of coccoid forms and straight rods decreases.[19] Also, the cellular infiltrate shows an increase in B lymphocytes and plasma cells.

TABLE 3–1. DISTINGUISHING FEATURES OF SUPRABONY AND INFRABONY POCKETS

Suprabony Pocket	Infrabony Pocket
1. The base of the pocket is coronal to the level of the alveolar bone.	1. The base of the pocket is apical to the crest of the alveolar bone, so that the bone is adjacent to the soft tissue wall (Fig. 3–2).
2. The pattern of destruction of the underlying bone is horizontal.	2. The bone destructive pattern is vertically angular.
3. Interproximally, the transseptal fibers that are restored during progressive periodontal disease are arranged horizontally in the space between the base of the pocket and the alveolar bone.	3. Interproximally, the transseptal fibers are oblique rather than horizontal. They extend from the cementum beneath the base of the pocket along the bone, and over the crest to the cementum of the adjacent tooth.
4. On the facial and lingual surfaces, the periodontal ligament fibers beneath the pocket follow their normal horizontal-oblique course between the tooth and the bone.	4. On the facial and lingual surfaces, the periodontal ligament fibers follow the angular pattern of the adjacent bone. They extend from the cementum beneath the base of the pocket along the bone and over the crest to join with the outer periosteum.

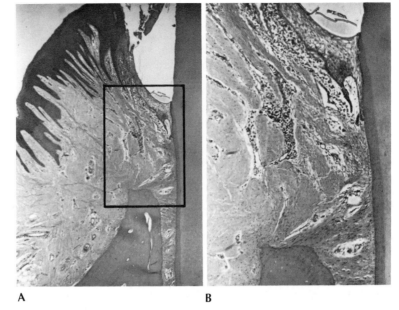

Figure 3–12. *A,* Area of inflammation extending from the gingiva into the suprabony area. *B,* Detailed view of rectangle in Figure 3–12*A,* showing extension of inflammation along blood vessels in between collagen bundles.

A   B

Pathways of Gingival Inflammation

Gingival inflammation extends to the supporting structures through the loosely arranged tissues around the blood vessels, into the alveolar bone.[39] *The pathway of the spread of inflammation is critical, because it affects the pattern of bone destruction in periodontal disease.*

Bacterial plaque causes inflammation in the marginal gingiva and interdental papillae. The inflammation penetrates and destroys the gingival fibers, usually at a short distance from their attachment to the cementum. It then spreads into the supporting tissues around all the surfaces of the teeth (Fig. 3–12).

Inflammation from the gingiva spreads *along the outer periosteal surface of the bone* and

Figure 3–13. Pathways of inflammation from the gingiva into the supporting periodontal tissues in periodontitis. *A,* **Interproximally.** (1) From the gingiva into the bone, (2) from the bone into the periodontal ligament, (3) from the gingiva into the periodontal ligament. *B,* **Facially and Lingually.** (1) from the gingiva along the outer periosteum, (2) from the periosteum into the bone, (3) from the gingiva into the periodontal ligament.

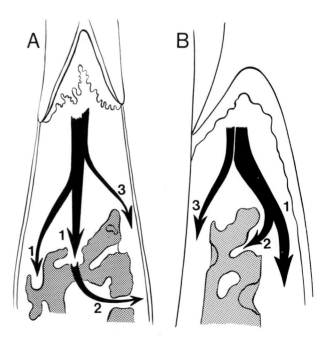

penetrates into the marrow spaces through *vessel channels in the outer cortex* on the facial and lingual surfaces (Fig. 3–13).

Interproximally, inflammation spreads in the loose connective tissue around the blood vessels, through the transseptal fibers, and then into the bone through vessel channels which perforate the crest of the interdental septum. After reaching the marrow spaces, the inflammation may return from the bone into the periodontal ligament or, less frequently, spread from the gingiva directly into the periodontal ligament and then into the interdental septum.[1]

Along its course from the gingiva to the bone, the inflammation reduces the transseptal fibers to disorganized granular fragments surrounded by inflammatory cells and edema.[28] However, there is a continuous tendency to recreate transseptal fibers across the crest of the interdental septum farther along the root as the bone destruction progresses. As a result, transseptal fibers are present even in cases of extreme periodontal bone loss.

Clinical Aspects of Inflammation in the Periodontal Ligament

Regardless of whether it extends directly from the gingiva or indirectly through the alveolar bone, inflammation is often present in the periodontal ligament in periodontal disease and contributes to *tooth mobility and pain.*

The inflammatory exudate reduces tooth support by causing degeneration and destruction of the principal fibers and breaks in the continuity between the roots and the bone. The extent to which inflammation in the periodontal ligament causes mobility is dramatically demonstrated when the inflammation is eliminated by treatment and the tooth becomes firm.

Inflammation in the periodontal ligament is usually chronic and asymptomatic. However, superimposed acute inflammation is frequently the cause of considerable pain. With the influx of the acute exudate, the tooth becomes elevated in the socket and the patient may wish to "grind" on it. Repeated contact with opposing teeth can cause sensitivity to percussion. The condition may develop into an acute periodontal abscess unless the inflammation is reduced.

BONE LOSS IN PERIODONTAL DISEASE

The crux of the problem of chronic destructive periodontal disease is that changes occur in the bone. Changes in the other tissues of the periodontium are important, but it is the destruction of bone that is responsible for the loss of teeth.

The height of the alveolar bone is normally maintained by an equilibrium between bone formation and bone resorption, regulated by local and systemic influences. When resorption exceeds formation, bone height is reduced (Fig. 3–14).

In periodontal disease the equilibrium is altered so that bone resorption exceeds bone formation. Bone loss may result from increased resorption in the presence of normal formation, decreased formation in the presence of normal resorption, or increased resorption combined with decreased formation.

Bone destruction is caused by local factors, gingival inflammation, and trauma from occlusion. Bone loss caused by extension of gingival inflammation is responsible for reduction in height of the alveolar bone, whereas trauma from occlusion causes bone loss lateral to the root surface.

Chronic inflammation is the most common cause of bone destruction in periodontal disease. The rate of bone loss has been found to average about 0.2 mm a year for facial surfaces and about 0.3 mm a year for interproximal surfaces when periodontal disease is allowed to progress untreated.[21]

This destruction is not a process of bone necrosis; it involves the activity of living cells along viable bone. When tissue necrosis and pus are present in periodontal disease, they occur in the soft tissue walls of periodontal pockets and are reflective of current inflammatory conditions. The level of bone is the consequence of past pathologic experiences. Therefore, *the degree of bone loss is not necessarily correlated with the depth of periodontal pockets, the severity of ulceration of the pocket wall, or the presence or absence of pus.*

Inflammation reaches the bone by extension from the gingiva. It spreads into the marrow spaces and replaces the marrow with a leukocytic and fluid exudate, new blood vessels, and proliferating fibroblasts. Multinuclear osteoclasts and mononuclear phagocytes are increased in number, and the bone

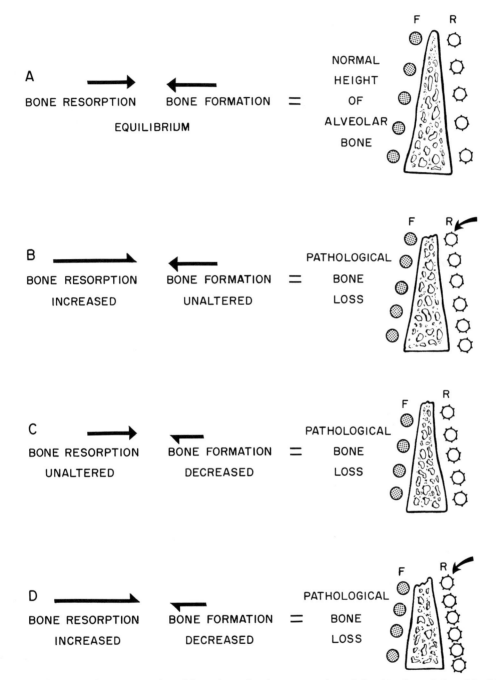

Figure 3–14. Diagrammatic representation of bone formative–bone resorptive relationships in periodontal health and disease. *A,* Physiologic equilibrium between bone resorption (R) and bone formation (F) responsible for the maintenance of normal alveolar bone height. *B,* Pathologic bone loss produced when bone resorption is increased *(arrow). C,* Pathologic bone loss produced when bone formation is decreased. *D,* Pathologic bone loss produced when bone resorption is increased *(arrow)* and formation is decreased.

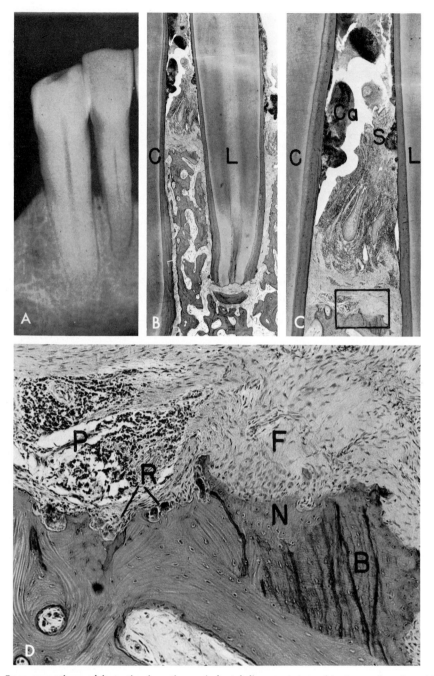

Figure 3–15. Bone resorption and formation in active periodontal disease. *A,* Lateral incisor and canine with bone loss. *B,* Survey section of lateral incisor (L) and canine (C). *C,* Interdental space between lateral incisor (L) and canine (C), showing calculus (Ca) and periodontal pockets with suppuration (S). A detailed view of the bone margin within the rectangle is shown in *D. D,* Bone margin beneath the periodontal pockets. Note the following: osteoclastic resorption (R) beneath the inflammation (P) and newly formed bone (N) with a thin surface layer of osteoid and osteoblasts adjacent to the resorption. The new bone is separated from the lamellated bone (B) by an irregular resorption line. An area of fibrosis is shown at F.

surfaces are lined with cove-like resorption lacunae.

Inflammation also stimulates bone formation immediately adjacent to active bone resorption and along trabecular surfaces at a distance from the inflammation in an apparent effort to reinforce the remaining bone (buttressing bone formation) (Fig. 3–15). Normally fatty bone marrow is partially or totally replaced by a fibrous type of marrow in the vicinity of the resorption.

Autopsy specimens from patients with untreated disease occasionally show areas where bone resorption had ceased and new bone was being formed on the previously eroded bone margin. *This finding indicates that bone resorption in periodontal disease may occur as an intermittent process, with periods of remission and exacerbation.* This is consistent with the varied rates of progression observed clinically in untreated periodontal disease. These periods of activity and inactivity appear to coincide with the quiescence or exacerbation of gingival inflammation, manifested by changes in the bleeding index, in the amount of exudate, and in the composition of bacterial plaque.

Although many investigations have been conducted and explanations considered, the exact mechanisms of bone destruction

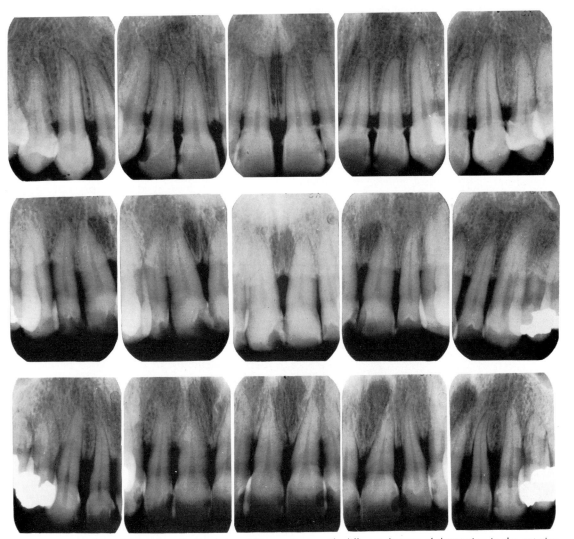

Figure 3–16. Horizontal bone loss. Radiographs of three patients with different degrees of destruction in the anterior maxilla.

in inflammatory periodontal disease are not known.

Bone Destructive Patterns in Periodontal Disease

In addition to reducing bone height, periodontal disease alters the morphology of the bone. An understanding of the nature and pathogenesis of these alterations is essential for an understanding of the periodontal disease process.

Horizontal Bone Loss

This is the most common pattern of bone loss in periodontal disease. The bone is reduced in height, and the bone margin is roughly perpendicular to the tooth surface (Fig. 3–16). The interdental septa and the facial and lingual plates are affected, but not necessarily equally around all surfaces of the same tooth.

Bone Deformities (Osseous Defects)

There are several types of bone deformities produced by periodontal disease. The presence of deformities may be suggested by radiographs, but *careful probing and surgical exposure of the areas are required to confirm their conformation and dimensions.*

Vertical or Angular Defects. Vertical or angular defects are those that occur in an oblique direction, leaving a hollowed-out trough in the bone alongside the root; the base of the defect is located apical to the surrounding bone (Fig. 3–17). In most instances angular defects have accompanying infrabony pockets; infrabony pockets always have an underlying angular defect.

Infrabony pockets are classified on the basis of the number of walls[13] and the depth and width of their underlying osseous defects. Angular defects have one wall, two walls, or three walls (Fig. 3–18). The number of walls in the apical portion of the defect may be greater than that in its occlusal portion; with these cases the term *combined osseous defect* is used. Angular defects can be shallow and narrow; shallow and wide; deep and narrow; or deep and wide. They generally occur in forms which represent gradients of these types.

Vertical defects occurring interdentally can generally be seen in the radiograph, although sometimes thick bony plates may obscure them. They also appear on facial, lingual, and palatal surfaces but are not seen on radiographs. Surgical exposure is the only sure way to determine the presence and configuration of vertical osseous defects.

Vertical defects increase with age, and approximately 60 per cent of individuals with interdental angular defects present only a single defect. The most common location of these defects, viewed radiographically, is on distal surfaces of molar teeth.[27]

The three-wall vertical defect has also been called an *intrabony defect*. These appear most frequently on the mesial aspects of second and third maxillary and mandibular molars. The one-wall vertical defect is also called a *hemiseptum*.

Vertical or angular destruction of alveolar bone is found in juvenile periodontitis. The cause of bone destruction in this type of periodontal disease is unknown.

Osseous Craters. Osseous craters are concavities in the crest of the interdental bone confined within the facial and lingual walls (Fig. 3–19). Craters have been found to make up about one third of all defects (35.2 per cent) and about two thirds (62 per cent) of all mandibular defects. They are twice as common in posterior segments as in anterior segments.[24, 25]

The facial and lingual crests of craters have been found to be identical in height in 85 per cent of cases, with the remaining 15 per cent

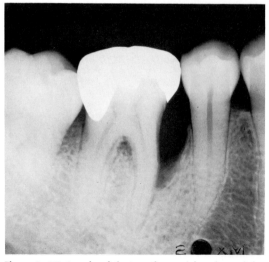

Figure 3–17. Angular defect on the mesial surface of the first molar. Note also the furcation involvement.

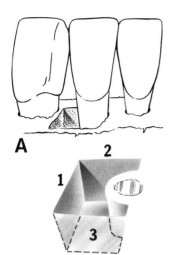

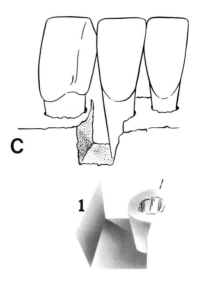

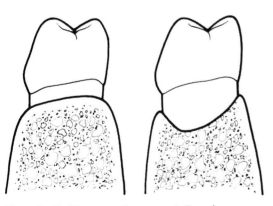

Figure 3–18. One-, two-, and three-walled infrabony defects on right lateral incisor. *A*, Three bony walls: (1) distal, (2) lingual, and (3) facial walls. *B*, Two-wall defect; (1) distal and (2) lingual walls. *C*, One-wall defect: (1) distal wall only.

Figure 3–19. Diagrammatic representation of an osseous crater in a faciolingual section between two lower molars. *Left*, Normal bone contour. *Right*, Osseous crater.

being nearly equally divided between higher facial and higher lingual crests.[31] The high frequency of interdental craters probably occurs because the interdental area collects more plaque and is more difficult to clean, the normal flat or even concave faciolingual shape of the interdental septum in lower molars may favor crater formation, and vascular patterns from the gingiva to the center of the crest may provide a convenient pathway for inflammation.[24, 31, 55]

Bulbous Bone Contours. These are bony enlargements caused by exostoses, adaptation to function, or buttressing bone formation. They are found more frequently in the maxilla than in the mandible.

Inconsistent Margins. These are angular or U-shaped defects produced by resorption of the facial or lingual alveolar plate or abrupt differences between the height of the facial or lingual margins and the height of the interdental septa. These defects have also been termed *reversed architecture.* They are more frequent in the maxilla[24] (Fig. 3–20).

Ledges. Ledges are plateau-like bone margins caused by resorption of thickened bony plates.

FURCATION INVOLVEMENT

The term *furcation involvement* refers to commonly occurring conditions in which the bifurcation or trifurcation of multirooted teeth are denuded by periodontal disease. The mandibular first molars are the most common sites and the maxillary first premolars the least common; the number of furcation involvements increases with age[18] (Fig. 3–21).

The denuded bifurcation or trifurcation may be visible clinically or obscured by the inflamed wall of a periodontal pocket. The extent of involvement is determined by exploration with a blunt probe; a simultaneous blast of warm air may facilitate visualization. The tooth may or may not be mobile and is usually symptom-free, but the patient may describe *sensitivity to thermal changes,* caused by caries or lacunar resorption of the root in the furcation area; *recurrent or constant throbbing pain,* caused by pulp changes; or *sensitivity to percussion,* caused by acute inflammatory involvement of the periodontal ligament. Furcation involvement may also result in acute periodontal or periapical abscess formation.

Microscopically, furcation involvement presents no unique pathologic features. It is simply a phase in the rootward extension of the periodontal pocket. In its early stages, it presents a widening of the periodontal space, with cellular and fluid inflammatory exudation, followed by epithelial proliferation into the bifurcation area from an adjoining periodontal pocket. Extension of the inflammation into the bone leads to resorption and reduction in bone height. Plaque, calculus, and bacterial debris occupy the denuded furcation space.

PERIODONTAL ABSCESS

A periodontal abscess is a localized purulent inflammation in the periodontal tissues. It is also known as a *lateral or parietal abscess.* Periodontal abscesses are most often caused by deep extension of infection from periodontal pockets into the supporting periodontal tis-

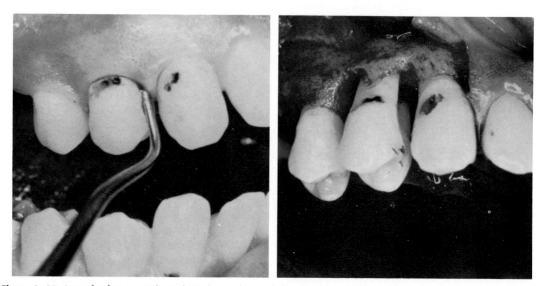

Figure 3–20. Irregular bone margin. *Left,* Probe in deep infrabony pocket on the mesial surface of maxillary premolar. *Right,* Elevated flap shows irregular bone margin with notching of interdental bone, reversed architecture.

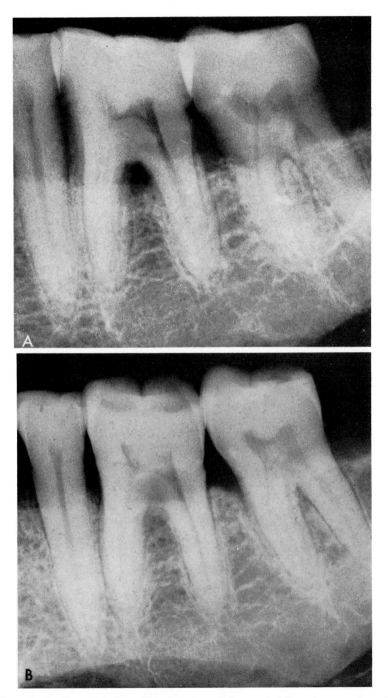

Figure 3–21. *A,* **Bifurcation involvement** indicated by triangular radiolucence in bifurcation area of mandibular first molar. The second molar presents only a slight thickening of the periodontal space in the bifurcation area. *B,* Same area, different angulation. The triangular radiolucence in the bifurcation of the first molar is obliterated, and involvement of the second molar bifurcation is apparent.

sues or into the connective tissue of the pocket wall. Localization of the abscess results when drainage into the pocket space is impaired. In complex pockets that describe tortuous courses around the roots, periodontal abscesses may form in the cul-de-sac, shut off from drainage to the surface. Incomplete removal of calculus during treatment of periodontal pockets may cause shrinkage of the gingival wall, occluding the pocket orifice, and allow periodontal abscesses to form in sealed-off pocket bottoms. Periodontal abscesses may also occur in the absence of periodontal disease, following trauma to the tooth or perforation of the lateral wall of the root in endodontic therapy.

Classification

Periodontal abscesses are classified according to location as follows:

1. *Abscess in the supporting periodontal tissues* along the lateral aspect of the root, generally causing a sinus in the bone, which extends laterally from the abscess to the external surface.

2. *Abscess in the soft tissue wall of a deep periodontal pocket.*

3. Periodontal abscesses may be *acute* or *chronic*. Acute lesions often subside but persist in the chronic state, whereas chronic lesions may exist without having been acute. Chronic lesions frequently undergo acute exacerbations.

Acute Abscess

The acute abscess is accompanied by symptoms such as *throbbing, radiating pain, exquisite tenderness of the gingiva, swelling, sensitivity of the tooth to percussion, tooth mobility, lymphadenitis, and possible systemic effects such as fever, leukocytosis, and malaise.*

The acute periodontal abscess appears as an ovoid elevation of the gingiva along the lateral aspect of the root. The gingiva is edematous and red, with a smooth, shiny surface. The shape and consistency of the elevated areas vary. They may be dome-like and relatively firm or pointed and soft (Fig. 3–22). In most instances, pus may be expressed from the gingival margin by gentle digital pressure. Occasionally, the patient may present symptoms of an acute periodontal abscess *without any notable clinical lesion or radiographic changes.* The microorganisms that colonize the periodontal abscess are primarily gram-negative anaerobic rods.[26]

Chronic Abscess

The chronic abscess usually presents a sinus that comes onto the gingival mucosa somewhere along the length of the root. There may be a history of intermittent exudation. The orifice of the sinus is often a difficult-to-detect pinpoint opening, which when probed reveals a sinus tract deep in

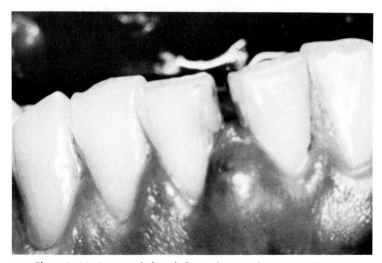

Figure 3–22. Acute periodontal abscess between lower central incisors.

the periodontium. The sinus may be covered by a small, pink, beadlike mass of granulation tissue.

The chronic periodontal abscess is usually asymptomatic. However, the patient may report episodes of dull, gnawing pain, slight elevation of the tooth, and a desire to bite down on and grind the tooth. The chronic periodontal abscess often undergoes acute exacerbations, including the associated symptoms.

Evaluation of Periodontal Abscess

Radiographic Appearance. *The "typical" radiographic appearance of the periodontal abscess is of a discrete area of radiolucence along the lateral aspect of the root.* However, the radiographic picture is often not typical because of the following reasons:

1. In the early stages the acute periodontal abscess is extremely painful but may present no radiographic changes.

2. Extensive bone destruction may already be present.

3. Lesions located in the soft tissue wall of a periodontal pocket are less likely to produce radiographic changes than those deep in the supporting tissues.

4. Abscesses on the facial or lingual surface are obscured by the radiopacity of the root; interproximal lesions are more likely to be visualized radiographically.

Therefore, the recognition of the periodontal abscess requires correlation of the history, clinical findings, and radiographic findings. Continuity of the lesion with the gingival margin is clinical evidence of a periodontal abscess. The suspected area should be probed carefully along the gingival margin in relation to each tooth surface to detect a channel from the marginal area to the deeper periodontal tissues. *Because complex pockets are often involved, the abscess is not necessarily located on the same surface of the root as the pocket from which it formed.*

References

1. Akiyoshi, M., and Mori, K.: Marginal periodontitis: a histological study of the incipient stage. J. Periodontol., *38*:45, 1967.
2. Aleo, J. J., DeRenzis, F. A., and Farber, P. A.: In vitro attachment of human gingival fibroblasts to root surfaces. J. Periodontol., *46*:639, 1975.
3. Aleo, J. J., DeRenzis, F. A., Farber, P. A., and Varboncoeur, A. P.: The presence and biologic activity of cementum bound endotoxin. J. Periodontol., *45*:672, 1974.
4. Armitage, G. C., and Christie, T. M.: Structural changes in exposed cementum. I. Light microscopic observations. J. Periodont. Res., *8*:343, 1973. II. Electronmicroscopic observations. J. Periodont. Res., *8*:356, 1973.
5. Bass, C. C.: A previously undescribed demonstrable pathologic condition in exposed cementum and the underlying dentine. Oral Surg., *4*:641, 1951.
6. Carranza, F. A., Jr., and Glickman, I.: Some observations on the microscopic features of the infrabony pockets. J. Periodontol., *28*:33, 1957.
7. Daly, C. G., Seymour, G. J., Kieser, J. B., and Corbet, E. F.: Histological assessment of periodontally involved cementum. J. Clin. Periodontol., *9*:266, 1982.
8. Davenport, R. H., Jr., Simpson, D. M., and Hassell, T. M.: Histometric comparison of active and inactive lesions of advanced periodontitis. J. Periodontol., *53*:285, 1982.
9. Deporter, D. A., and Brown, D. J.: Fine structural observations on the mechanisms of loss of attachment during experimental periodontal disease in the rat. J. Periodont. Res., *15*:304, 1980.
10. Frank, R. M.: Bacterial penetration in the apical wall of advanced human periodontitis. J. Periodont. Res., *15*:563, 1980.
11. Glickman, L., and Smulow, J. B.: Alterations in the pathway of gingival inflammation into the underlying tissues induced by excessive occlusal forces. J. Periodontol., *33*:7, 1962.
12. Glickman, I., and Smulow, J. B.: The combined effects of inflammation and trauma from occlusion in periodontitis. Int. Dent. J., *19*:393, 1969.
13. Goldman, H. M., and Cohen, D. W.: The intrabony pocket: classification and treatment. J. Periodontol., (*29*):272, 1958.
14. Graham, J. W.: Toxicity of sterile filtrate from parodontal pockets. Proc. R. Soc. Med., *30*:1165, 1937.
15. Hatfield, C. G., and Baumhammers, A.: Cytotoxic effects of periodontally involved surfaces of human teeth. Arch. Oral Biol., *16*:465, 1971.
16. Herting, H. C.: Electron microscope studies of the cementum surface structures of periodontally healthy and diseased teeth. J. Dent. Res., *46*(Suppl.):1247, 1967.
17. Katz, R. V., Hazen, S. P., Chilton, N. W., and Mumma, R. D., Jr.: Prevalence and intraoral distribution of root caries in an adult population. Caries Res., *16*:265, 1982.
18. Larato, D. C.: Some anatomical factors related to furcation involvements. J. Periodontol., (*46*):608, 1975.
19. Lindhe, J., Liljenberg, B., and Listgarten, M. A.: Some microbiological and histopathological features of periodontal disease in man. J. Periodontol., *51*:264, 1980.
20. Listgarten, M. A., and Hellden, L.: Relative distributions of bacteria at clinically healthy and periodontally diseased sites in humans. J. Clin. Periodontol., *5*:665, 1978.
21. Löe, H., Anerud, A., Boysen, H., and Smith, M.: The natural history of periodontal disease in man.

The rate of periodontal destruction before 40 years of age. J. Periodontol., (49):607, 1978.

22. Lopez, N. J., Belvederessi, M., and de la Sotta, R.: Inflammatory effects of periodontally diseased cementum studied by autogenous dental root implants in humans. J. Periodontol., 51:582, 1980.

23. McMillan, L., Burrill, D. Y., and Fosdick, L. S.: An electron microscope study of particulates in periodontal exudate. Abstract. Dent. Res., 37:51, 1958.

24. Manson, J. D.: Bone morphology and bone loss in periodontal disease. J. Clin. Periodontol., (3):14, 1976.

25. Manson, J. D., and Nicholson, K.: The distribution of bone defects in chronic periodontitis. J. Periodontol., (45):88, 1974.

26. Newman, M. G., and Sims, T. N.: The predominant cultivable microbiota of the periodontal abscess. J. Periodontol., 50:350, 1979.

27. Nielsen, J. I., Glavind, L., and Karring, T.: Interproximal periodontal intrabony defects. Prevalence, localization and etiological factors. J. Clin. Periodontol., (7):187, 1980.

28. Ooya, K., and Yamamoto, H.: A scanning electron microscopic study of the destruction of human alveolar crest in periodontal disease. J. Periodont. Res., 13:498, 1978.

29. Orban, B., and Ray, A. G.: Deep necrotic foci in the gingiva. J. Periodontol., 19:91, 1948.

30. Page, R. C., and Schroeder, H. H.: Structure and pathogenesis. In Schluger, S., Yuodelis, R., and Page, R.: Periodontal Disease. Philadelphia, Lea & Febiger, 1977.

31. Saari, J. T., Hurt, W. C., and Briggs, N. L.: Periodontal bony defects on the dry skull. J. Periodontol., (39):278, 1968.

32. Saglie, R., Carranza, F. A., Jr., Newman, M. G., and Pattison, G. L.: Scanning electron microscopy of the gingival wall of deep periodontal pockets in humans. J. Periodont. Res., 17:284, 1982.

33. Saglie, R., Newman, M. G., Carranza, F. A., Jr., and Pattison, G. L.: Bacterial invasion of gingiva in advanced periodontitis in humans. J. Periodontol., 53:217, 1982.

34. Schroeder, H. E.: Quantitative parameters of early human gingival inflammation. Arch. Oral Biol., 15:383, 1970.

35. Schroeder, H. E., and Listgarten, M. A.: Fine Structure of the Developing Epithelial Attachment of Human Teeth. Monographs in Developmental Biology. Vol. 2. Basel, S. Karger, 1971.

36. Selvig, K. A.: Biological changes at the tooth-saliva interface in periodontal disease. J. Dent. Res., 48(Suppl.):846, 1969.

37. Sottosanti, J. S.: A possible relationship between occlusion, root resorption, and the progression of periodontal disease. J. Western Soc. Periodontol., 25:69, 1977.

38. Waerhaug, J.: The angular bone defect and its relationship to trauma from occlusion and downgrowth of subgingival plaque. J. Clin. Periodontol., 6:61–82, 1979.

39. Weinmann, J. P.: Progress of gingival inflammation into the supporting structures of the teeth. J. Periodontol., 12:71, 1941.

40. Zander, H. A.: The attachment of calculus to root surfaces. J. Periodontol., 24:16, 1953.

Chapter 4

Gingival and Periodontal Disease in Children and Adolescents

THE PERIODONTIUM OF THE DECIDUOUS DENTITION

The effects of periodontal disease observed in adults have their inception earlier in life. The gingival disease of childhood may progress to jeopardize the periodontium of the adult. The increasing awareness of the prevalence of gingival and periodontal disease in children, coupled with the need for more information regarding the early stages of periodontal disease, has focused attention upon the periodontium in childhood.[6, 7]

The *gingiva* of the deciduous dentition is pale pink, firm, and shown to be stippled in 35 per cent of children from 5 to 13 years of age.[33] The interdental gingiva is comparable to that of adults, consisting of facial and lingual papillae with intervening depressions or *cols*. The mean gingival sulcus depth for the primary dentition is 2.1 mm + 0.2 mm.[29]

The *periodontal ligament* of the deciduous teeth is wider than that of the permanent dentition. During eruption the principal fibers are parallel to the long axis of the teeth; the bundle arrangement seen in the adult dentition occurs when the teeth encounter their functional antagonists.

The *alveolar bone* around deciduous teeth, seen radiographically, shows a prominent lamina dura. The trabeculae are fewer but thicker and the marrow spaces tend to be larger than in the adult. The crests of the interdental septa are flat.[7]

Physiologic Gingival Changes Associated With Tooth Eruption

During the transitional period of tooth eruption, physiologic changes occur in the gingiva that must be differentiated from gingival disease. Several physiologic changes are associated with tooth eruption.

Pre-eruption Bulge

Before the crown appears in the oral cavity, the gingiva presents a bulge which is firm, may be slightly blanched, and conforms to the contour of the underlying crown.

Formation of the Gingival Margin

The marginal gingiva and sulcus develop as the crown enters the oral mucosa. The area usually is edematous, rounded, and slightly reddened during eruption.

Normal Prominence of the Gingival Margin

When the mixed dentition is present, the marginal gingiva around the permanent teeth

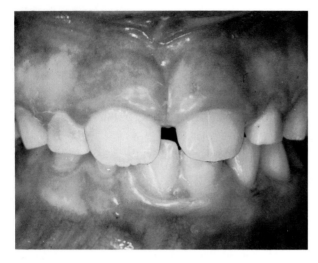

Figure 4–1. Developmental gingival enlargement caused by the normal prominence of the gingiva at this stage of tooth eruption.

may be quite prominent, particularly in the maxillary anterior region. This occurs because the gingiva is still attached to the crown, and appears prominent when superimposed upon the bulk of the underlying enamel (Fig. 4–1).

GINGIVAL DISEASES

Chronic Marginal Gingivitis

Chronic marginal gingivitis is the most prevalent gingival change in childhood. The gingiva presents the same changes in color, size, consistency, and surface texture characteristic of adult gingivitis. A fiery red surface discoloration is often superimposed upon underlying chronic changes. Gingivitis in children, as in adults, is caused by bacterial plaque; materia alba and poor oral hygiene favor the accumulation of plaque. *Calculus* is uncommon in infants and young children but occurs in 33 to 43 per cent of older children, between 10 and 15 years of age.[12]

Gingivitis Associated with Tooth Eruption

Gingivitis commonly occurs around erupting teeth and is termed *eruption gingivitis*. However, *tooth eruption does not cause gingivitis*; the inflammation results from plaque accumulation. Inflammatory changes may accentuate the normal prominence of the gingival margin and create the impression of a marked gingival enlargement.

Loose, Carious, and Malposed Teeth

Partially exfoliated, carious, or malposed deciduous teeth frequently cause gingivitis. Eroded margins of partially resorbed teeth favor plaque accumulation that causes gingival changes varying from slight discoloration and edema to abscess formation with suppuration. Large carious lesions favor plaque build-up and frequently lead to *unilateral chewing habits*, aggravating the accumulation of plaque on the nonchewing side. *Malposed teeth* also cause an increased tendency to accumulate plaque and materia alba. Severe changes include gingival enlargement, bluish-red discoloration, ulceration, and the formation of deep pockets from which pus can be expressed (Fig. 4–2). Gingival health and contour are restored by correction of the malposition, elimination of local irritants, and, when necessary, surgical removal of the enlarged gingiva. *Gingivitis is increased in children with excessive overbite and overjet, with nasal obstruction, and with mouth breathing.*

Localized Gingival Recession

Gingival recession is commonly seen in children. The gingiva may or may not be inflamed depending upon the presence of local irritants. In children, the *position of the tooth in the arch* is the most important cause of gingival recession[27] (Fig. 4–3). It occurs on teeth in labial version or on those tilted or rotated so that the roots project labially. The recession may correct itself if the teeth attain

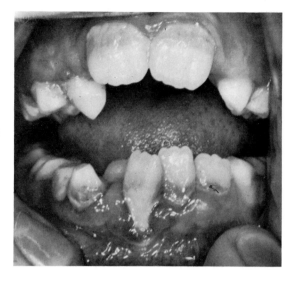

Figure 4–2. **Severe gingivitis** associated with accumulation of plaque around malposed teeth.

proper alignment, or the teeth may need to be realigned orthodontically.

Acute Gingival Infections

Acute Herpetic Gingivostomatitis

This is the most common type of acute gingival infection in childhood. It often occurs as a sequel to upper respiratory tract infection. (For a full discussion, see Chapter 2.)

Acute Necrotizing Ulcerative Gingivitis

The incidence of acute necrotizing ulcerative gingivitis in childhood is low. (For a full discussion, see Chapter 2.) In children living in areas where chronic malnutrition occurs and in children with Down's syndrome, the incidence and severity of acute necrotizing ulcerative gingivitis seems to increase.[19, 28]

Acute herpetic gingivostomatitis, more common in childhood, is easily misdiagnosed as acute necrotizing ulcerative gingivitis. Therefore, the ability to differentiate between the two diseases is important.

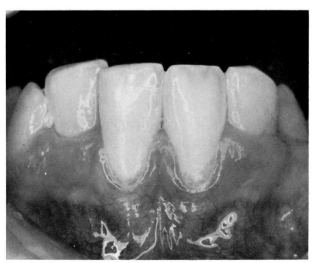

Figure 4–3. **Gingival recession** on labially positioned mandibular central incisors.

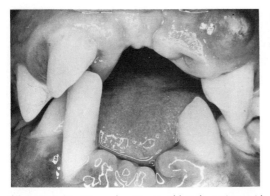

Figure 4–4. Dentition of a 17-year-old male patient with **Papillon-Lefèvre syndrome.** The missing teeth were exfoliated.

Traumatic Changes in the Periodontium

In shedding deciduous teeth, resorption of teeth and bone weakens the periodontal support so that the existing functional forces are injurious to the remaining supporting tissues.[4] Excessive occlusal forces may be produced by malalignment, mutilation, loss or extraction of teeth, or by dental restorations.

Most injuries are repaired and tooth loss does not result. However, traumatized teeth may be sore or loose and repair may result in *ankylosis* of the tooth to the bone. When the permanent dentition erupts, ankylosed deciduous teeth appear to be *submerged*.

JUVENILE PERIODONTITIS

There are cases of severe rapid periodontal destruction and premature tooth loss in children and teenagers, the etiology of which is not well understood. These cases occur infrequently and are referred to as "juvenile periodontitis." The term "periodontosis" has been used to designate this condition in the past but the term "juvenile periodontitis" is preferred. The term "localized" refers to periodontal destruction limited to some areas of the mouth; generally, no health complications are present. Individuals with overlying systemic illness have "generalized juvenile periodontitis," and the entire dentition is usually involved.

Generalized Form

This type of juvenile periodontitis attacks the whole dentition and is associated with

systemic disturbances. Generalized juvenile periodontitis appears associated with the following diseases:

Papillon-Lefèvre Syndrome. This syndrome is characterized by hyperkeratotic skin lesions and severe destruction of the periodontium.[2, 9, 13, 17, 22, 26] The skin and periodontal changes usually appear together before the age of 4 years. The skin lesions consist of hyperkeratosis and ichthyosis of localized areas in the palms, soles, knees, and elbows (Figs. 4–4 and 4–5).

Periodontal lesions consist of early inflammatory involvement leading to bone loss and exfoliation of teeth. Primary teeth are lost by age 5 or 6. The permanent dentition erupts normally, but the teeth are lost within a few years from destructive periodontal disease. Patients are usually edentulous by the age of 15, except for the third molars, which are lost a few years after eruption.

This syndrome is inherited and appears to follow an autosomal recessive pattern[14]; parents are not affected, but both must carry the autosomal genes. It may occur in siblings; males and females are equally affected. The estimated frequency is one to four cases per million.[15]

Down's Syndrome (Mongolism, Trisomy 21). This is a congenital disease caused by a chromosomal abnormality and characterized by mental deficiency and growth retardation. The prevalence of periodontal disease in Down's syndrome is high, and although plaque, calculus, and periodontal pockets are present, the severity of periodontal destruction exceeds that explainable by local factors alone.[11, 20, 34] It is usually characterized by generalized formation of deep periodontal pockets, with high plaque scores, but only moderate gingivitis (Fig. 4–6). Acute necrotizing lesions are a frequent finding. The reasons for the increased prevalence and severity of periodontal destruction in children with Down's syndrome is not known.

Congenital Heart Disease. Gingival disease and other oral symptoms may occur in children with congenital heart disease.[21, 22] The oral changes may include a purplish-red discoloration of the lips and severe marginal gingivitis and periodontal destruction.

Diabetes. In childhood, uncontrolled diabetes may be accompanied by marked destruction of alveolar bone. Although gingival inflammation is also a frequent finding, the extent of the alveolar bone loss exceeds that

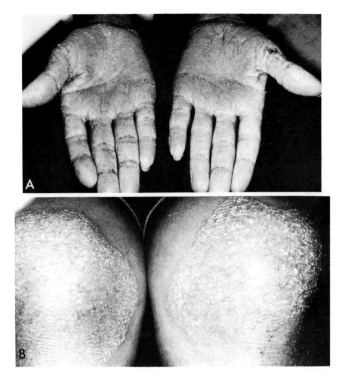

Figure 4–5. Palms (A) and knees (B) of the patient in Figure 4–4. Note the hyperkeratotic scaly lesions.

generally seen in children with comparable gingival inflammation.

Prepubertal Periodontitis, Generalized Form

Children with advanced periodontal destruction and no systemic diseases have also been described.[25] These cases are rare, start during or immediately following eruption of the primary teeth, and exhibit acute inflammation and proliferation of the gingival tissues, with very rapid destruction of bone.

Defects in peripheral blood neutrophils and monocytes have been found in these children and they have frequent respiratory infections. All primary teeth are affected, but not necessarily the permanent dentition.

Localized Form

Historical Background

The localized form of juvenile periodontitis was first described by Gottlieb[16] in 1923, under the name "diffuse atrophy of the al-

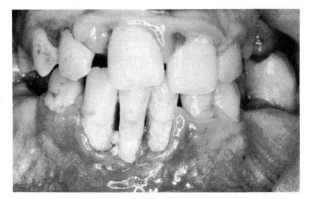

Figure 4–6. Down's syndrome patient, 14 years old, with severe periodontal destruction.

veolar bone." He described it as different from marginal atrophy; characterized by loss of collagen fibers and replacement by loose connective tissue in the periodontal ligament and by extensive bone resorption, resulting in a widened periodontal ligament space. The gingiva was apparently not involved. In 1938 Wannenmacher[36] described the incisor–first molar location of the disease, which he called "parodontitis marginalis progressiva." Contrary to others at that time, Wannenmacher considered this disease an inflammatory process. In 1942 Orban and Weinmann[24] introduced the term "periodontosis."

In 1971, Baer[1] defined "periodontosis" as a "disease of the periodontium occurring in an otherwise healthy adolescent which is characterized by a rapid loss of alveolar bone about more than one tooth of the permanent dentition. There are two basic forms in which it occurs. In one form, the teeth affected are the incisors and the first molars, in the other, more generalized form, most of the dentition can be affected. The amount of destruction manifested is not commensurate with the amounts of local irritants present."

The term "juvenile periodontitis" was introduced by Chaput et al. in 1967 in the French literature and by Butler[8] in 1969 in the English literature. It is the preferred name.

Prevalence

Differences of opinion with regard to the definition of and diagnostic criteria for the localized form of juvenile periodontitis make it very difficult to establish the prevalence of the disease. Saxen, in a study population of 8096 16-year-old adolescents from a geographically restricted area of Finland found a prevalence of 0.1 per cent.[30] Earlier studies do not offer clear evidence of sound criteria for differentiating juvenile periodontitis from other forms of the disease.

Age and Sex Distribution

Localized juvenile periodontitis affects both males and females and is seen most frequently in the period between puberty and the age of 25. It is more likely to be seen in females, particularly in the youngest age groups.[18]

Distribution of Lesions

The distribution of lesions in the mouth is characteristic and as yet unexplained. *The classic distribution is in the first molars and incisors, with the least destruction in the cuspid-premolar area. Frequently, bilateral symmetrical patterns of bone loss occur.*[10]

Clinical Findings

During the circumpubertal period (11 to 13 years of age), the onset of osseous destruction is insidious. The most striking feature of early juvenile periodontitis is the *lack of clinical inflammation.* Late in the incipient stages there is deep pocket formation around affected teeth, so that the *most common clinical symptoms first presented are mobility and migration of the incisors and first molars* (Fig. 4–7).

As the disease progresses, other symptoms usually arise. Denuded root surfaces may become sensitive to thermal changes, foods, and tactile stimuli such as toothbrushing. Deep, dull, radiating pain may be present upon mastication, probably due to irritation of the supporting structures by mobile teeth and impacted food. Periodontal abscesses may also form.

Radiographic Findings

Vertical loss of alveolar bone around the first molars and incisors in otherwise healthy young individuals is taken to be a diagnostic sign of classic juvenile periodontitis (Fig. 4–7C). Alveolar bone in patients in this age group develops normally with tooth eruption, and only subsequently does it undergo resorptive changes. *One also sees distolabial migration of the maxillary incisors, with diastema formation* (Fig. 4–7A). The lower incisors seem to migrate less than do maxillary ones, although occlusal patterns and tongue pressure can vary the changes. Apparent increases in the sizes of the clinical crowns, accumulations of plaque and calculus, and clinical inflammation appear.

Clinical Course

Juvenile periodontitis progresses rapidly. Evidence indicates that the *rate of bone loss is about three to four times faster* than in typical periodontitis.[1, 2] In affected persons, bone

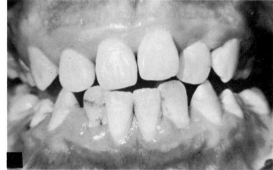

A

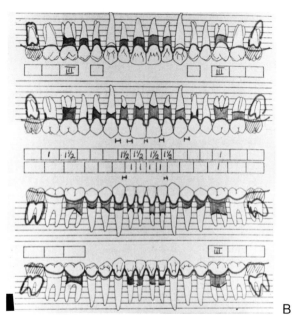

B

Figure 4–7. Idiopathic juvenile periodontitis in a 14-year-old male. *A,* Clinical picture showing gingival inflammation and migration of teeth with diastema formation. *B,* Diagram depicting pocket depth (shaded areas on teeth), tooth mobility (in boxes between upper and lower teeth), and furcation involvements (in boxes with Roman numerals adjacent to molars and first upper premolars). *C,* Radiographs demonstrating the typical molar-incisor distribution of bone loss. Note the higher bone level in canines and premolars and in second molars.

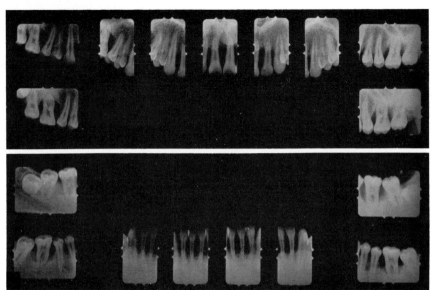

C

resorption progresses until the teeth are either treated, exfoliated, or extracted.

Role of Heredity

Several authors have described a familial pattern of alveolar bone loss and have implicated (without substantial evidence) a genetic factor in localized juvenile periodontitis.[8] Benjamin and Baer,[3] in the most comprehensive study on familial patterns, described the disease in identical twins, siblings, and first cousins, as well as in parents and offspring. Newman and Socransky[23] have also described a familial pattern and have suggested the possibility of a transmissible microbiologic component in the pathogenesis of the disease.

Subgingival plaque in juvenile periodontitis remains relatively thin (20 to 200 microns) and does not tend to mineralize.[35]

Bacteriology

In recent years the relationship of lesions of localized juvenile periodontitis to a bacterial flora different from that of adult periodontitis has been described.[25] This flora consists mainly of gram-negative anaerobic rods, along with a minimal amount of attached plaque with a larger unattached component. Suggested bacterial pathogens in juvenile periodontitis are *Actinobacillus actinomycetemcomitans*[31, 32] and *Capnocytophaga*.[23] These organisms have been found to invade the gingival tissues in this disease. (For a more complete discussion of this topic, see Chapter 5.)

Immunology

Some immune defects have been implicated in the pathogenesis of localized and generalized juvenile periodontitis. Impaired neutrophil chemotaxis and inhibition of macrophage migration[10] have been reported, although proofs are still lacking. (For a more complete discussion, see Chapter 5.)

Treatment

See Chapter 13.

References

1. Baer, P. N.: The case for periodontosis as a clinical entity. J. Periodontol., 42:516, 1971.
2. Baer, P. N., and Benjamin, S. D.: Periodontal Disease in Children and Adolescents. Philadelphia, J. B. Lippincott Company, 1974.
3. Benjamin, S. D., and Baer, P. N.: Familial patterns of advanced alveolar bone loss in adolescence (periodontosis). Periodontics, 5:82, 1967.
4. Bernick, S., and Freedman, N.: Microscopic studies of the periodontium of the primary dentitions of monkeys. II. Posterior teeth during the mixed dentitional period. Oral Surg., 7:322, 1954.
5. Blitzer, B., Sznajder, N., and Carranza, F. A., Jr.: Hallazgos clinicos periodontales en ninos con cardiopatias congenitas. Rev. Asoc. Odontol. Argent., 63:169, 1975.
6. Bradley, R. F.: Periodontal lesions of children—their recognition and treatment. Dent. Clin. North Am., 5:671, 1961.
7. Brauer, J. C., Highley, L. B., Massler, M., and Schour, I.: Dentistry for Children. 2nd ed. Philadelphia, Blakiston Company, 1947.
8. Butler, J. H.: A familial pattern of juvenile periodontitis (periodontosis). J. Periodontol., 40:115, 1969.
9. Carranza, F. A., Jr., Saglie, F. R., Newman, M. G., and Valentin, P. L.: Scanning and transmission electronmicroscopy of tissue-invading microorganisms in localized juvenile periodontitis. J. Periodontol., 54:598, 1983.
10. Cianciola, R.J., et al.: Defective polymorphonuclear leukocyte function in a human periodontal disease. Nature, 265:445, 1977.
11. Cohen, M. M., Winer, R. A., Schwartz, S., and Shklar, G.: Oral aspects of mongolism. Part I. Periodontal disease in mongolism. Oral Surg., 14:92, 1961.
12. Everett, F. G., Tuchler, H., and Lu, K. H.: Occurrence of calculus in grade school children in Portland, Oregon. J. Periodontol., 34:54, 1963.
13. Galanter, D. R., and Bradford, S.: Hyperkeratosis palmoplantaris and periodontosis: the Papillon-Lefèvre syndrome. J. Periodontol., 40:40, 1969.
14. Glickman, I.: Periodontosis: a critical evaluation. J. Am. Dent. Assoc., 44:706, 1952.
15. Gorlin, R. J., Sedano, H., and Anderson, V. E.: The syndrome of palmar-plantar hyperkeratosis and premature periodontal destruction of the teeth. A clinical and genetic analysis of the Papillon-Lefèvre syndrome. J. Pediatr., 65:895, 1964.
16. Gottlieb, B.: Die diffuse Atrophy des Alveolarknochens. Z. Stomatol., 21:195, 1923.
17. Haneke, E.: The Papillon-Lefèvre syndrome; keratosis palmoplantaris with periodontopathy. Hum. Genet., 51:1, 1979.
18. Hormand, J., and Frandsen, A.: Juvenile periodontitis. Localization of bone loss in relation to age, sex, and teeth. J. Clin. Periodontol., 6:407, 1979.
19. Jimenez, M., Ramos, J., Garrington, G., and Baer, P. N.: The familial occurrence of acute necrotizing gingivitis in Colombia. J. Periodontol., 40:414, 1969.
20. Johnson, N. P., and Young, M. A.: Periodontal disease in Mongols. J. Periodontol., 34:41, 1963.

21. Kaner, A., Losch, P., and Green, M.: Oral manifestations of congenital heart disease. J. Pediatr., *29*:269, 1946.

22. Martinez Lalis, R. R., Lopez Otero, R., and Carranza, F. A., Jr.: A case of Papillon-Lefèvre syndrome. Periodontics, *3*:292, 1965.

23. Newman, M. G., and Socransky, S. S.: Predominant cultivable microbiota in periodontosis. J. Periodont. Res., *12*:120, 1977.

24. Orban, B., and Weinmann, J. P.: Diffuse atrophy of alveolar bone. J. Periodontol., *13*:31, 1942.

25. Page, R. C., and Schroeder, H. E.: Periodontitis in Man and Other Animals. Basel, S. Karger, 1982.

26. Papillon, M. M., and Lefèvre, P.: Deux cas de keratodermie palmaire et plantaire symétrique familiale (maladie de Meleda) chez le frère et la soeur. Coexistance dans les deux cas d'alterations dentaires graves. Soc. Franc. Derm. Syph., *31*:82, 1924.

27. Parfitt, G. J., and Mjor, I. A.: A clinical evaluation of local gingival recession in children. J. Dent. Child., *31*:257, 1964.

28. Pindborg, J. J., Bhat, M., Devanath, K. R., Narayana, H. R., and Ramachandra, S.: Occurrence of acute necrotizing gingivitis in South India children. J. Periodontol., *37*:14, 1966.

29. Rosenblum, F. N.: Clinical study of the depth of the gingival sulcus in the primary dentition. J. Dent. Child., *5*:289, 1966.

30. Saxen, L.: Prevalence of juvenile periodontitis in Finland. J. Clin. Periodontol., *7*:177, 1980.

31. Slots, J., Reynolds, H. S., and Genco, R. J.: *Actinobacillus actinomycetemcomitans* in human periodontal disease: a cross-sectional microbiological investigation. Infect. Immun., *29*:1013, 1980.

32. Slots, J., Zambon, J. J., Rosling, B. C., Reynolds, H. S., Christersson, L. A., and Genco, R. J.: *Actinobacillus actinomycetemcomitans* in human periodontal disease. Association, serology, leukotoxicity, and treatment. J. Periodont. Res., *17*:447, 1982.

33. Soni, N. N., Silberkweit, M., and Hayes, R. L.: Histological characteristics of stippling in children. J. Periodontol., *34*:31, 1963.

34. Sznajder, N., Carraro, J. J., Otero, E., and Carranza, F. A., Jr.: Clinical periodontal findings in trisomy 21 (mongolism). J. Periodont. Res., *3*:1, 1968.

35. Waerhaug, J.: Subgingival plaque and loss of attachment in periodontosis as well as observed in autopsy material. J. Periodontol., *47*:636, 1976.

36. Wannenmacher, E.: Ursachen auf dem Gebiet der Paradentopathien. Zbl. Gesant. Zahn, Mund, Kieferheilk., *3*:81, 1938.

Chapter 5

Dental Plaque: Microbiology and Immunology

ETIOLOGY OF PERIODONTAL DISEASE

Etiologic factors of periodontal disease have customarily been classified into local and systemic factors, although their effects are interrelated. *Local factors* are those in the immediate environment of the periodontium, whereas *systemic factors* result from the general condition of the patient.

Local factors cause inflammation, which is the principal pathologic process in periodontal disease; systemic factors monitor the tissue response to local factors, so that the effect of local irritants may be dramatically aggravated by unfavorable systemic conditions. The following diagram, modified from that developed by Bahn,[3] shows in schematic form the role of the different factors:

AGGRESSION	$\longrightarrow$	HOST RESPONSE	$\longleftarrow$	DEFENSE

AGGRESSION
Plaque
Bacterial Products

HOST RESPONSE
↑   ↑   ↑
Factors That Upset Balance

—By increasing aggression:
Calculus
Faulty dentistry
Food impaction
Mouth breathing

—By decreasing defense:
Systemic factors (hormonal,
  nutritional, genetic, etc.)
Trauma from occlusion (?)

DEFENSE
Reparative tissue
  capacity
Humoral resistance

79

Plaque is necessary to initiate the disease. A small but variable amount of plaque can, however, be controlled by the body defense mechanisms, resulting in an equilibrium between aggression and defense. This equilibrium can be broken either by increasing the amount and/or the virulence of the bacteria or by reducing the defensive capacity of the tissues. Many factors favor the accumulation of plaque: calculus, faulty dentistry (inadequate restorations), food impaction, and mouth breathing.

Factors that reduce the defensive capacity of the tissues include all the systemic conditions that may disturb the tissue response to irritation. Their exact mechanism of action is in most cases obscure.

It should also be clearly understood that diseases besides periodontal disease can attack the periodontal tissues. These other diseases may result from a variety of causes, by direct extension from the oral mucosa or the jaw bones or owing to a systemic involvement. Included in this group of diseases showing periodontal manifestations are herpetic gingivostomatitis, bacterial infections like tuberculosis or syphilis, various dermatoses, blood diseases, and some benign and malignant tumors.

Systemic factors can act either by reducing tissue resistance to plaque or by initiating changes. In the first case, the resulting disease will be periodontal disease; in the second it will be a periodontal manifestation of the systemic disease.

ROLE OF MICROORGANISMS IN PERIODONTAL DISEASE

Numerous investigations have documented the fact that bacterial plaque is the etiologic agent in most forms of periodontal disease. However, the exact nature of the microbiota associated with periodontal health and disease has not yet been determined.

Earlier theories regarding the role of dental plaque suggested that plaque consisted of a complex and homogeneous bacterial mass which would lead to disease where allowed to overgrow. It was later found that the bacterial composition of plaque associated with healthy sites is different from that of the plaque associated with disease. The con-

cept of bacterial specificity, formally discussed by Loesche as the *"specific plaque hypothesis"* in 1976, suggests that specific forms of periodontal disease have specific bacterial etiologies.[34] Therefore, periodontal disease may be a group of diseases with different etiologies and clinical courses, but with similar symptomatologies. These findings opened a new era in periodontal bacteriology allowing more accurate clinical and laboratory diagnoses to be made.[59]

Many types of deposits exist on the tooth surface above and below the gingival margin. In the past these were designated by a variety of terms rarely differentiating among the aggregations.

The term "plaque" is used universally to describe the association of bacteria to the tooth surface. Based on its relationship to the gingival margin, plaque is considered to be *supragingival* and *subgingival*. Some authors have described the plaque near the gingival margin as *marginal plaque*. Recently the presence of bacteria within the gingival tissues has been confirmed.[15, 18, 53] These bacteria appear in the tissues either as isolated organisms or as bacterial aggregates. The applicability of the term "plaque" to these bacteria is not clear.

SUPRAGINGIVAL PLAQUE

Structure and Organization

Small amounts of supragingival plaque are not clinically visible unless they are disclosed by pigments from within the oral cavity or stained by disclosing dyes (Fig. 5–1). As plaque develops and accumulates, it becomes a visible mass with a pinpoint nodular surface that varies in color from gray to yellowish-gray to yellow. Supragingival plaque develops mostly on the gingival third of the teeth, with a predilection for surface cracks, defects, rough areas, and overhanging margins of dental restorations.

Supragingival plaque consists primarily of proliferating microorganisms and a scattering of epithelial cells, leukocytes, and macrophages in an adherent intercellular matrix. Bacteria constitute approximately 70 to 80 per cent of the solid material, and the rest is intercellular matrix. Organic and inorganic

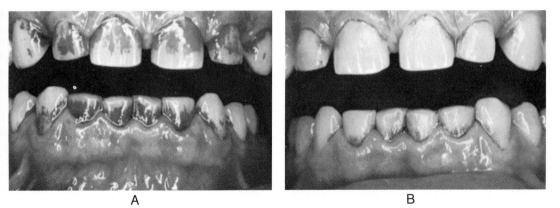

Figure 5–1. Supragingival plaque. *A,* Disclosed supragingival plaque covering one half to two thirds of the clinical crowns. (Courtesy of Dr. S. Socransky.) *B,* Supragingival plaque (same patient as in *A*) disclosed with an oxidation-reduction dye that indicates reduced (anaerobic) area of plaque. The supragingival anaerobic areas (purple stain) are located interproximally and along the gingival margin. (Courtesy of Dr. S. Socransky.)

solids form 20 per cent or more of the plaque; the remainder is water.

Formation begins with the adhesion of bacteria to the acquired pellicle or tooth surface, whether enamel, cementum, or dentin. Plaque mass grows by (1) the adhesion of new bacteria, (2) the multiplication of bacteria, and (3) the accumulation of bacterial and host products.

Measurable amounts of supragingival plaque may form within 1 hour after the teeth are thoroughly cleaned,[29] with maximum accumulation reached in 30 days or less. Rates of formation and locations vary among individuals, on different teeth in the same mouth, and on different areas of individual teeth.[35] These factors are influenced by diet, age, saliva composition, oral hygiene, tooth alignment, systemic disease, and host susceptibility.

Irreversible bacterial colonization of the pellicle does not appear to take place until 2 to 4 hours after enamel has been exposed to the bacteria. Organisms *initially* colonize smooth surfaces and pits and grooves as single cells rather than as aggregates, and they are mainly gram-positive cocci. Adhesion by means of polysaccharides produced by bacteria is mediated by cell surface glycosyltransferase, the enzyme that governs the production of these polysaccharides. Stagnation is the principal factor governing the retention of bacteria at periodontal disease-prone sites,[19] and there is clear evidence that some organisms adhere more readily than others.

Supragingival Plaque Matrix

Organic Content

The organic matrix consists principally of carbohydrates and proteins (approximately 30 per cent each), and lipids (approximately 15 per cent), with the nature of the remainder unclear. These components represent extracellular products of plaque bacteria, their cytoplasmic and cell membrane remnants, ingested foodstuff, and derivatives of salivary glycoproteins. The principal carbohydrate present in the matrix is *dextran,* a bacteria-produced polysaccharide forming approximately 9.5 per cent of the total plaque. Other matrix carbohydrates are levan, galactose, and methylpentose in the form of rhamnose. When *Streptococcus mutans* is present in the plaque, *mutan,* another type of extracellular carbohydrate, is found to contribute to the organic matrix. Bacterial remnants provide muramic acid, lipids, and some matrix protein, of which salivary glycoproteins are the principal source.

Inorganic Content

The principal inorganic components of the supragingival plaque matrix are calcium and phosphorus; there are also small amounts of magnesium, potassium, and sodium. The total inorganic content of early supragingival plaque is small, increasing when plaque is transformed to calculus. Fluoride topically applied to the teeth or added to drinking water, toothpaste, and mouthwash, or in the form of a coating on dental floss, becomes incorporated in the plaque and is thought to become incorporated on the tooth surface. The fluoride may act to deter the metabolism of plaque bacteria, kill them directly, or aid in remineralization of the tooth surface.

Diet and Supragingival Plaque Formation

Dental plaque is not food residue. Supragingival plaque forms more rapidly during sleep, when no food is ingested, than following meals. The mechanical action of food and the increased salivary flow caused by mastication are thought to deter plaque formation. Saliva and salivary flow are major ecologic influences on supragingival plaque. Individuals with dry mouths have increased amounts of supragingival plaque. Also, supragingival plaque forms more rapidly in patients on soft diets, whereas hard, chewy foods retard formation.

Dietary supplements of sucrose increase supragingival plaque formation and affect its bacterial composition. This effect is attributed to extracellular polysaccharides produced by bacteria; glucose supplements do not have a similar effect. Plaque formation also occurs in people on high-protein, low-fat diets and those on carbohydrate-free diets, but in smaller amounts.

The etiologic role of supragingival plaque in periodontal disease is still not well understood, but it is quite clear that supragingival and subgingival plaque are directly responsible for the initiation and progression of

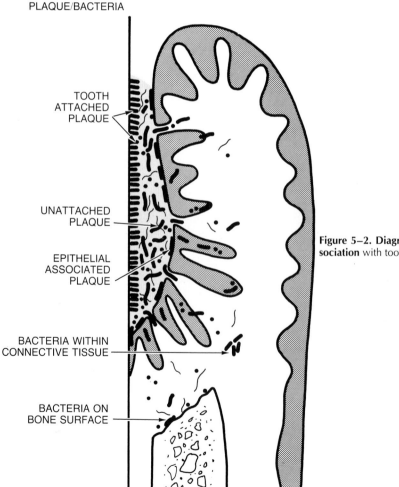

PLAQUE/BACTERIA

TOOTH ATTACHED PLAQUE

UNATTACHED PLAQUE

EPITHELIAL ASSOCIATED PLAQUE

BACTERIA WITHIN CONNECTIVE TISSUE

BACTERIA ON BONE SURFACE

Figure 5–2. Diagram depicting plaque-bacteria association with tooth surface and periodontal tissues.

periodontal diseases. It is probable that supragingival plaque strongly influences the growth, accumulation, and pathogenic potential of subgingival plaque, especially in the early stages of gingivitis and periodontitis. Once the disease has progressed and periodontal pocket formation has taken place, the influence of supragingival plaque on all but the most coronally located subgingival plaque is minimal.

SUBGINGIVAL PLAQUE

Structure and Organization

The gingival sulcus and periodontal pocket harbor a diverse collection of bacteria. The nature of the organisms that colonize these retentive sites differs from that of organisms found in supragingival plaque. The morphology of the gingival sulcus and periodontal pocket makes them less subject to the cleansing activities of the mouth. Thus, these retentive areas form a relatively stagnant environment in which organisms that cannot readily adhere to a tooth surface have the opportunity to colonize. It is not surprising, therefore, to find that the majority of the motile bacteria colonize these sites. These organisms may also adhere to other bacteria, to the teeth, and/or to the subgingival pocket epithelium. In addition, organisms within these retentive sites have direct access to the nutrients and immunoglobulins present in sulcular fluid. The anaerobic nature of the area permits organisms that can exist only in areas of low oxygen concentration to survive.

Subgingival plaque can be described as *tooth-associated* plaque, and *epithelium-associated* plaque (Fig. 5–2). It has now been demonstrated that bacteria and other microorganisms from the epithelium-associated plaque may penetrate, invade, and colonize the gingival connective tissue. These may be referred to as *connective tissue–associated* bacteria.

Tooth-Associated (Attached) Subgingival Plaque

Plaque bacteria are attached to the tooth surface in the gingival sulcus and periodontal pocket. The organisms are thought to be gram-positive rods and cocci, such as *Streptococcus mitis*, *S. sanguis*, *Eubacterium*, *Bifidobacterium*, *Actinomyces viscosus*, *A. naeslundii*, *Propionibacterium*, *Bacterionema matruchotii*, and other species. In addition, some gram-negative cocci and rods can always be found in this attached subgingival plaque. The apical border of tooth-associated plaque is always found some distance away from the junctional epithelium. The tooth (attached) component of subgingival plaque is associated with the deposition of mineral salts, with the formation of calculus, and with root caries and root resorption areas (Fig. 5–3).

Epithelium-Associated Subgingival Plaque

A loosely adherent component of the subgingival plaque is in direct association with the subgingival epithelium and extends from the gingival margin to the junctional epithelium. In the past this zone has been called the zone of unattached subgingival plaque. It contains one portion that is in contact with the epithelium and another that is loose in the pocket lumen. Conceptually, the term "unattached" plaque is reserved for the latter portion. However, little is known about differences between the unattached plaque and the epithelium-associated plaque, so they will be considered together.

Epithelium-associated plaque contains predominantly but not exclusively motile and gram-negative organisms (Table 5–1), which are in direct contact with the epithelium and the surface of the tooth coronal to the junctional epithelium. Removal of teeth for study disturbs the plaque loosely adherent to the tooth surface and leaves what has been termed a "plaque-free zone" immediately coronal to the junctional epithelium. In vivo, this is a zone of unattached plaque.

The relative proportions of the subgingival plaque zones appear to be related to the nature and activity of the disease that is present in a particular pocket. In rapidly advancing lesions, such as those of localized juvenile periodontitis, the tooth-associated component of subgingival plaque appears to be minimal. Instead, the periodontal pocket contains predominantly loosely adherent gram-negative rods and spirochetes that make up the larger epithelium-associated subgingival plaque zone. A similar pattern of subgingival bacterial colonization has been demonstrated in patients with a rapidly progressing form of periodontitis. In the case of chronic, longstanding, and slowly progressing periodontal

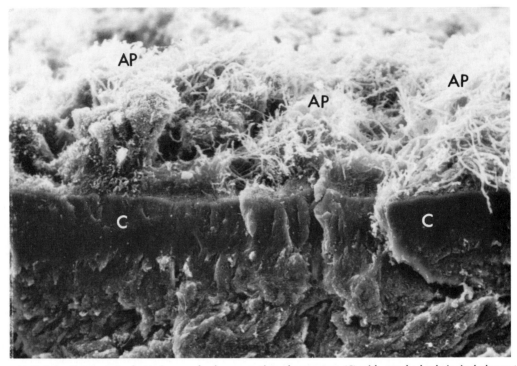

Figure 5–3. Scanning electron photomicrograph of cross section of cementum (C) with attached subgingival plaque (AP). Area shown is within a periodontal pocket. (Courtesy of Dr. J. Sottosanti.)

pockets, the proportion of tooth-associated subgingival plaque is much larger.

Connective Tissue–Associated Plaque

Direct invasion of the periodontal tissues (Fig. 5–4) occurs in gingivitis,[12] *in the lateral walls of periodontal pockets in advanced chronic periodontitis*[15, 53] *and juvenile periodontitis*[5, 18] *in humans.*

Invasive bacteria have been found in the intercellular spaces of the stratum spinosum. Coccal forms, short rods, filaments, and spirochetes have been found occupying spaces between intercellular connections. Accumulations of bacteria are found on the epithelial side of the basal lamina, and penetration into the connective tissue is found where perforations or interruptions exist. Bacteria can also gain access to the epithelium through ulcerations in the pocket wall or through spaces on the surface created by emigrating polymorphonuclear leukocytes. This pattern of gingival epithelial invasion is similar to that of the invasion of other epithelial surfaces of man.

Mechanisms of Bacteria-Mediated Destruction

Periodontal health is maintained as long as the balance between host resistance and bacterial virulence is in favor of the host. Perio-

TABLE 5–1. CHARACTERISTICS OF SUBGINGIVAL PLAQUE

Attached to Tooth	Unattached	Attached to Epithelium
Gram-positive bacteria predominate	Gram variable	Gram variable
Does not extend to junctional epithelium	Extends to junctional epithelium	Extends to junctional epithelium
May penetrate the cementum	—	May penetrate epithelium and connective tissue
Associated with calculus formation and root caries	Associated with gingivitis	Associated with gingivitis and periodontitis

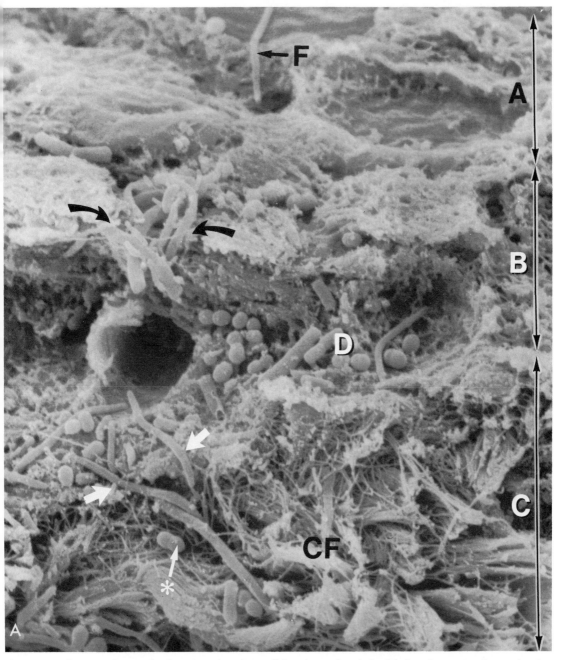

Figure 5–4. Electron micrograph of section of pocket wall in advanced periodontitis in a human specimen, showing bacterial penetration into the epithelium and connective tissue. *A,* Scanning electron microscope view of surface of pocket wall (A), sectioned epithelium (B), and sectioned connective tissue (C). Curved arrows point to areas of bacterial penetration into the epithelium. Thick white arrows point to bacterial penetration into the connective tissue through a break in the continuity of the basal lamina. F, filamentous organism on surface of epithelium; D, accumulation of bacteria (rods, cocci, filaments) on basal lamina; CF, connective tissue fibers. Asterisk points to coccobacillus in connective tissue.

Illustration continued on following page

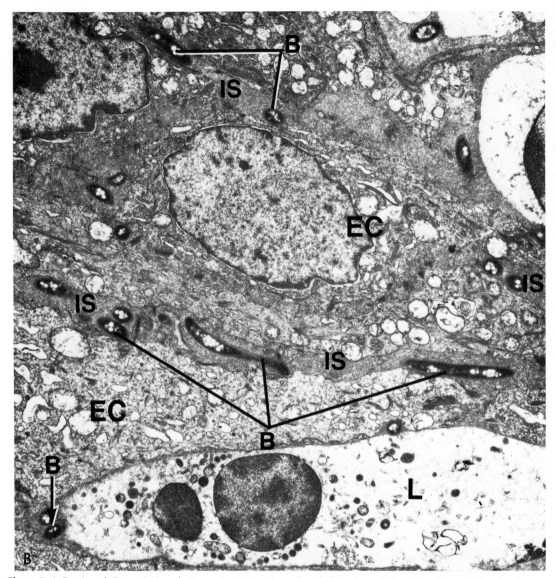

Figure 5–4 *Continued.* Transmission electron microscope view of epithelium in periodontal pocket wall showing bacteria in intercellular spaces. EC, epithelial cell; IS, intercellular space; B, bacteria; L, leukocyte about to engulf bacteria. × 8000.

dontopathic microorganisms produce a variety of pathogenic and virulence factors which are undoubtedly involved in all stages of the disease process.

Bacteria can cause disease *indirectly* by minimizing the host defense mechanisms, and/or triggering immunopathologic processes.[36] They can also cause tissue destruction *directly* by producing lytic enzymes or toxic products that may be responsible for destroying the periodontal tissues.

The pathogenic potential of organisms isolated in periodontal lesions has been demonstrated in other ways. For example, bacteria colonizing the mouths of humans can initiate dangerous infections in other parts of the body.[13, 14] Infections initiated by oral organisms can occur accidentally, through skin punctures with dental probes, or from human bite wounds. Organisms associated with periodontal disease have been found in infected surgical wounds and in lung abscesses caused by aspiration[13]; bacterial endocarditis due to pathogenic oral organisms is a constant concern of dental clinicians.

MICROBIOLOGY OF PERIODONTAL HEALTH AND DISEASE

The oral cavity is sterile at birth, but a simple, primarily facultative flora becomes established within 6 to 10 hours.[60] Anaerobes appear in saliva within the first 10 days and are present in most mouths by five months of age, and in 100 per cent of mouths when the incisors appear. Anaerobes increase with age of the host, but the facultative types remain numerically predominant.

Most of the salivary bacteria are derived from the dorsum of the tongue, from which they are detached by mechanical action; lesser amounts come from the remainder of the oral mucous membrane. The number of microorganisms increases temporarily during sleep and decreases after eating and toothbrushing.

These organisms initiate plaque growth by means of their ability to adhere to the tooth surface (pellicle) and then to proliferate in that particular ecologic niche. The colonization of the tooth surface by supragingival plaque bacteria appears to be quite specific and apparently depends upon the interaction of the bacterial surface with the salivary glycoprotein of the pellicle. *Streptococcus sanguis* and gram-positive rods have been shown to be the major bacteria which initiate supragingival plaque.[17]

Once supragingival plaque is initiated, secondary growth and maturation take place (Fig. 5–5). During this phase, bacterial population shifts occur *(bacterial succession)*. Filamentous organisms and gram-negative bacteria increase in proportion. In general, this plaque appears more compact. Bacterial cohesive interactions are also more evident.

Health

To date there have been few technically acceptable studies that have specifically documented the nature of the sulcular microbial flora associated with periodontal health. In general terms, the healthy periodontal tissues of humans appear to be associated with a minimal supragingival and subgingival microbial flora.

Subgingivally, the nature of the microbiota apparently conforms to the architectural arrangement previously described. Electron microscopic studies of in situ plaque located near the marginal gingiva and in the gingival crevice area at healthy sites have revealed a relatively thin layer (less than 60 microns) of predominantly gram-positive coccoid cells. Cultural studies have shown a predominance of streptococci (mainly *S. sanguis*); *Actinomyces viscosus*, *A. naeslundii*, and *A. israelii* are frequently present, sometimes in relatively high numbers. Gram-negative organisms such as *Capnocytophaga*, *Bacteroides* species, *Campylobacter*, and *Fusobacterium* can be isolated. *Mycoplasma* colonizes the gingival sulcus regularly.[11] Very few motile forms and spirochetes are present in this relatively scanty microflora. There appears to be no marked difference in bacterial composition between the supragingival and subgingival microflora associated with healthy sites.

In the healthy host, bacteria colonize in a predictable sequence. As one group of bacteria colonizes, the environment changes to allow new organisms to become established or different existing species to become dominant. Thus, supragingival plaque affects the establishment of the subgingival flora by lowering the oxidation-reduction potential, providing essential growth factors, and altering the gingival tissues; these features in turn influence the numbers and types of subgingival microorganisms. In addition, the supragingival bacteria may provide sites of attachment for subgingival organisms.

Clinical studies indicate that supragingival plaque control in periodontally healthy persons appears to be sufficient to prevent the maturation of a simple, health-compatible plaque to a complex, disease-associated plaque.[1] In patients with existing periodontal disease, the influence of supragingival microorganisms and plaque control (oral hygiene) procedures appears to be limited to approximately 4 mm into the pocket.

Gingivitis

The initial development of gingivitis is thought to be a major consequence of the bacteria associated with an increase in supragingival plaque formation.[33] Increases in gram-positive filaments and rods, mainly *Actinomyces*, appear to be of major significance in the sequence of development of supragin-

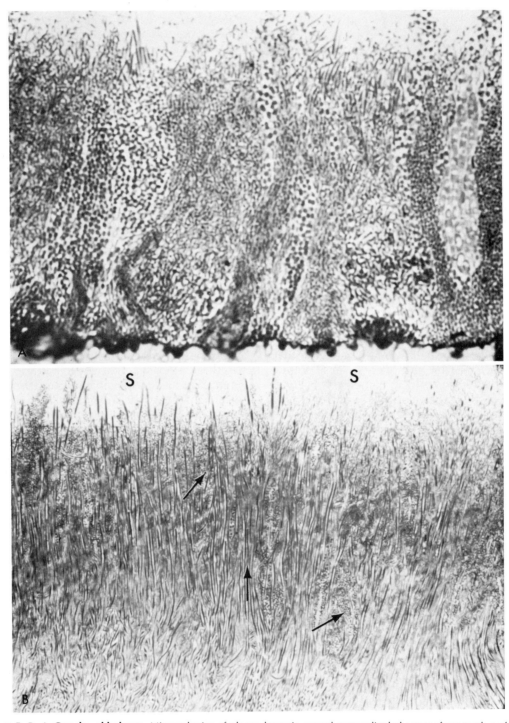

Figure 5–5. *A,* **One-day-old plaque.** Microcolonies of plaque bacteria extend perpendicularly away from tooth surfaces. (From Listgarten, M.: J. Periodontol., 46:10, 1975.) *B,* **Developed supragingival plaque** showing overall filamentous nature and microcolonies *(arrows)* extending perpendicularly away from tooth surface. Saliva-plaque interface shown (S). (Courtesy of Dr. Max Listgarten.)

gival plaque. The appearance of gram-negative forms, such as spirochetes, *Bacteroides*, *Fusobacterium*, vibrios, and other motile forms, in the late stages of the development of gingival redness (clinical inflammation) clearly indicates a sequential process in the development of gingivitis, since these organisms are associated with subgingival plaque. However, the initial insult to the periodontal structures in gingivitis may be associated with noxious elements of large masses of gram-positive bacteria from supragingival plaque. In the early stages of gingivitis, edematous changes in the marginal gingiva may contribute to the successional acquisition of pathogenic subgingival species by providing mechanical retention and nutrients from increased amounts of gingival fluid.

It has been suggested by many investigators that repeated episodes of gingivitis can lead to periodontal bone loss (periodontitis). This fact is a generally accepted clinical observation (see Chapter 2). It stems from many epidemiologic studies that have demonstrated that the continued presence of bacterial plaque is associated with alveolar bone loss. *However, it is quite clear that some individuals may have recurrent episodes of gingivitis without developing periodontitis, and that gingivitis alone is reversible when plaque is removed.*[1, 33]

Recently the epithelial invasion of gram-positive and gram-negative bacteria was reported in some cases of advanced gingivitis.[12] It is possible that this is the initiating event in the progression of gingivitis to periodontitis.

Periodontitis

Limited data suggest that specific organisms, or groups of organisms, are associated with different forms of human periodontal diseases. However, important observations suggest that trends or patterns of bacterial colonization in periodontal pockets exist. The nature of the microbiota depends upon the state of periodontal destruction, disease activity, and host resistance. Whether the lesion is associated with chronic disease or with a more rapid form of periodontal destruction is also an important consideration.[56, 57]

In the *most common chronic forms of periodontitis*, there is a large component of attached subgingival plaque. Filamentous organisms such as *Actinomyces israelii*, *A. naeslundii*, and *A. viscosus* are numerous.[10] These organisms may constitute 30 to 40 per cent of the bacteria present. In almost all cases this attached plaque is associated with varying degrees of calculus formation.[54] *A. naeslundii* and *A. israelii* demonstrate a characteristic pathogenicity when implanted as monocontaminants in germ-free rats.[20] These organisms form large accumulations of bacterial plaque and cause root caries. Alveolar bone loss appears to be associated with suppression of osteoblasts.

The unattached component of the subgingival plaque in chronic periodontitis has not been adequately studied. However, electron microscopic observations suggest that this zone contains numerous gram-negative rods and spirochetes. Limited information from cultural studies also suggests that *Bacteroides melaninogenicus*, *Fusobacterium*, *Capnocytophaga*, *Campylobacter*, and *Selenomonas* species are present in various concentrations.

In *rapidly destructive forms of periodontitis*, the unattached component of the pocket flora predominates at the apical portion of the periodontal pocket.[42] The microbiota is characterized by gram-negative microorganisms, including *Bacteroides gingivalis*, *B. melaninogenicus*, *Wolinella recta*, *Haemophilus*, and spirochetes. In addition, *Capnocytophaga* organisms and *Selenomonas sputigena* are found in periodontitis lesions.[9]

Localized Juvenile Periodontitis

Since the disease entity of localized juvenile periodontitis (LJP) can be sharply defined, it is considered a good model in which disease activity and bone destruction can be accurately predicted and studied.[30] (See Chapter 4 for a complete discussion of the clinical aspects of this type of periodontal disease.)

Although many details of the microbiota of LJP lesions have not been well defined, a number of observations are consistent (Table 5–2). The number of organisms in LJP lesions is less than in most forms of destructive periodontal disease, and it is one to three orders of magnitude lower than in comparable adult periodontitis pockets.

TABLE 5–2. MICROBIOLOGIC FEATURES ASSOCIATED WITH LOCALIZED JUVENILE PERIODONTITIS

Fewer bacteria (gram-negative rods)
Major proportion of subgingival plaque loosely adherent to tooth surface
Bacterial invasion demonstrated
Pathogenic potential in animal models
Immunologic response
Antibacterial treatment

The predominant cultivable microbiota of the LJP lesion is dominated by gram-negative rods.[37–41, 43, 55] Most of the isolates from such lesions have been saccharolytic and capnophilic, as well as anaerobic.

At present, three groups of organisms appear to be most frequently encountered in lesions of LJP patients. One group, which initially received considerable attention, consists of fusiform-shaped, capnophilic rods that have the ability to glide on agar surfaces. Members of this group had been called *Bacteroides ochraceus*, but now are designated by the genus name *Capnocytophaga*.[13] These organisms are not anaerobic but require increased carbon dioxide tension for their growth; they are referred to as capnophilic ("carbon dioxide loving").

Some strains of *Capnocytophaga* produce a substance that inhibits the proliferation of human fibroblasts. These strains may also cause distinctive abnormalities in host white blood cells.

A second group of capnophilic, gram-negative rods frequently isolated from LJP lesions includes the species *Actinobacillus actinomycetemcomitans*. Strains of this species produce a protein exotoxin capable of destroying polymorphonuclear leukocytes and gingival fibroblasts, and the endotoxin it becomes appears to be a potent stimulator of bone resorption, macrophage cytotoxicity, and platelet aggregation.[2] Both the exotoxin and the endotoxin may be associated with membrane vesicles shed during the growth of these organisms. Serologic studies have demonstrated a significant host response to *Actinobacillus* in LJP patients.

A third group of organisms frequently encountered appears to fit descriptions of the species *Eubacterium saburreum*. This species is gram-positive in very young cultures and gram-negative in older preparations; cells are long, blunt-ended rods which often produce filaments.

These three groups of organisms are not solely confined to LJP lesions. However, their frequency of isolation and their proportions when isolated are clearly much higher in LJP lesions than in lesions of adult destructive diseases or in healthy sites of adult patients or age-matched control subjects.

Anatomic studies of the subgingival microbiota in LJP lesions revealed that the majority of the subgingival bacteria are loosely adherent to the tooth surface.[31, 32] Electron microscopic studies have shown many of those microorganisms to be gram-negative. Bacterial penetration of the gingival epithelium and connective tissue by spirochetes, gram-negative fusiform rods, *Mycoplasma*, and *A. actinomycetemcomitans*[5, 52] has also been documented.

The cultural and anatomic association of microorganisms with LJP lesions provides the basis for research which may clarify the exact role of these bacteria. Such observations are prerequisite to a more accurate assessment of the response (or failure of response) of the host to potentially pathogenic bacteria and/or their products.

THE HOST RESPONSE IN PERIODONTAL DISEASE

It is now recognized that host response plays a role in most forms of periodontal disease. In gingivitis, periodontitis, and juvenile periodontitis, the development of the disease depends upon the interaction between the resident microbiota and the host response. In other types of periodontal disease, such as desquamative gingivitis, the lesions frequently result from the host response.

The nature and severity of periodontal pathology are now thought to be dependent on specific microorganisms and modified by factors such as white blood cell defects,[6] mechanical and traumatic forces, drug ingestion, nutritional deficiencies, systemic disease, and age.

The histopathology of gingivitis and periodontitis suggests that an immunologic response occurs in the pathogenesis of these diseases. Inflammation in the periodontal tissues is triggered to some extent by the host response to the continuous bacterial anti-genic exposure and the direct nonimmuno-logic effects of bacterial products from the dental plaque microorganisms. In disease, the gingival tissues are infiltrated with all the elements necessary to elicit immune re-sponses: *plasma cells*, which produce immu-noglobulins that can participate in immediate hypersensitivity and immune complex dis-ease; *lymphocytes*, including T-cells actively responsible for cell-mediated immunity and B-cells responsible for antibody-mediated re-actions; *mast cells*; *polymorphonuclear leuko-cytes*; and *macrophages*.

Although inflammation is a host defense mechanism to localize and destroy foreign materials, the host's own tissues may also be destroyed in the process.[51] Thus, *inflammation may account for part of the soft tissue destruction and alveolar bone loss seen in the course of human periodontal disease.*

Antibodies

The host can respond to the presence of oral bacteria and their products by the pro-duction of *antibodies*, primarily by mature plasma cells. The possible role of antibodies in periodontal and gingival disease is sum-marized in Table 5–3. These proteins, de-rived from the blood and functioning as an-tibodies, are the effectors of humoral immunity. They are referred to as *immuno-globulins*. Human immunoglobulin is divided into five classes on the basis of structural differences that are responsible for different biologic effects subsequent to antigen bind-ing. These five classes are IgG, IgM, IgA, IgE, and IgD.

The reaction of antibodies and bacterial antigens within the gingival tissues creates the potential for adverse tissue responses. The host, in the process of attempting to destroy or remove foreign antigens, may ex-hibit an inflammatory response excessive for elimination of the antigens. Such responses occur in immediate hypersensitivity and in immune complex or Arthus reactions.

The general concept that develops from studies of antibody titers to oral bacteria is that most humans with clinically healthy periodontal tissues have a spectrum of antibodies to plaque organisms. In periodontitis, antibody titers vary in concentra-tion depending on the specific organism to which antibodies have been detected.

Immune Mechanisms

Immune mechanisms are usually protec-tive responses of the host to the presence of foreign substances such as bacteria and vi-ruses, but they may, at the same time, also cause local tissue destruction by triggering several types of overreaction or *hypersensitiv-ity*. Tissue damage (immunopathology) may occur in a sensitized host upon subsequent exposure to the sensitizing antigen.

Three antibody-mediated responses poten-tially of importance to periodontal disease are classified as *hypersensitivity reactions*[4, 16]: They are anaphylaxis or immediate hyper-sensitivity (Type I), cytotoxic reactions (Type II), and immune complex or Arthus reactions (Type III). In addition, reactions to transfused blood are involved with immediate hypersen-sitivity reactions. Another type of hypersen-sitivity, which depends upon the interaction of immunocompetent cells, is the delayed

TABLE 5–3. POSSIBLE ROLE OF ANTIBODIES IN PERIODONTAL AND GINGIVAL DISEASE*

Reaction or Process	Effects
Activation of C' by Ag-Ab complexes	Protective early changes in inflammation
Phagocytosis of Ag-Ab complexes by PMNs with release of lysosomes	Destructive
Enhanced lymphocyte stimulation by Ag-Ab complexes	Release of lymphokines with protective and destructive effects
Blocking of lymphocytes by free antibody or by Ag-Ab complexes	Suppression of cell-mediated immune reactions
Neutralization of bacterial allergens, toxins, or histolytic enzymes	Protective
Enhanced opsonization or bacteriolysis of plaque bacteria	Protective

*Adapted from Genco, R., et al.: J. Periodontol., 45:336, 1974.
PMN's = polymorphonuclear leukocytes. Ag-Ab complexes = antigen-antibody complexes.

and Ivanyi, L.: Immunopotentiation by dental microbial plaque and its relationship to oral disease in man. Arch. Oral Biol., 21:749, 1976.

26. Lehner, T., Wilton, J. M. A., Ivanyi, L., and Manson, J. B.: Immunologic aspects of juvenile periodontitis (periodontosis). J. Periodont. Res., 9:261, 1974.

27. Lehner, T., et al.: Sequential cell-mediated immunoresponse in experimental gingivitis in man. Clin. Exp. Immunol., 16:481, 1974.

28. Lerner, C.: Arthus reaction in the oral cavity of laboratory animals. J. Periodontol., 3:18, 1965.

29. Lie, T.: Early dental plaque morphogenesis. J. Periodont. Res., 12:73, 1977.

30. Liljenberg, B., and Lindhe, J.: Juvenile periodontitis. J. Clin. Res., 7:48, 1980.

31. Listgarten, M. A.: Structure of surface coatings on teeth. A review. J. Periodontol., 47:139, 1976.

32. Listgarten, M. A., Mayo, H. E., and Tremblay, R.: Development of dental plaque on epoxy resin crowns in man. A light and electron microscopic study. J. Periodontol., 46:10, 1975.

33. Löe, H. E., Theilade, E., and Jensen, S. B.: Experimental gingivitis in man. J. Periodontol., 36:177, 1965.

34. Loesche, W.: Chemotherapy of dental plaque infections. Oral Sci. Rev., 9:65, 1976.

35. Manganiello, A. D., Socransky, S. S., Smith, C., Propas, D., Oram, V., and Dogan, I. L.: Attempts to increase viable count recovery of human supragingival dental plaque. J. Periodont. Res., 12:107, 1977.

36. Mims, C.: The pathogenesis of infectious disease. 2nd ed. New York, Academic Press, 1982.

37. Newman, M. G.: Periodontosis. J. West. Soc. Periodontol., 24:5, 1976.

38. Newman, M. G., and Socransky, S. S.: Predominant cultivable microbiota in periodontosis. J. Periodont. Res., 12:120, 1977.

39. Newman, M. G., Socransky, S. S., and Listgarten, M. A.: Relationship of microorganisms to the etiology of periodontosis. J. Dent. Res., 53:290, 1974.

40. Newman, M. G., Williams, R. C., and Crawford, A.: Predominant cultivable microbiota of periodontosis. III. J. Dent. Res., 54:211, 1975.

41. Newman, M. G., Socransky, S. S., Savitt, E. D., Propas, D. A., and Crawford, A.: Studies of the microbiology of periodontosis. J. Periodontol., 47:373, 1976.

42. Newman, M. G., Angel, I., Karge, H., Weiner, M., Grinenko, V., and Schusterman, L.: Bacterial studies of Papillon-Lefèvre syndrome. J. Dent. Res., 56:220, 1977.

43. Newman, M. G., Socransky, S. S., Savitt, E., Krichevsky, M., Listgarten, M., and Lai, W.: Characterization of bacteria isolated from periodontosis. J. Dent. Res., 53:325, 1974.

44. Nisengard, R. J.: The role of immunology in periodontal disease. J. Periodontol., 48:505, 1977.

45. Nisengard, R. J., and Beutner, E. H.: Relation of immediate hypersensitivity to periodontitis in animals and man. J. Periodontol., 41:223, 1970.

46. Nisengard, R. J., Beutner, E. H., and Hazen, S. P.: Immunologic studies of periodontal disease. III. Bacterial hypersensitivity and periodontal disease. J. Periodontol., 39:329, 1968.

47. Nisengard, R. J., Beutner, E. H., Neugeboren, N., Neiders, M., and Asaro, J.: Experimental induction of periodontal disease with Arthus-type reactions. Clin. Immunol. Immunopathol., 8:97, 1977.

48. Patters, M. R., Sedransk, N., and Genco, R. J.: The lymphoproliferative response during human experimental gingivitis. J. Periodont. Res., 14:269, 1979.

49. Piper, P. J., and Vane, J. R.: Release of additional factors in anaphylaxis and its antagonism by antiinflammatory drugs. Nature, 223:29, 1971.

50. Ranney, R. R., and Zander, H. A.: Allergic periodontal disease in sensitized squirrel monkeys. J. Periodontol., 41:12, 1970.

51. Rizzo, A. A., and Mergenhagen, S. E.: Host responses in periodontal disease. Proceedings of the International Conference on Research on the Biology of Periodontal Disease. Chicago, 1977.

52. Saglie, R., Newman, M. G., Carranza, F. A., Jr., et al.: Immunochemical localization of *Actinobacillus actinomycetemcomitans* in sections of gingival tissue in localized juvenile periodontitis. Acta Odont. Lat.-Am., 7:41, 1984.

53. Saglie, R., Newman, M. G., Carranza, F. A., Jr., and Pattison, G. A.: Bacterial invasion of gingiva in advanced periodontitis in humans. J. Periodontol., 53:217, 1982.

54. Sidaway, D. A.: A microbiological study of dental calculus. J. Periodont. Res., 15:240, 1980.

55. Slots, J.: The predominant cultivable organisms in juvenile periodontitis. Scand. J. Dent. Res., 84:1, 1976.

56. Slots, J.: The predominant cultivable microflora of advanced periodontitis. Scand. J. Dent. Res., 85:114, 1977.

57. Slots, J.: Subgingival microflora and periodontal disease. J. Clin. Periodontol., 6:351, 1979.

58. Smith, F. N., Lang, N. P., and Löe, H.: Cell-mediated immune responses to plaque antigens during experimental gingivitis in man. J. Periodont. Res., 13:232, 1978.

59. Socransky, S. S.: Microbiology of periodontal disease. Present status and future considerations. J. Periodontol., 48:497, 1977.

60. Socransky, S. S., and Manganiello, A. D.: The oral microbiota of man from birth to senility. J. Periodontol., 42:485, 1971.

61. Wahl, S. M., Iverson, G. M., and Oppenheim, J. J.: Induction of guinea pig B-cell lymphokine synthesis by mitogenic and nonmitogenic signals to Fe, Ig and C3 receptors. J. Exp. Med., 140:1631, 1974.

Chapter 6

Calculus

The cause of gingival inflammation is bacterial plaque. Factors such as calculus, faulty restorations, partial removable prostheses, and food impaction were previously considered to be etiologic agents in periodontal disease but are now recognized to act only by favoring plaque accumulation. Although *the primary effect of calculus is due to the fact that it is always covered by bacteria*, it plays a major role in maintaining and accentuating periodontal disease by keeping plaque in close contact with the gingival tissue and creating areas where plaque removal is impossible. *When calculus is present, the gingival tissues are inflamed; when it is present in deep subgingival lesions, the potential for repair and new attachment is nonexistent. Therefore, the therapeutic importance of acquiring competence in the ability to remove calculus cannot be overemphasized.*

SUPRAGINGIVAL AND SUBGINGIVAL CALCULUS

Calculus is composed of mineralized bacterial plaque that adheres to the surfaces of natural teeth and dental prostheses. It usually appears in the early teen years of life and increases in amount with age.[9, 15, 26] It is uncommon in children and occurs in almost 100 per cent of the population by age 40.[1] It is classified according to its relation to the gingival margin as subgingival or supragingival calculus. Supragingival calculus and subgingival calculus generally occur together, but one may be present without the other. Supragingival calculus has also been referred to as *salivary*, and subgingival calculus as *serumal*, because the minerals for the formation of supragingival calculus come from the saliva, whereas the gingival fluid, which resembles serum, is the main mineral source of subgingival calculus.[11, 38]

Supragingival calculus (visible calculus) refers to calculus coronal to the crest of the gingival margin and visible in the oral cavity (Fig. 6–1). Supragingival calculus is usually white or whitish yellow, of hard, clay-like consistency, and easily detached from the tooth surface. Its recurrence after removal may be rapid, especially in the lingual area of the mandibular incisors. The color is affected by such factors as tobacco smoke and food pigments. It may localize on a single tooth or a group of teeth or be generalized throughout the mouth. Supragingival calculus occurs most frequently and in greatest quantity on the buccal surfaces of the maxillary molars opposite Stensen's duct (Fig. 6–2), and on the lingual surfaces of the mandibular anterior teeth opposite Wharton's

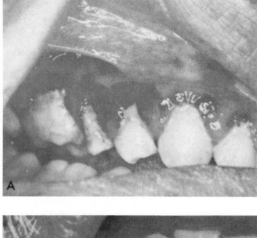

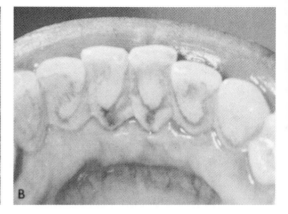

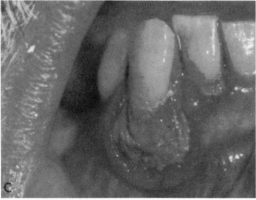

Figure 6–1. Supragingival calculus. *A,* Heavy calculus deposits on facial surfaces of upper first molar and second premolar. Note the severe gingival inflammation in the entire quadrant. *B,* Calculus deposits on lingual surfaces of lower incisors forming a bridge over the interdental papillae. Gingival inflammation can also be seen. *C,* Heavy calculus deposit on facial surface of lower cuspid with associated gingival recession.

Figure 6–2. Calculus on molar opposite Stensen's duct.

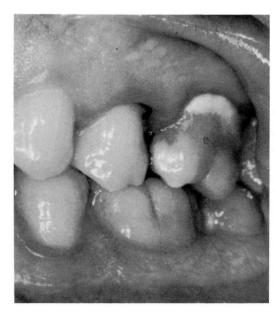

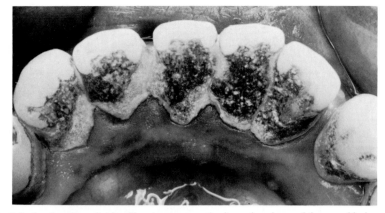

Figure 6–3. Calculus forming a bridge-like structure on the lingual surfaces of the mandibular anterior teeth.

duct. In extreme cases calculus may form a bridge-like structure along adjacent teeth or cover the occlusal surfaces of teeth (Fig. 6–3) without functional antagonists.

Subgingival calculus refers to calculus below the crest of the marginal gingiva, usually in periodontal pockets, and is not visible upon oral examination. Determination of the location and extent of subgingival calculus requires careful exploration with an instrument (Fig. 6–4). It is usually dense and hard, dark brown or greenish black, flintlike in consistency, and firmly attached to the tooth surface (Fig. 6–5).

When the gingival tissues recede, subgingival calculus becomes exposed and is classified as supragingival. Thus, supragingival calculus can be composed of both the supragingival and subgingival types.

Radiographic Signs

Supragingival and subgingival calculus are sometimes seen in radiographs (Fig. 6–6). Supragingivally, well-calcified deposits are readily detectable, forming irregular contours on the roentgenographic crown. Supragingival and subgingival interproximal calculus is easily detectable because it forms irregularly shaped projections into the interdental space. Normally the location of calculus does not indicate the depth of the periodontal pocket,

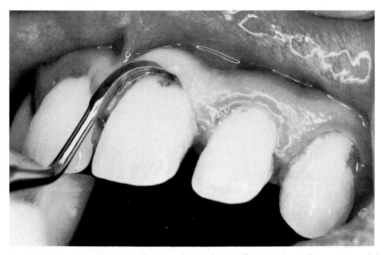

Figure 6–4. Subgingival calculus revealed by deflecting the pocket wall. Note the inflammation of the marginal gingiva on adjacent lateral incisor and canine associated with supra- and subgingival calculus.

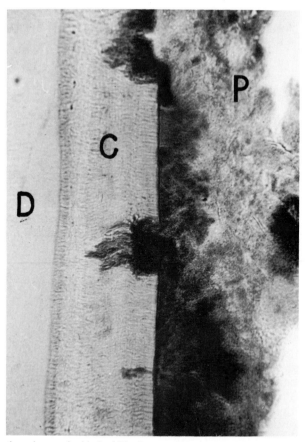

Figure 6–5. Calculus on tooth surface embedded within the cementum (C). Note the early stage of penetration shown in the lower portion of the illustration. The dentin is at D. P, plaque attached to calculus.

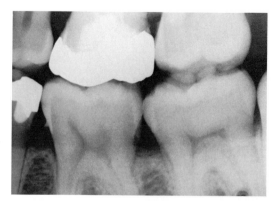

Figure 6–6. Radiographic appearance of subgingival calculus. Note the interproximal spicules.

since the most apical plaque is not calcified enough to be radiographically evident.

COMPOSITION OF CALCULUS

Inorganic Content

Supragingival calculus consists of 70 to 90 per cent inorganic components,[6] and the remainder is composed of organic constituents. The inorganic portion consists of 75.9 per cent calcium phosphate, 3.1 per cent calcium carbonate, and traces of magnesium phosphate and other metals. The percentage of inorganic components of calculus is similar to that of other calcified tissues of the body. At least two thirds of the inorganic component is crystalline in structure.[14] The four main crystal forms are hydroxyapatite (approximately 58 per cent); magnesium whitlockite and octacalcium phosphate (approximately 21 per cent each);[29] and brushite (approximately 9 per cent). Generally two or more crystal forms occur in calculus, with hydroxyapatite and octacalcium phosphate being the most common (in 97 to 100 per cent of all supragingival calculus) and in the greatest amounts. Brushite is more common in the mandibular anterior region and magnesium whitlockite in the posterior areas. The incidence of the four crystal forms varies with the age of the deposit.[32]

Organic Content

The organic component of calculus consists of a mixture of protein-polysaccharide complexes, desquamated epithelial cells, leukocytes, and various types of microorganisms; 1.9 to 9.1 per cent of the organic component is carbohydrate. Protein derived from the saliva accounts for 5.9 to 8.2 per cent of the organic component of calculus and includes most of the amino acids.[18, 20, 36] Lipids account for 0.2 per cent of the organic content.[17]

Subgingival Calculus

The composition of subgingival calculus is slightly different from that of supragingival.

It has the same hydroxyapatite content,[39] more magnesium whitlockite, and less brushite and octacalcium phosphate.[29] The ratio of calcium to phosphate is higher subgingivally, and the sodium content increases in calculus located in deep periodontal pockets.[16] Salivary proteins present in supragingival calculus are not found subgingivally.[2] Dental calculus, salivary duct calculus, and calcified dental tissues are similar in inorganic composition.

ATTACHMENT OF CALCULUS TO THE TOOTH SURFACE

Differences in the manner in which calculus is attached to the tooth surface affect the relative ease or difficulty encountered in its removal. Calculus is attached by organic pellicle; penetration of calculus bacteria into cementum (this theory is not accepted by some investigators);[12] mechanical locking into surface irregularities, such as resorption lacunae and caries; and close adaptation of calculus undersurface depressions to the gently sloping mounds of the unaltered cementum surface (Fig. 6–7).[37, 44] Calculus embedded deeply in cementum may appear morphologically similar to cementum and has been termed "calculocementum."[33, 35]

CALCULUS FORMATION

Calculus is attached dental plaque that has undergone mineralization. The soft plaque is hardened by precipitation of mineral salts, usually starting between the first and fourteenth day of plaque formation; however, calcification has been reported in as few as 4 to 8 hours.[40] Calcifying plaques may become 50 per cent mineralized in 2 days and 60 to 90 per cent mineralized in 12 days.[22, 30, 34]

All plaque does not necessarily undergo calcification. Early plaque contains a small amount of inorganic material, which increases as the plaque develops into calculus. Plaque that does not develop into calculus reaches a plateau of maximum mineral content by 2 days.[22, 31, 34] Microorganisms are not always essential in calculus formation, since formation occurs readily in germ-free rodents.[5, 10]

Calcification entails the binding of calcium

calculus to root planed surfaces. Periodontics, 6:78, 1968.

13. Leach, S. A., and Saxton, C. A.: An electron microscopic study of the acquired pellicle and plaque formed on the enamel of human incisors. Arch. Oral Biol., 11:1081, 1966.

14. Leung, S. W., and Jensen, A. T.: Factors controlling the deposition of calculus. Int. Dent. J., 8:613, 1958.

15. Lilienthal, B., Amerena, V., and Gregory, G.: An epidemiological study of chronic periodontal disease. Arch. Oral Biol., 10:553, 1965.

16. Little, M. F., and Hazen, S. P.: Dental calculus composition. 2. Subgingival calculus: ash, calcium, phosphorus and sodium. J. Dent. Res., 43:645, 1964.

17. Little, M. F., Bowman, L. M., and Dirksen, T. R.: The lipids of supragingival calculus. J. Dent. Res., 43:836, 1964.

18. Little, M. F., Bowman, L., Casciani, C. A., and Rowley, J.: The composition of dental calculus. III. Supragingival calculus—the amino acid and saccharide component. Arch. Oral Biol., 11:385, 1966.

19. Mandel, I. D.: Calculus formation. The role of bacteria and mucoprotein. Dent. Clin. North Am., 4:731, 1960.

20. Mandel, I. D.: Histochemical and biochemical aspects of calculus formation. Periodontics, 1:43, 1963.

21. Moskow, B. S.: Calculus attachment in cemental separations. J. Periodontol., 40:125, 1969.

22. Muhlemann, H. R., and Schroeder, H.: Dynamics of supragingival calculus formation. Adv. Oral Biol., 1:175, 1964.

23. Muhlemann, H. R., and Villa, P. R.: The Marginal Line Calculus Index. Helv. Odontol. Acta, 11:175, 1967.

24. Muhler, J. C., and Ennever, J.: Occurrence of calculus through several successive periods in a selected group of subjects. J. Periodontol., 33:22, 1962.

25. Mukherjee, S.: Formation and prevention of supragingival calculus. J. Periodont. Res., 3(Suppl. 2), 1968.

26. Ramfjord, S. P.: The periodontal status of boys 11 to 17 years old in Bombay, India. J. Periodontol., 32:237, 1961.

27. Rizzo, A. A., Scott, D. B., and Bladen, H. A.: Calcification of oral bacteria. Ann. N.Y. Acad. Sci., 109:14, 1963.

28. Rizzo, A. A., Martin, G. R., Scott, D. B., and Mergenhagen, E. E.: Mineralization of bacteria. Science, 135:439, 1962.

29. Rowles, S. L.: The inorganic composition of dental calculus. In Blackwood, H. J. J. (ed.): Bone and Tooth. Oxford, Pergamon Press, 1964, pp. 175-183.

30. Schroeder, H. E.: Inorganic content and histology of early dental calculus in man. Helv. Odontol. Acta, 7:17, 1963.

31. Schroeder, H. E.: Crystal morphology and gross structures of mineralizing plaque and of calculus. Helv. Odontol. Acta, 9:73, 1965.

32. Schroeder, H. E., and Bambauer, H. U.: Stages of calcium phosphate crystallization during calculus formation. Arch. Oral Biol., 11:1, 1966.

33. Selvig, J.: Attachment of plaque and calculus to tooth surfaces. J. Periodont. Res., 5:8, 1970.

34. Sharawy, A., Sabharwal, K., Socransky, S., and Lobene, R.: A quantitative study of plaque and calculus formation in normal and periodontally involved mouths. J. Periodontol., 37:495, 1966.

35. Sottosanti, J. S.: A possible relationship between occlusion, root resorption, and the progression of periodontal disease. J. Western Soc. Periodontol. 25:69, 1977.

36. Standford, J. W.: Analysis of the organic portion of dental calculus. J. Dent. Res., 45:128, 1966.

37. Stanton, G.: The relation of diet to salivary calculus formation. J. Periodontol., 40:167, 1969.

38. Stewart, R. T., and Ratcliff, P. A.: The source of components of subgingival plaque and calculus. Periodont. Abstr., 14:102, 1966.

39. Theilade, J., and Schroeder, H. E.: Recent results in dental calculus research. Int. Dent. J., 16:205, 1966.

40. Tibbetts, L. S., and Kashiwa, H. K.: A histochemical study of early plaque mineralization. I.A.D.R. Abst. 1970, No. 616, p. 202.

41. Turesky, S., et al.: Effects of changing the salivary environment on progress of calculus formation. J. Periodontol., 33:45, 1962.

42. Volpe, A. R., Kupczak, L. J., King, W. J., Goldman, H., and Schulmann, S. M.: In vivo calculus assessment. Part IV. Parameters of human clinical studies. J. Periodontol., 40:76, 1969.

43. Wasserman, B. H., Mandel, J. D., and Levy, B. M.: In vitro calcification of calculus. J. Periodontol., 29:145, 1958.

44. Zander, H. A.: The attachment of calculus to root surfaces. J. Periodontol., 24:16, 1953.

45. Zander, H. A., Hazen, S. P., and Scott, D. B.: Mineralization of dental calculus. Proc. Soc. Exp. Biol. Med., 103:257, 1960.

Chapter 7

Local Irritants

Many factors in the oral environment favor the accumulation of bacterial plaque and therefore contribute to the etiology of periodontal disease. These are discussed in detail in this chapter.

MATERIA ALBA

Materia alba is primarily an acquired bacterial coating, which is a yellow or grayish-white, soft, sticky deposit somewhat less adherent than dental plaque (Fig. 7–1).[54] Materia alba is clearly visible without the use of disclosing solutions and forms on tooth surfaces, restorations, calculus, and gingiva.[36, 39] It tends to accumulate on the gingival third of the teeth and on malposed teeth. It can form on previously cleaned teeth within a few hours and during periods when no food is ingested.[45] Materia alba can be flushed away with a water spray, but mechanical cleansing is required to ensure complete removal.

Long considered to consist of stagnant food debris, materia alba is now recognized to be a *concentration of microorganisms, desquamated epithelial cells, leukocytes, and a mixture of salivary proteins and lipids,*[36, 54, 65] *with few or no food particles.*[45] It lacks a regular internal pattern such as is observed in plaque. The irritating effect of materia alba upon the gingiva is most likely caused by bacteria and their products, but materia alba has also been demonstrated to be toxic when injected into experimental animals after the bacterial component has been destroyed by heat.[6]

FOOD DEBRIS

Most food debris is rapidly liquefied by bacterial enzymes and cleared from the oral cavity within 5 minutes after eating, but some remains on

103

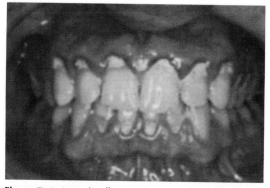

Figure 7–1. Materia alba can be generalized throughout the mouth, with heaviest accumulation near the gingiva. Note the gingivitis present.

the teeth and mucosa.[8, 45] Salivary flow; mechanical action of the tongue, cheeks, and lips; and form and alignment of the teeth and jaws all affect the rate of food clearance. Clearance is accelerated by increased chewing and low viscosity of saliva.[32] Although it contains bacteria, food debris is different from plaque and materia alba. *Dental plaque is not a derivative of food debris, nor is food debris an important cause of gingivitis.*[15] Fibrous strands of food trapped interproximally in areas of food impaction are not considered to be food debris.

The clearance rates of food from the oral cavity varies with the type of food and the individual. Liquids are cleared more readily than solids. For example, traces of sugar ingested in aqueous solution remain in the saliva for approximately 15 minutes, whereas sugar consumed in solid form is present for as long as 30 minutes after ingestion.[63] Sticky foods, such as figs, toffee, and caramel, may adhere to tooth surfaces for over 1 hour, whereas coarse foods like raw carrots and apples are quickly cleared. Plain bread is cleared faster than bread with butter,[8, 22] brown rye bread faster than white,[32] and cold foods slightly faster than hot. The chewing of apples and other fibrous foods can effectively remove most of the food debris from the oral cavity, although it has no significant effect on the reduction of plaque.[9, 34]

FAULTY DENTISTRY

Faulty dental restorations and prostheses are common causes of gingival inflammation

and periodontal destruction. Inadequate dental procedures may also injure the periodontal tissues. Margins, contours, occlusion, materials, and design of removable partial dentures are of importance in maintaining periodontal health.

Margins of Restorations

Overhanging margins provide ideal locations for the accumulation of plaque and the multiplication of bacteria (Fig. 7–2). Removal of overhangs permits more effective plaque control, resulting in the disappearance of gingival inflammation and increased alveolar bone support.[21, 23] Numerous studies[20, 26, 27, 49] have shown a positive correlation between subgingival margins and gingival inflammation. It has also been shown that even high-quality restorations, if placed subgingivally, will increase plaque accumulation, gingival inflammation,[33, 50] and the rate of gingival fluid flow.[42]

Roughness in the subgingival area is considered the major cause of plaque buildup and the resultant inflammatory response.[56] The subgingival zone is made up of the crown and the margin of the restoration, the luting material, and the prepared tooth surface. Silness[58] has described the following sources of roughness: stripes and scratches in the surface of carefully polished acrylic resin, porcelain, or gold restorations; separation of the cervical crown margin and the cervical margin of the finishing line by the luting material, exposing the rough surface of the prepared tooth; dissolution and disintegra-

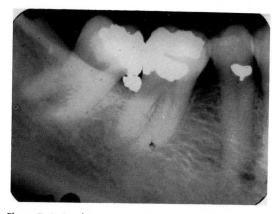

Figure 7–2. Amalgam excess, which is a source of irritation to the gingiva.

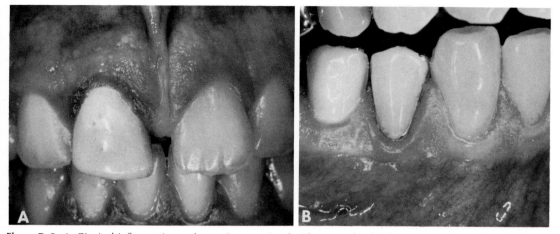

Figure 7–3. *A,* Gingival inflammation and recession associated with accumulated irritants on **rough margin of crown.** *B,* **Inadequate mesioproximal contour** on first premolar restoration leads to accumulation of irritants and gingival inflammation.

tion of the luting material, causing crater formation between the preparation and the restoration; and inadequate marginal fit of the restoration.

The undersurface of pontics in fixed bridges should barely touch the mucosa. When this contact is excessive, it will prevent cleaning. Plaque will accumulate, causing inflammation and possibly pseudopocket formation.

Contours

Over-contoured crowns and restorations tend to accumulate plaque (Fig. 7–3*A*) and limit the self-cleaning mechanisms of the adjacent cheek, lips, and tongue.[1, 31, 38, 66] Claims that under-contouring of crowns may also have a deleterious effect due to lack of protection of the gingival margin during mastication have not been proven.[66]

Inadequate or improperly located proximal contacts and failure to reproduce the normal protective anatomy of the occlusal marginal ridges and developmental grooves lead to food impaction (Fig. 7–3*B*). Failure to reestablish adequate interproximal embrasures fosters the accumulation of irritants.

Occlusion

Restorations that do not conform to the occlusal patterns of the mouth cause occlusal disharmonies that may be injurious to the supporting periodontal tissues by causing trauma from occlusion (see Chapter 8).

Materials

Restorative materials are not by themselves injurious to the periodontal tissues.[1, 28] One exception to this may be self-curing acrylics.[64]

Restorative materials differ in their capacity to retain plaque,[64] but all can be adequately cleaned if they are polished[41, 52] and accessible to brushing. The composition of plaque formed on all types of restorative materials is similar, with the exception of that formed on silicate.[41] Plaque formed at the margins of restorations is similar to that formed on adjacent tooth surfaces.

Design of Removable Partial Dentures

Several investigations have shown that after the insertion of partial dentures there is an increase in mobility of the abutment teeth, in gingival inflammation, and in periodontal pocket formation.[10, 12, 55] This is due to the fact that partial dentures favor the accumulation of plaque, particularly if they cover the gingival tissue. Partial dentures that are worn night and day induce more plaque formation than those used only during the day.[10] The presence of removable partial dentures induces not only quantitative changes in dental plaque[18] but also qualitative changes, promoting the development of spirilla and spirochetes.[19]

These observations emphasize the need for careful and personalized oral hygiene instruction in order to avoid harmful effects of partial dentures on the remaining teeth.[7]

Dental Procedures

The use of rubber dam clamps, copper bands, matrix bands, and disks in such a manner as to lacerate the gingiva results in varying degrees of inflammation. Although for the most part such transient injuries undergo repair, they are needless sources of discomfort to patients. Injudicious tooth separation and excessively vigorous condensing of gold foil restorations can also injure the supporting tissues of the periodontium and may cause acute symptoms such as pain and sensitivity to percussion.

PROBLEMS ASSOCIATED WITH ORTHODONTIC THERAPY

Retention of Plaque

Orthodontic appliances tend to retain bacterial plaque and food debris, resulting in gingivitis (Fig. 7–4). Proper oral hygiene methods should be taught when appliances are inserted, and the importance of these techniques must be stressed. The condition of the periodontium should be checked regularly during orthodontic treatment, and periodontal care should be instituted at the earliest sign of disease. Water irrigation devices are helpful oral hygiene aids for these patients.

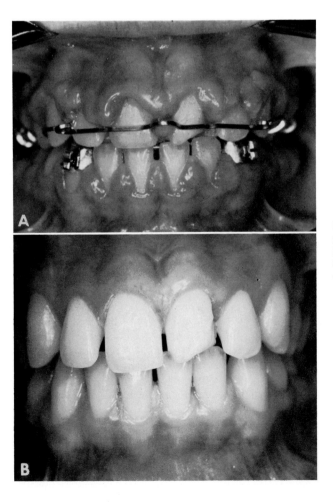

Figure 7–4. Gingival inflammation and enlargement associated with orthodontic appliance and poor oral hygiene. *A*, Gingival disease with orthodontic appliance in place. *B*, After removal of the appliance and periodontal treatment.

Irritation from Orthodontic Bands

Orthodontic treatment is often started at a stage of tooth eruption when the junctional epithelium is still on the enamel. The bands should not extend into the gingival tissues beyond the level of attachment. Forceful detachment of the gingiva from the tooth followed by apical proliferation of the junctional epithelium results in the increased gingival recession sometimes seen in orthodontically treated patients.[46] If gingival inflammation is present, the gingival margin is prevented from following the migrating epithelium, and pocket formation results.

Tissue Injury from Orthodontic Forces

To assure periodontal health, it is important to avoid excessive force and too rapid tooth movement in orthodontic treatment. Excessive force may produce necrosis of the periodontal ligament and adjacent alveolar bone. These ordinarily undergo repair; however, destruction of the periodontal ligament at the crest of the alveolar bone may lead to irreparable damage. If the periodontal fibers beneath the junctional epithelium are destroyed by excessive force and the epithelium is stimulated to proliferate along the root by local irritants, the epithelium will cover the root and prevent re-embedding of the periodontal fibers in the course of repair. Ab-

sence of functional stimulation from the periodontal fibers may result in atrophy of the crest of the alveolar bone. Excessive orthodontic forces also increase the risk of apical root resorption.

FOOD IMPACTION

Food impaction is the forceful wedging of food into the periodontium by occlusal forces. It may occur interproximally or in relation to the facial or lingual tooth surfaces. Food impaction is a very common cause of gingival inflammation (Fig. 7–5). Far too frequently, failure to recognize and eliminate food impaction is responsible for the unsuccessful outcome of an otherwise well-treated case of periodontal disease.

Mechanism of Food Impaction

The forceful wedging of food normally is prevented by the integrity and location of the proximal contacts, the contour of the marginal ridges and developmental grooves, and the contour of the facial and lingual surfaces. The location of the contact point is also important in protecting the tissues against food impaction. The optimal cervicoocclusal location of the contact is at the longest mesiodistal diameter of the tooth, close to the crest of the marginal ridge. The prox-

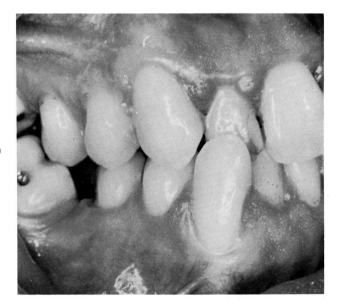

Figure 7–5. Malposed teeth with food impaction areas and gingival inflammation

imity of the contact point to the occlusal plane reduces the tendency toward food impaction in the smaller occlusal embrasure. The absence of contact or the presence of an unsatisfactory proximal relationship is conducive to food impaction.

The contour of the occlusal surface established by the marginal ridges and related developmental grooves normally serves to deflect food away from the interproximal spaces. As the teeth wear down and are flattened, the wedging effect of the opposing cusp into the interproximal space is exaggerated and food impaction results. Cusps that tend to forcibly wedge food interproximally are known as *plunger cusps*. The plunger cusp effect may occur with wear, or as the result of shifts in tooth positions from unreplaced missing teeth.

Excessive anterior overbite is a common cause of food impaction. The forceful wedging of food into the gingiva on the facial surfaces of the mandibular anterior teeth and the lingual surfaces of the maxillary teeth produces varying degrees of periodontal involvement. Gingival changes in the mandibular anterior region, associated with excessive anterior overbite, are easily detectable. Unless they are severe, however, the effects of food impaction on the lingual surface of the maxilla are often overlooked. It should be stressed that inflammation caused by lingual food impaction may spread to the contiguous facial gingival margin. The possibility that lingual food impaction may be a contributory factor should always be explored when the etiology of gingival disease in the anterior maxilla is being considered.

Hirschfeld's classic analysis[24] of the factors leading to food impaction implicates uneven occlusal wear, opening of the contact points due to loss of proximal support or extrusion, congenital morphologic abnormalities, and improperly constructed restorations. However, the presence of these abnormalities does not necessarily lead to food impaction and periodontal disease. A study of interproximal contacts and marginal ridge relationships in three groups of periodontally healthy males revealed that from 61.7 to 76 per cent of the proximal contacts were defective and 33.5 per cent of adjacent marginal ridges were uneven.[43]

Lateral Food Impaction

In addition to food impaction due to occlusal forces, lateral pressure from the lips, cheeks, and tongue may force food interproximally. This is more likely to occur when the gingival embrasure is enlarged by tissue destruction in periodontal disease or by recession. Impaction results when food forced into such an embrasure during mastication is retained instead of passing through.

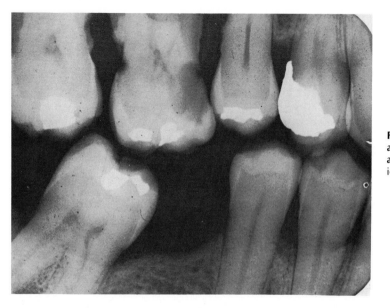

Figure 7–6. Tilted mandibular molar and extruded maxillary molar associated with unreplaced tooth. Note caries in maxillary molar.

UNREPLACED MISSING TEETH

Failure to replace extracted teeth initiates a series of changes often resulting in periodontal disease.[14, 25] In isolated cases, spaces created by tooth extraction may not cause undesirable sequelae. However, the high frequency with which periodontal disease results from the failure to replace one or more missing teeth suggests the advisability and prophylactic value of early prosthesis.

The ramifications of the failure to replace the first molar are sufficiently consistent to be recognized as a clinical entity (Fig. 7–6). When the mandibular first molar is missing, the initial change is a mesial drifting and tilting of the mandibular second and third molars and extrusion of the maxillary first molar. The distal cusps of the mandibular second molar are elevated and act as plungers, impacting food into the interproximal space between the extruded maxillary first molar and the maxillary second molar. If there is no maxillary third molar, the distal cusps of the mandibular second molar act as wedges which break the contact between the maxillary first and second molars and deflect the maxillary second molar distally. This results in food impaction, gingival inflammation, and bone loss in the interproximal area between the maxillary first and second molars. Tilting of the mandibular molars and extrusion of the maxillary molars alter the respective contact relationships of these teeth, thereby favoring food impaction. Bone loss and pocket formation are commonly seen in relation to the extruded and tilted teeth.

Tilting of the posterior teeth also results in reduction in vertical dimension and accentuation of the anterior overbite. The mandibular anterior teeth slide gingivally along the palatal surfaces of the maxillary anterior teeth, resulting in a distal shift in the position of the mandible. In addition, there is food impaction and pocket formation in relation to the anterior teeth and a tendency toward labial migration and diastema formation in the maxilla. Further complications are distal drifting of the second premolar with food impaction and pocket formation in the opened interproximal space between the premolars. These changes are also accompanied by alterations in the functional relationships of the inclined cusps, with resultant occlusal disharmonies injurious to the periodontium.

The combination of changes associated with unreplaced mandibular first molars does not occur in all cases, nor do all the identified changes occur with failure to replace other teeth in the arch. *In general, however, drifting and tilting of the teeth, and alterations in proximal contact, result from unreplaced teeth. These changes are common factors in the etiology of periodontal disease.*

MALOCCLUSION

Depending upon its nature, malocclusion exerts a varied effect in the etiology of gingivitis and periodontal disease.[37, 51] Irregular alignment of teeth will make plaque control difficult or even impossible. Gingival recession is associated with facially displaced teeth.

Occlusal disharmony associated with malocclusion results in injury to the periodontium.[40, 44] The incisal edges of the anterior teeth can cause irritation to the gingiva in the opposing jaw where severe overbite exists. Open bite relationships can also lead to unfavorable periodontal changes caused by accumulation of plaque and diminution in function.[11, 29]

MOUTH BREATHING

Gingivitis is often associated with mouth breathing[35] (Fig. 7–7). The gingival changes include erythema, edema, enlargement, and a diffuse surface shininess in the exposed areas. The maxillary anterior region is the common site of such involvement. In many cases the altered gingiva is clearly demarcated from the adjacent unexposed normal mucosa. The exact manner in which mouth breathing affects gingival changes has not been demonstrated. Its harmful effect is generally attributed to irritation from surface dehydration. However, comparable changes could not be produced by air drying the gingivae of experimental animals.[30]

ORAL HABITS

Oral habits are important factors in the initiation and progression of periodontal disease. Frequently, the presence of an unsuspected habit is revealed in patients who have

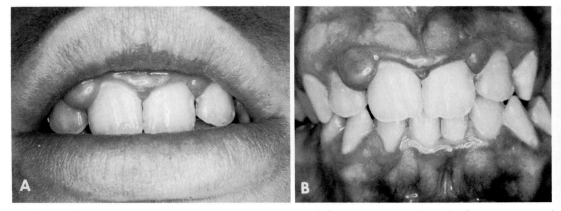

Figure 7–7. **Gingivitis in mouth breather.** *A*, High lip line in mouth breather. *B*, Gingivitis and inflammatory gingival enlargement in exposed area of gingiva.

failed to respond to periodontal therapy. Habits of significance in the etiology of periodontal disease have been classified as follows:[60]

1. *Neuroses*. Habits such as lip biting and cheek biting can lead to extra-functional positioning of the mandible. Toothpick biting and wedging between the teeth, "tongue thrusting" (see the following section), fingernail biting, and pencil and fountain pen biting are occlusal neuroses.

2. *Occupational habits*. These include the holding of nails in the mouth as practiced by cobblers, upholsterers, and carpenters; thread biting; and pressure of reeds during the playing of certain musical instruments.

3. *Miscellaneous habits*. Other habits include pipe or cigarette smoking, tobacco chewing, incorrect methods of toothbrushing, mouth breathing, and thumb sucking.

Tongue-Thrusting

Special mention should be made of tongue-thrusting because it is so frequently undetected. It entails persistent, forceful wedging of the tongue against the teeth, particularly in the anterior region. Instead of the dorsum of the tongue being placed against the palate with the tip behind the maxillary teeth during swallowing, the tongue is thrust forward against the mandibular anterior teeth, which tilt and also spread laterally.

Tongue-thrusting is generally associated with abnormal swallowing habits (reverse swallow), which develop in infancy. Nasopharyngeal disease and allergy have been implicated as possible causes of tongue-thrusting.

Tongue-thrusting causes excessive lateral pressure, which may be traumatic to the periodontium.[13, 57] It also causes spreading and tilting of the anterior teeth, with an open bite anteriorly, posteriorly, or in the premolar area (Fig. 7–8).

TOBACCO

Ordinarily, smoking does not lead to striking gingival changes. However, heat and the accumulated products of combustion are local irritants that are particularly undesirable in periods of post-treatment healing. The following oral changes may occur in smokers:

1. Brownish, tar-like deposits and discoloration of tooth structure.

2. Diffuse grayish discoloration and leukoplakia of the gingiva.

3. "Smoker's palate," characterized by prominent mucous glands with inflammation of the orifices and a diffuse erythema or by a wrinkled "cobblestone" surface.

The correlation between tobacco smoking and acute necrotizing ulcerative gingivitis has been clearly shown,[3] although a cause-and-effect relationship has not been proven. Both smoking and acute necrotizing ulcerative gingivitis may be the result of underlying anxiety and tension.

The influence of tobacco smoking on chronic gingivitis and plaque accumulation is still controversial. When smokers and nonsmokers are matched with regard to age and

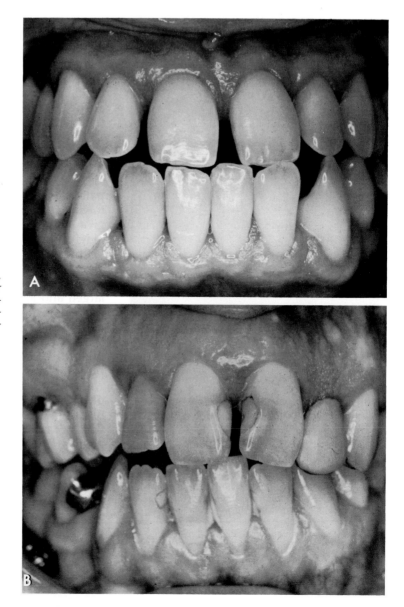

Figure 7–8. Tongue-thrusting. *A*, Tilting and spreading of anterior teeth associated with tongue-thrusting. *B*, Hypo-occlusion of lateral incisor, canine, and premolar associated with tongue-thrusting.

oral hygiene levels, no difference is found in the degree of gingival inflammation and periodontal breakdown.[33, 48, 56] Several authors, however, have reported more severe gingivitis and periodontitis in smokers,[2, 17, 62] probably because of increased plaque accumulation, but others have found that tobacco smoking has little or no effect on the rate of plaque formation.[5]

It has been noted that women from the ages of 20 to 39 and men from 30 to 59 years of age who smoke cigarettes have about twice the chance of having periodontal disease or becoming edentulous as do nonsmokers.[59]

A specific type of gingivitis termed "gingivitis toxica,"[47] characterized by destruction of the gingiva and underlying bone, has been attributed to the chewing of tobacco.

TOOTHBRUSH TRAUMA

Alterations in the gingiva as well as abrasions of the teeth may result from aggressive

23. Highfield, J. E., and Powell, R. N.: Effects of removal of posterior overhanging metallic margins of restorations upon the periodontal tissues. J. Clin. Periodontol., 5:169, 1978.

24. Hirschfeld, I.: Food impaction. J. Am. Dent. Assoc., 17:1504, 1930.

25. Hirschfeld, I.: Individual missing tooth. J. Am. Dent. Assoc., 24:67, 1937.

26. Hüttner, G.: Follow-up study of crowns and abutments with regard to the crown edge and the marginal periodontium. Dtsch. Zahnaerztl. Z., 26:724, 1971.

27. Karlsen, K.: Gingival reactions to dental restorations. Acta Odontol. Scand., 28:895, 1970.

28. Kawakara, H., Yamagani, A., and Nakamura, M., Jr.: Biological testing of dental materials by means of tissue culture. Int. Dent. J., 18:443, 1968.

29. King, J. D., and Gimson, A. P.: Experimental investigations of paradontal disease in the ferret and related lesions in man. Br. Dent. J., 83:126, 1947.

30. Klingsberg, J., Cancellaro, B. A., and Butcher, E. O.: Effects of air drying on rodent oral mucous membrane: a histologic study of simulated mouth breathing. J. Periodontol., 32:38, 1961.

31. Koivumaa, K. K., and Wennstrom, A.: A histological investigation of the changes in gingival margins adjacent to gold crowns. Odont. T., 68:373, 1960.

32. Lanke, L. S.: Influence on salivary sugar of certain properties of foodstuffs and individual oral conditions. Acta Odontol. Scand., 15(Suppl. 23):3, 1957.

33. Leon, A. R.: Amalgam restorations and periodontal disease. Br. Dent. J., 140:377, 1976.

34. Lindhe, J., and Wicen, P.: The effects on the gingivae of chewing fibrous foods. J. Periodont. Res., 4:193, 1969.

35. Lite, T., et al.: Gingival pathosis in mouth breathers. A clinical and histopathologic study and a method of treatment. Oral Surg., 8:382, 1955.

36. Mandel, I. D.: Dental plaque: Nature, formation, and effects. J. Periodontol., 37:357, 1966.

37. Miller, J., and Hobson, P.: The relationship between malocclusion, oral cleanliness, gingival conditions and dental caries in school children. Br. Dent. J., 111:43, 1961.

38. Morris, M. L.: Artificial crown contours and gingival health. J. Prosthet. Dent., 12:1146, 1962.

39. Mühlemann, H. R., and Schroeder, H.: Dynamics of supragingival calculus formation. Adv. Oral Biol., 1:175, 1964.

40. Mühlemann, H. R., et al.: Okklusion und Artikulation im Atiologiekomplex Parodontaler Erkrankungen. Parodontologie, 11:20, 1957.

41. Norman, R. D., Mehia, R. V., Swartz, M. L., and Phillips, R. W.: Effect of restorative materials on plaque composition. J. Dent. Res., 51:1596, 1972.

42. Normann, W., Regolati, B., and Renggli, H. H.: Gingival reaction to well-fitted subgingival proximal gold inlays. J. Clin. Periodontol., 1:120, 1974.

43. O'Leary, T. J., and Sosa, C. E.: Signs of periodontal breakdown in patients with malocclusion. J. Dent. Educ., 10:172, 1955.

44. O'Leary, T. J., Badell, M., and Bloomer, R.: Interproximal contact and marginal ridge relationships in periodontally healthy young males classified as to orthodontic status. J. Periodontol., 46:6, 1975.

45. Parfitt, G. J.: Summary of the problem of the prevention of periodontal disease. Ala. J. Med. Sci., 5:305, 1968.

46. Pearson, L. E.: Gingival height of lower central incisors, orthodontically treated and untreated. Angle Ortho., 38:337, 1968.

47. Pindborg, J. J.: Tobacco and gingivitis. II. Correlation between consumption of tobacco, ulceromembranous gingivitis and calculus. J. Dent. Res., 28:461, 1949.

48. Preber, H., Kant, T., and Bergstrom, J.: Cigarette smoking, oral hygiene and periodontal disease in Swedish army conscripts. J. Clin. Periodontol., 7:106, 1980.

49. Renggli, H. H.: The influence of subgingival proximal filling borders on the degree of inflammation of the adjacent gingiva. A clinical study. Schweiz. Monatsschr Zahnheilkd., 84:181, 1974.

50. Renggli, H. H., and Regolati, B.: Gingival inflammation and plaque accumulation by well-adapted supragingival and subgingival proximal restorations. Helv. Odontol. Acta, 16:99, 1972.

51. Rosenzweig, K. A., and Langer, A.: Oral disease in yeshiva students. J. Dent. Res., 40:993, 1961.

52. Sanchez-Sotres, L., Van Huysen, G., and Gilmore, H. W.: A histologic study of gingival tissue response to amalgam, silicate and resin restorations. J. Periodontol., 42:8, 1969.

53. Schour, I., and Sarnat, B. G.: Oral manifestations of occupational origin. J.A.M.A., 120:1197, 1942.

54. Schroeder, H. E.: Formation and Inhibition of Dental Calculus. Berne, Stuttgart, and Vienna, Hans Huber Publ., 1969, pp. 12–15.

55. Seeman, S.: Study of the relationship between periodontal disease and the wearing of partial dentures. Aust. Dent. J., 8:206, 1963.

56. Sheiham, A.: Periodontal disease and oral cleanliness in tobacco smokers. J. Periodontol., 42:259, 1971.

57. Sheppard, I. M.: Tongue dynamics. Dent. Digest, 59:117, 1953.

58. Silness, J.: Fixed prosthodontics and periodontal health. Dent. Clin. North Am., 24:317, 1980.

59. Solomon, H., Priore, R., and Bross, I.: Cigarette smoking and periodontal disease. J. Am. Dent. Assoc., 77:1081, 1968.

60. Sorrin, S.: Habit: An etiologic factor of periodontal disease. Dent. Digest, 41:290, 1935.

61. Stafne, E. C., and Bowing, H. H.: The teeth and their supporting structures in patients treated by irradiation. Am. J. Orthod., 33:567, 1947.

62. Summers, C. J., and Oberman, A.: Association of oral disease with twelve selected variables. I. Periodontal disease. J. Dent. Res., 47:457, 1968.

63. Volker, J. F., and Pinkerton, D. M.: Acid production in saliva-carbohydrates. J. Dent. Res., 26:229, 1947.

64. Waerhaug, J., and Zander, H. A.: Reaction of gingival tissue to self-curing acrylic restorations. J. Am. Dent. Assoc., 54:760, 1957.

65. World Health Organization: Periodontal disease: report of an expert committee on dental health. Int. Dent. J., 11:544, 1961.

66. Yuodelis, R. A., Weaver, J. D., and Sapkos, S.: Facial and lingual contours of artificial complete crowns and their effect on the periodontium. J. Prosthet. Dent., 29:61, 1973.

Chapter 8

Occlusion and Periodontal Disease

CONCEPTS OF OCCLUSION

Recognition of occlusal relationships that are injurious to the periodontium and that may be associated with disorders of the masticatory musculature and temporomandibular joints requires an understanding of the principles of occlusion and masticatory function.

The term *occlusion* refers to the contact relationships of the teeth resulting from neuromuscular control of the masticatory system (musculature, temporomandibular joints, mandible, and periodontium).[39] Physiologic occlusion exists in individuals with no signs of occlusion-related pathosis. Traumatic occlusion is one judged to be a causal factor in the formation of traumatic lesions or disturbances in the supporting structures of the teeth, muscles, and temporomandibular joints. *The criterion that determines whether an occlusion is traumatic is whether it produces injury, not how the teeth occlude.*

The following definitions are necessary for the understanding of this topic:

Intercuspal position (ICP). This is the position of the mandible in which there is maximum intercuspation of the teeth; it is also the most cranial point of all functional contact. Synonyms: centric occlusion (CO), habitual occlusion, acquired centric, habitual centric.

Muscular contact position (MCP). The position of the mandible when it has been lifted by a minimum of muscular effort from its resting posture to the very first occlusal contact.

Retruded position (RP). Any position of the mandible on the terminal hinge path. Synonyms: centric relation (CR), terminal hinge position.

Retruded contact position (RCP). The end point of terminal hinge closure. Synonym: centric relation contact (CRC).

Excursive movement. Movement occurring when the mandible moves away from the intercuspal position. This movement is related to the direction in which the mandibular teeth move from ICP during excursion. The Latin word *trudere*, meaning "to thrust," is used with appropriate prefixes denoting the direction of movement.

Protrusion. Movement occurring when the mandible moves anteriorly from the intercuspal position.

Retrusion. Movement occurring when the

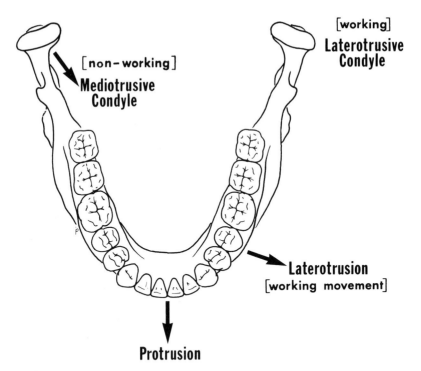

Figure 8–1. Mandibular movement is named after the direction of movement the mandible takes when it moves away from the intercuspal position. Functional parts of the mandible can also be identified by reference to the movement to which they are related.

mandible moves posteriorly from the intercuspal position.

Laterotrusion. Movement occurring when the mandible moves away from the midline (Fig. 8–1). Synonym: working movement.

Laterotrusive side. The side that moves away from the midline in laterotrusion. Synonyms: working side, functional side (see Fig. 8–1).

Mediotrusive side. The side that moves toward the midline in laterotrusion. Synonyms: non-working side, balancing side, non-functional side, idling side (see Fig. 8–1).

Contacts and Movements

Intercuspal Contact

The teeth make contact in a variety of patterns, with fewer contacts than frequently believed. This suggests that generalized tooth contact relationships in natural dentitions are not common.[1] In almost all asymptomatic individuals, simultaneous posterior contacts on the existing posterior teeth are normal during firm ICP closure.

Supracontacts and Occlusal Interferences

Supracontact is a general term for any contact that hinders the remaining occlusal surfaces from achieving a many-pointed, stable contact. A supracontact is a morphologic relationship and is not necessarily correlated with a dysfunctional situation. Moreover, a supracontact in relation to one mandibular contact situation is not necessarily a supracontact in relation to other contact situations.[22] *Occlusal interferences* are supracontacts capable of injuring the supporting periodontal tissues or complicating mandibular movement. Interferences that deflect closure in the retruded position are referred to as *retrusive prematurities*; those that interfere with closure in ICP are called *intercuspal prematurities*.

Occlusal interferences and occlusal disorders tend to destabilize the occlusion. They promote reduced muscle contraction at the involved occlusal position, muscle hyperactivity at the postural position and incoordination in the timing and length of muscle contraction during function.[27, 37] Occlusal interferences may incite muscle activity in an effort to wear away the obstructing tooth surfaces; this activity may possibly develop into bruxing, clamping, or clenching habits.[10, 21, 38] These habits may increase the magnitude and/or modify the direction and frequency of the forces exerted upon the teeth, resulting in traumatic periodontal lesions and loosening of the teeth. They also deflect the pathway of the mandible.[53]

Mandibular Movement

Jaw movement can be classified as border, contact, and intraborder movement (Figs. 8–2 and 8–3).

Border movements are the limits to which the mandible can move in any direction. Posselt[35] developed a rhomboid figure that represents border movement of the mandible (Fig. 8–2).

Contact movement is the movement of the mandible with one or more of the opposing occlusal surfaces in contact (Fig. 8–3).

Intraborder movement is any mandibular movement within the perimeter of border movement. Intraborder movement is chiefly associated with free movement, chewing, and phonation.

Condyle Movements

In opening and closing the jaw, the condyles are capable of rotation, translation, or combinations of the two motions. On full opening, the condyles glide along the posterior slope of the articular eminence to an average of 1 mm anterior to the inferior crest of the eminence.[40] The jaws ordinarily open and close into ICP, rather than into RCP. Opening involves simultaneous rotation and downward translation of the condyle. Movements of the mandible with the teeth in contact, which are termed excursions, may be laterotrusive, protrusive, lateroprotrusive, or retrusive.

Forces of Occlusion

The forces of occlusion are created by the musculature in chewing, swallowing, and speech and are transmitted through the teeth to the periodontium. These forces function in synchronized balance. They guide the alignment of the teeth as they erupt and participate in maintaining the position of the teeth in the arches. Tooth position and arch form are not static; they are maintained by the balance among the various forces of occlusion. Disturbance of this balance may lead to altered tooth positions and changes in the functional environment that may be injurious to the periodontium.

Postural Position of the Mandible and the Free Way Space

When the teeth are not in contact in mastication, swallowing, or speech, the lips are

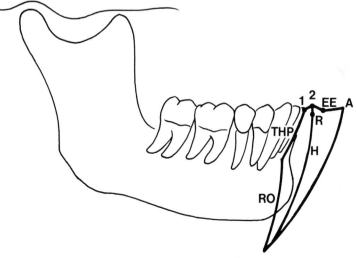

Figure 8–2. Rhomboid figure of mandibular movements in the sagittal plane (Posselt). 1, Retruded contact position. 2, Intercuspal position. THP, Terminal hinge path. EE, Edge-to-edge position. RO, retruded path beyond terminal hinge opening. The condyles undergo both rotation and translation at this point. A, Border movement with maximum protrusion. H, Habitual (functional) pathway of the mandible. R, The rest (postural) position of the mandible. H and R are intraborder.

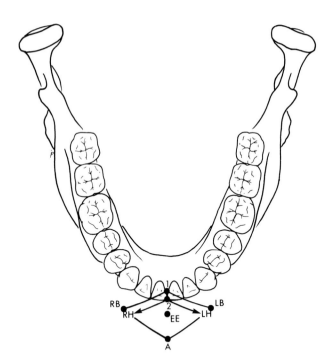

Figure 8–3. Movements of the mandible at the incisal point (infradental). 1, Retruded contact position. 2, Intercuspal position. EE, Edge-to-edge position. A, Contact at maximal protrusion. RH and LH, Right and left habitual movement positions. RB and LB, Right and left border positions. Jaw undergoes maximum lateral movement at RB and LB.

at rest and the jaws are apart. This is termed the *postural position of the mandible*[28] and is also referred to as the "*physiologic rest position.*"[54] In order to maintain the mandible in this position, it is necessary to support it against the force of gravity; the muscles, especially the temporal muscle, are in a mild state of contraction.[26]

The space between the mandibular and maxillary teeth when the mandible is in the postural position is called the *free way space* or the vertical dimension of rest.

Vertical Dimension of Occlusion

The term vertical dimension of occlusion designates the distance between the maxilla and mandible when the teeth are in occlusion. The vertical dimension is maintained by a balance between the rates of occlusal wear and continuous tooth eruption.

Types of Occlusion

Balanced Occlusion

Balanced occlusion refers to simultaneous contact between the right and left posterior segments of the arch in lateral excursion of the mandible and simultaneous contact between the posterior and anterior segments of the arch in protrusive excursion. Although at one time considered to be an ideal type of functional relationship, balanced occlusion is rarely encountered in the natural dentition.[16]

Canine-Protected Occlusion

According to the concept of *canine-protected occlusion,*[8] the maxillary canines act to guide the mandible in lateral and protrusive excursions so that the posterior teeth come into closure with a minimum of horizontal forces (Fig. 8–4A). The mandibular canines and first premolars engage the lingual surfaces of the maxillary canines so as to disclude the incisors, premolars, and molars (Fig. 8–4B). This hypothesis is that the maxillary canines are especially equipped to absorb lateral forces because of the size of the roots, great radicular bone support, and an especially sensitive proprioceptive mechanism which by reflex reduces muscle forces when the canines make occlusal contact. In a recent study, the teeth of persons having canine-protected occlusions had significantly lower mean Periodontal Disease Index scores than those of individuals having progressive disclusion or group function.

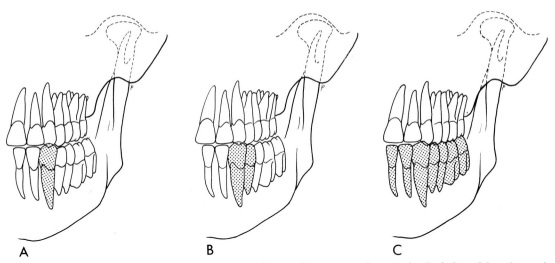

Figure 8–4. Types of occusion. *A,* Canine-protected occlusion. The canine teeth act as the discluders of the other teeth. *B,* Canine-premolar disclusion as found in normal young adults.[33] *C,* Group function.

Group Function

Group function is the simultaneous gliding contact of teeth on the laterotrusive side during laterotrusion (Fig. 8–4C). Group function is physiologically acceptable as a disclusion system.

Malocclusion

Abnormalities in the position of the teeth are not the same as occlusal interferences. In fact, malocclusions often result in an adaptive functional state free of obvious occlusal interferences. These situations are most often caused by loss of teeth; faulty restorations, orthodontics, or occlusal adjustment; or occlusal habits.

Dental Wear and Tear

Attrition is the term used for wear and tear caused by *teeth against teeth* (Fig. 8–5).[51] Physical wearing patterns may occur on incisal, occlusal, and approximal tooth surfaces. A certain amount of tooth wear is physiologic, but intensified or even pathologic wear may prevail with abnormal anatomic or unusual functional factors. *Abrasion* is wear caused by *teeth against foreign substances,* such as wear from hard toothbrushes, coarse toothpowders, or excessive use of toothpicks.[51] It is independent of masticatory function (see Chapter 9).

Excessive attrition may result in obliteration of the cusps and the formation of either a flat or a cupped-out occlusal surface and reversal of the occlusal plane of the premolars

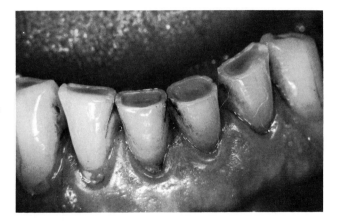

Figure 8–5. Occlusal wear (attrition). Flat, shiny, discolored surfaces produced by occlusal wear.

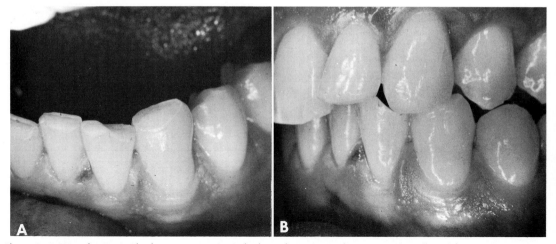

Figure 8–6. Wear facets. *A,* Flat facets worn on incisal edges of anterior teeth. Note notch on lateral incisor also produced by wear. *B,* Maxillary canine fits into notch on lateral incisor produced by parafunctional mandibular movements.

and first and second molars. Occlusal wear increases with age and is characterized by a reduction in cusp height and inclination and by the formation of facets. Tooth surfaces worn by attrition are hard, smooth, and shiny (facets), and if dentin is exposed, a yellowish-brown discoloration is frequently present. Facets generally represent occlusal wear from parafunctional (non-functional) tooth contacts such as bruxism and from premature tooth contacts, but may also be produced through mastication.

Facets vary in size and location, depending upon whether they are produced by physiologic or abnormal wear (Fig. 8–6).[2, 3, 56] They are usually not sensitive to thermal and tactile stimulation.

Erosion and *abrasion* are not related to occlusal trauma and are described on page 129.

Bruxism

Bruxism is clenching or grinding of the teeth when the individual is not chewing or swallowing. *Clenching* is the continuous or intermittent closure of the jaws under vertical pressure. *Tapping* and *toothsetting* involve repetitive mandibular movement or placement at isolated contact locations. Bruxism often occurs without any neurologic disorders or defects and can be viewed as a phenomenon present in healthy individuals, provided some other factors eliciting this behavior are present.

Most people are not aware of a bruxism habit until it is brought to their attention. Bruxing can be very loud, or it can be silent.

Not enough is known to say conclusively whether occlusal factors are a direct cause of bruxism. It has been suggested that occlusal malrelationships or interferences may precipitate bruxism when combined with nervous tension.[48]

In bruxism, the muscles move the mandible over tooth contacts where there is a potential for large forces. Most subjects brux by just "playing" on the teeth, without much forceful contraction. However, under general neuromuscular tension, increased tooth contact pressure will result. Over an extended period, this pressure may exceed the threshold of the periodontal pressor-receptors, and the patient will no longer be aware of increased muscle activity.[22] The muscles involved will be unable to relax, resulting in fatigue, tenderness, and limited opening of the mouth.

Treatment

Bruxism, including clamping and clenching habits, is common, but not all individuals with these habits are injured by them. Injuries that occur are microtrauma to the periodontium, musculature,[5–7, 29] and temporomandibular joints.

There are three general modalities by which the patient with bruxism can be treated. The *behavioral modality* is initiated by the dentist through *explanation* and *arousal* of the patient to awareness of the habit. Specific behavioral therapies such as biofeedback, hypnosis, and negative practice may be prescribed.[41] The *emotional modality* may be initiated in the form of psychologic guidance.[29, 47, 50, 52] The *interceptive modality* consists of prescribing a bite guard appliance (maxillary stabilization splint) to protect the tooth surfaces and to dissipate forces built up in the musculoskeletal system through bruxism.[36]

Occlusal adjustment plays a role in the treatment of bruxism when premature tooth contacts are obvious, especially when they occur in connection with recently placed dental restorations. More invasive occlusal alterations, in the form of reconstruction or orthodontic treatment, are sometimes necessary.

TRAUMA FROM OCCLUSION

The periodontium tries to accommodate to increased functional demands. Adaptive capacity varies among individuals and in the same person at different times. The effects of occlusal forces upon the periodontium are influenced by their magnitude, direction, duration, and frequency.

When the *magnitude of occlusal forces* is increased, the periodontium responds with a thickening of the periodontal ligament, an increase in the number and width of periodontal ligament fibers, and an increase in the density of alveolar bone.

Changing the *direction of occlusal forces* causes a reorientation of the stresses and strains within the periodontium.[15] The principal fibers of the periodontal ligament are arranged so that they can best accommodate occlusal forces in the long axis of the tooth. When *axial forces* are increased, there is distortion of the periodontal ligament, compression of the periodontal fibers, and resorption of bone in the apical areas. The fibers in relation to the remainder of the root are placed under tension, and new bone is formed.[49] Dental restorations and prostheses should be designed to direct occlusal forces axially to take advantage of the greater tolerance of the periodontium to forces in this direction.[20]

Lateral or *horizontal forces* are ordinarily accommodated by bone resorption in areas of pressure and by bone formation in areas of tension. The most advantageous point of application of a lateral force is near the cervical line. As the point of application is moved coronally, the distance from the center of rotation is lengthened and the force upon the periodontal ligament increases.[55]

Torques or *rotational forces* cause both tension and pressure. This force, under physiologic conditions, results in bone formation and bone resorption.[46] Torques are the type of force most likely to injure the periodontium.

The *duration* and *frequency of occlusal forces* affect the response of alveolar bone. Constant pressure on the bone causes resorption, whereas intermittent force favors bone formation. The time lapse between pressure applications apparently influences the bone response. Recurrent forces over short intervals of time have essentially the same resorbing effect as constant pressure.

An inherent "margin of safety" common to all tissues permits some variation in occlusion without adversely affecting the periodontium. However, *when occlusal forces exceed the adaptive capacity of the tissues, tissue injury results.*[12, 17, 30, 31] *The injury is called trauma from occlusion*. The occlusion which produces such injury is called a traumatic occlusion. Excessive occlusal forces may also disrupt the function of the masticatory musculature and cause painful spasms, injure the temporomandibular joints, or produce excessive tooth wear, but the term *trauma from occlusion* refers to injury of the periodontium.

Any occlusion which produces periodontal injury is traumatic. Normal appearing occlusions as well as obvious malocclusions can be associated with trauma from occlusion. The dentition may be anatomically and esthetically acceptable, but functionally injurious. Conversely, not all malocclusions are necessarily injurious to the periodontium.

Acute trauma from occlusion results from an abrupt change in occlusal force such as those produced by restorations or prosthetic appliances which interfere with or alter the direction of occlusal forces on the teeth. The results are tooth pain, sensitivity to percussion, and increased mobility. If the force is dissipated by a shift in the position of the tooth or by wearing away or correction of the restoration, the injury heals and the symptoms subside. Otherwise, periodontal injury may worsen and develop into necrosis, cause periodontal abscess formation, or persist as a symptom-free chronic condition. Acute trauma can also produce cemental tears.

Chronic trauma from occlusion is more common than the acute form and is of greater clinical significance. It most often develops from gradual changes in the occlusion produced by tooth wear, drifting, and extrusion of teeth, combined with parafunctional habits such as bruxism and clenching, rather than as a sequel to acute periodontal trauma.

Causes of Trauma from Occlusion

Trauma from occlusion may be caused by (1) alterations in occlusal forces, (2) reduced capacity of the periodontium to withstand occlusal forces, or (3) a combination of the two. When trauma from occlusion is the result of alterations in the occlusal forces, it is called *primary trauma from occlusion*. When it results from reduced ability of the tissues to resist the occlusal forces, it is known as *secondary trauma from occlusion*.

Primary Trauma From Occlusion

Trauma from occlusion may be considered the primary etiologic factor in periodontal destruction if the only alteration to which a tooth is subjected is occlusal. Examples are periodontal injury produced around teeth with a previously healthy · periodontium caused by: (1) insertion of a "high filling," (2) insertion of a prosthetic replacement that creates excessive forces on abutment and antagonistic teeth, (3) drifting or extrusion of teeth into spaces created by unreplaced missing teeth, and (4) the orthodontic movement of teeth into functionally unacceptable positions. Most of the studies of the effects of trauma from occlusion on experimental animals have been on primary trauma. *These changes do not alter the level of connective tissue attachment and do not initiate pocket formation.*

Secondary Trauma From Occlusion

Trauma from occlusion is considered a secondary cause of periodontal destruction when the adaptive capacity of the tissues to withstand occlusal forces is impaired. The periodontium becomes vulnerable to injury, and previously well-tolerated occlusal forces become traumatic. Bone loss due to marginal inflammation reduces the periodontal attachment area. This increases the burden upon the remaining tissues, because there is less tissue to support the forces and there is altered leverage upon the remaining tissues. *Advanced bone loss is the most common cause of secondary trauma and is very difficult to remedy.*

Stages of Trauma from Occlusion

Trauma from occlusion occurs in three stages.[4, 9] The first is injury, the second is repair, and the third is adaptive remodeling of the periodontium.

Stage I: Injury

The severity, location, and pattern of tissue damage depend on the severity, frequency, and direction of the injurious forces. *Slightly excessive pressure* stimulates resorption of the alveolar bone, with a resultant widening of the periodontal ligament space. *Slightly excessive tension* causes elongation of the periodontal ligament fibers and apposition of alveolar bone. In areas of increased pressure the blood vessels are numerous and reduced in size; in areas of increased tension they are enlarged.[57]

Greater pressure produces a gradation of changes in the periodontal ligament, starting with compression of the fibers, which produces areas of hyalinization.[43, 44] Subsequent injury to the fibroblasts and other connective tissue cells leads to necrosis of areas of the ligament.[42, 45] Vascular changes are also produced.

Severe tension causes widening of the periodontal ligament, thrombosis, hemorrhage, tearing of the periodontal ligament, and resorption of alveolar bone. *Pressure severe enough to force the root against bone causes necrosis of the periodontal ligament and bone.* The bone is resorbed from viable periodontal ligament adjacent to necrotic areas and from marrow spaces, a process called "undermining resorption."[30] The bifurcation and trifurcation areas are the most susceptible to injury from excessive occlusal forces.[14]

Stage II: Repair

Repair is constantly occurring in the normal periodontium. During trauma from occlusion the injured tissues stimulate increased reparative activity. The damaged tissues are removed, and new connective tissue cells and fibers, bone, and cementum are formed in an attempt to restore the injured periodontium. Forces remain traumatic only as long as the damage produced exceeds the reparative capacity of the tissues.

When bone is resorbed by excessive occlusal forces, nature attempts to compensate by forming new bone, termed *buttressing bone formation.* This is an important feature of the reparative process associated with trauma from occlusion.[13] Buttressing bone formation occurs within the jaw (central buttressing) and on the bone surface (peripheral buttressing). In *central buttressing* the endosteal cells deposit new bone, which restores the bony trabeculae and reduces the size of the marrow spaces. *Peripheral buttressing* occurs on the facial and lingual surfaces of the alveolar plate. Depending upon its severity, it may produce a shelf-like thickening of the alveolar margin, referred to as *lipping,* or a pronounced bulge in the contour of the facial and lingual bone.[9, 11]

Stage III: Adaptive Remodeling of the Periodontium

If the repair cannot keep pace with the destruction caused by the occlusion, the periodontium is remodeled in an effort to create a structural relationship in which the forces are no longer injurious to the tissues.

Changes Produced by Trauma from Occlusion

Trauma from occlusion may cause excessive loosening of teeth, widening of the periodontal ligament, and angular (vertical) defects in the alveolar bone without pockets.[9, 23] The most common sign of trauma to the periodontium is *increased tooth mobility.* Tooth mobility produced by trauma occurs in two phases. The *initial phase* is the result of alveolar bone resorption increasing the width of the periodontal ligament and reducing the number of periodontal fibers. The *second phase* occurs after repair of the traumatic lesion and adaptation to the increased forces, which results in permanent widening of the periodontal ligament space (see page 131).

Effects of Insufficient Occlusal Force

Insufficient occlusal force may also be injurious to the supporting periodontal tissues. Insufficient stimulation causes degeneration of the periodontium, manifested by thinning of the periodontal ligament, atrophy of the fibers, osteoporosis of the alveolar bone, and reduction in bone height. Hypofunction may result from open bite relationships, absence of functional antagonists, or unilateral chewing habits.

Influence of Trauma from Occlusion on the Progression of Marginal Periodontitis

Animal studies[19, 24, 25, 32] have shown that trauma from occlusion, in association with marginal periodontitis, *increases the amount of alveolar bone loss and changes the shape of the alveolar crest.* The changes in shape consist of widening of the marginal periodontal ligament space and narrowing of the interproximal alveolar bone.[24, 25] Loss of connective tissue was not a consistent finding. When trauma from occlusion was eliminated, a significant reversibility of bone loss occurred, except in the presence of periodontitis. This indicates that inflammation inhibits the potential for bone regeneration[18, 33, 34] and emphasizes the importance of eliminating the marginal inflammatory component.

Trauma from occlusion does not alter the inflammatory process but changes the tissue

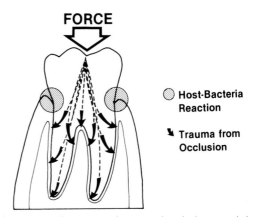

Figure 8–7. The reaction between dental plaque and the host takes place in the gingival sulcus region. **Trauma from occlusion** appears in the supporting tissues of the tooth.

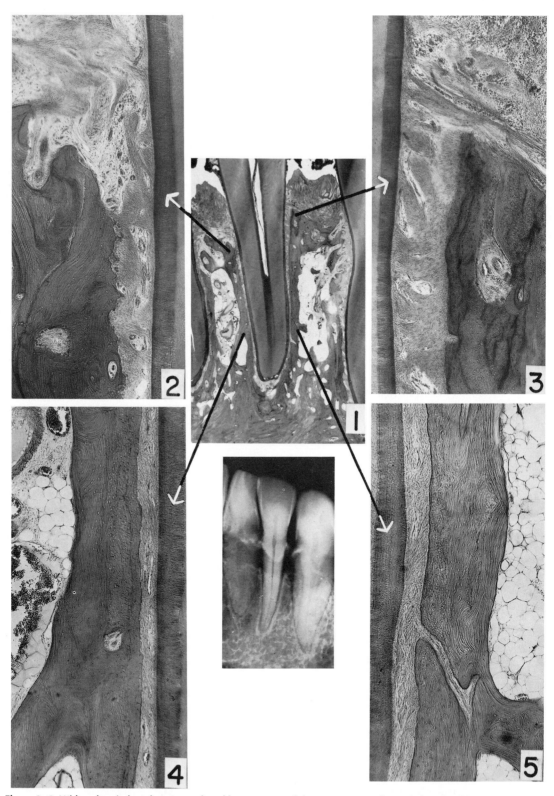

Figure 8–8. Widened periodontal space produced by two types of tissue response to increased occlusal forces. Radiograph shows thickening of periodontal space and lamina dura around the lateral incisor. *1,* Survey microscopic section of lateral incisor. *2,* Mesial surface widening of the periodontal space has resulted from thickening of the periodontal ligament, which is a favorable response to increased tension. *4* and *5,* Thinned periodontal ligament at axis of rotation, one third the distance from the apex.

environment and the architecture of the area around the inflamed sites (Fig. 8–7).[9, 24] In the absence of inflammation the response to trauma from occlusion is adaptive. However, in the presence of inflammation the changes in the shape of the alveolar crest may be conducive to angular bone loss, permitting existing pockets to become infrabony.

Radiographic Signs of Trauma from Occlusion

The radiographic signs of trauma from occlusion include (1) widening of the periodontal space, often with thickening of the lamina dura along the lateral aspect of the root, in the apical region, and in bifurcation areas; (2) "vertical" rather than "horizontal" destruction of the interdental septum, with the formation of infrabony defects; (3) radiolucence and condensation of the alveolar bone; and (4) root resorption (Fig. 8–8).

Widening of the periodontal space and thickening of the lamina dura do not necessarily indicate destructive changes. They may result from thickening and strengthening of the periodontal ligament and alveolar bone, which represent an adaptive response to increased occlusal forces.

References

1. Anderson, J. R., and Myers, G. E.: Natural contacts in centric occlusion in 32 adults. J. Dent. Res., 50:7, 1971.
2. Arstad, T.: The Capsular Ligaments of the Temporomandibular Joint and Retrusion Facets of the Dentition in Relationship to Mandibular Movements. Oslo, Academisk Forlag, 1954.
3. Beyron, H. L.: Occlusal changes in the adult dentition. J. Am. Dent. Assoc., 48:674, 1954.
4. Carranza, F. A., Jr.: Histometric evaluation of periodontal pathology. J. Periodontol., 38:741, 1970.
5. Christensen, L. V.: Facial pain from the masticatory system induced by experimental bruxism. Tandlaegebladet, 71:1171, 1967.
6. Christensen, L. V.: Facial pain from experimental tooth clenching. Tandlaegebladet, 74:175, 1970.
7. Christensen, L. V.: Facial pain in negative and positive work of human jaw muscles. Scand. J. Dent. Res., 84:327, 1976.
8. D'Amico, A.: The canine teeth: normal functional relation of the natural teeth of man. J. South. Cal. Dent. Assoc., 26:6, 49, 127, 175, 194, 239, 1958.
9. Dotto, C. A., Carranza, F. A., Jr., and Itoiz, M. E.: Efectos mediatos del trauma experimental en ratas. Rev. Asoc. Odontol. Argent., 54:48, 1966.
10. Funakoshi, M., Fujita, N., and Takehama, S.: Relations between occlusal interference and jaw muscle activities in responses to changes in head position. J. Dent. Res., 55:684, 1976.
11. Glickman, I., and Smulow, J. B.: Buttressing bone formation in the periodontium. J. Periodontol., 36:365, 1965.
12. Glickman, I., and Smulow, J. B.: Effect of excessive occlusal forces upon the pathway of gingival inflammation in humans. J. Periodontol., 36:141, 1965.
13. Glickman, I., and Smulow, J. B.: Adaptive alterations in the periodontium of the Rhesus monkey in chronic trauma from occlusion. J. Periodontol., 39:101, 1968.
14. Glickman, I., Stein, R. S., and Smulow, J. B.: The effects of increased functional forces upon the periodontium of splinted and nonsplinted teeth. J. Periodontol., 32:290, 1961.
15. Glickman, I., Roeber, F., Brion, M., and Pameijer, J.: Photoelastic analysis of internal stresses in the periodontium created by occlusal forces. J. Periodontol., 41:30, 1970.
16. Ingervall, B.: Tooth contacts on the functional and nonfunctional side in children and young adults. Arch. Oral Biol., 17:191, 1972.
17. Itoiz, M. E., Carranza, F. A., Jr., and Cabrini, R. L.: Histologic and histometric study of experimental occlusal trauma in rats. J. Periodontol., 34:305, 1963.
18. Kantor, M., Polson, A. N., and Zander, H. A.: Alveolar bone regeneration after removal of inflammatory and traumatic factors. J. Periodontol., 46:687, 1976.
19. Kaufman, H., Carranza, F. A., Jr., Endres, B., Newman, M. G., and Murphy, N. C.: The influence of trauma from occlusion on the bacterial repopulation of periodontal pockets in dogs. J. Periodontol., 55:86, 1984.
20. Kemper, W. W., Johnson, J. F., and Van Huysen, G.: Periodontal tissue changes in response to high artificial crowns. J. Prosthet. Dent., 20:160, 1968.
21. Kloprogge, M. J., and van Griethuysen, A. M.: Disturbances in contraction and coordination pattern of the masticatory muscles due to dental restoration. J. Oral Rehabil., 3:207, 1976.
22. Krogh-Poulsen, W. G., and Olsson, A.: Management of the occlusion of the teeth. In Schwarz, L., and Chayes, C. (eds.): Facial Pain and Mandibular Dysfunction. Philadelphia, W. B. Saunders Company, 1968.
23. Lindhe, J., and Ericsson, I.: The influence of trauma from occlusion on reduced but healthy periodontal tissues in dogs. J. Clin. Periodontol., 3:110, 1976.
24. Lindhe, J., and Svanberg, G.: Influence of trauma from occlusion on progression of experimental periodontitis in the beagle dog. J. Clin. Periodontol., 1:3, 1974.
25. Meitner, S.: Codestructive factors of marginal periodontitis and repetitive mechanical injury. J. Dent. Res., 54:C78, 1975.
26. Moller, E.: Evidence that the rest position is subject to servocontrol. In Anderson, D. J., and Mathew, B. (eds.): Mastication. Bristol, John Wright and Sons, 1976, pp. 72–80.
27. Moller, E.: The myogenic factor in headache and facial pain. In Kawamura, Y., and Dubner, R. (eds.): Oral-facial Sensory and Motor Functions. Tokyo, Quintessence, 1982, p. 225.

28. Moyers, R. E.: Some physiologic considerations of centric and other jaw relations. J. Prosthet. Dent., 6:183, 1956.

29. Nadler, S.: The importance of bruxism. J. Oral Med., 23:142, 1968.

30. Orban, B.: Tissue changes in traumatic occlusion. J. Am. Dent. Assoc., 15:2090, 1928.

31. Orban, B., and Weinmann, J.: Signs of traumatic occlusion in average human jaws. J. Dent. Res., 13:216, 1933.

32. Polson, A. M.: Trauma and progression of marginal periodontitis in squirrel monkeys. II. Codestructive factors of periodontitis and mechanically produced injury. J. Periodont. Res., 9:108, 1974.

33. Polson, A. M., Meitner, S. W., and Zander, H. A.: Trauma and progression of marginal periodontitis in squirrel monkeys. III. Adaption of interproximal alveolar bone to repetitive injury. J. Periodont. Res. 11:279, 1976.

34. Polson, A. M., Meitner, S. W., and Zander, H. A.: Trauma and progression of marginal periodontitis in squirrel monkeys. IV. Reversibility of bone loss due to trauma alone and trauma superimposed upon periodontitis. J. Periodont. Res., 11:290, 1976.

35. Posselt, V.: Studies in the mobility of the human mandible. Acta Odontol. Scand., 10(Suppl. 10):1, 1952.

36. Posselt, V., and Wolff, I. B.: Treatment of bruxism by bite guards and bite plates. J. Can. Dent. Assoc., 29:773, 1963.

37. Pruzansky, S.: Applicability of electromyographic procedures as a clinical aid in the detection of occlusal disharmony. Dent. Clin. North Am., 4:117, 1960.

38. Ramfjord, S. P.: Bruxism, a clinical and electromyographic study. J. Am. Dent. Assoc., 62:21, 1961.

39. Ramfjord, S. P., Kerr, D. A., and Ash, M. M.: World Workshop in Periodontics. Ann Arbor, University of Michigan Press, 1966.

40. Ricketts, R. M.: Variations of the temporomandibular joint as revealed by cephalometric laminagraphy. Am. J. Orthod., 36:877, 1950.

41. Rugh, J. D., and Solberg, W. K.: Electromyographic evaluation of bruxist behavior before and after treatment. Can. Dent. Assoc. J., 3:56, 1975.

42. Rygh, P.: Ultrastructural cellular reactions in pressure zones of rat molar periodontium incident to orthodontic movement. Acta Odontol. Scand., 30:575, 1972.

43. Rygh, P.: Ultrastructural changes in pressure zones of human periodontium incident to orthodontic tooth movement. Acta Odontol. Scand., 31:109, 1973.

44. Rygh, P.: Ultrastructural changes of the periodontal fibers and their attachment in rat molar periodontium incident to orthodontic tooth movement. Scand. J. Dent. Res., 81:467, 1973.

45. Rygh, P.: Elimination of hyalinized periodontal tissues associated with orthodontic tooth movement. Scand. J. Dent. Res., 82:57, 1974.

46. Rygh, P., and Selvig, K. A.: Erythrocytic crystallization in rat molar periodontium incident to tooth movement. Scand. J. Dent. Res., 81:62, 1973.

47. Sadowski, C., and BeGole, E. A.: Long-term effects of orthodontic treatment on periodontal health. Am. J. Orthod., 80(2):156, 1981.

48. Scharer, P.: Bruxism. Front. Oral Physiol., 1:293, 1974.

49. Schwarz, A. M.: Movement of teeth under traumatic stress. Dental Items Intern., 52:96, 1930.

50. Shapiro, S., and Shannon, J.: Bruxism—as an emotional reactive disturbance. Psychosomatics, 6:427, 1965.

51. Sognnaes, R.: Periodontal significance of intraoral frictional ablation. J. Western Soc. Periodontol., 25:112, 1977.

52. Thaller, J. L., Rosen, G., and Saltzman, S.: Study of the relationship of frustration and anxiety to bruxism. J. Periodontol., 38:193, 1967.

53. Thielemann, L. K.: Biomechanik der Paradentose ins besondere Artikulationsausgleich durch Einschleifen. 2nd ed. Munchen, Barth, 1956.

54. Thompson, J. R.: The rest position of the mandible and its significance to dental science. J. Am. Dent. Assoc., 33:151, 1946.

55. Thurow, R. C.: The periodontal membrane in function. Angle Orthod., 15:8, 1945.

56. Weinberg, L. A.: Diagnosis of facets in occlusal equilibration. J. Am. Dent. Assoc., 52:26, 1956.

57. Zaki, A. E., and Van Huysen, G.: Histology of the periodontium following tooth movement. J. Dent. Res., 42:1373, 1956.

Chapter 9

Clinical Examination

Although the dental hygienist is not responsible for diagnosing the periodontal status of patients, critical examination and judgment of changes occurring in the periodontium is required. This chapter presents a recommended sequence of procedures for examination of patients to be used at initial visits or at recall visits. It includes the health history, dental history, oral examination, dental examination, and periodontal and radiographic evaluation of patients.

HEALTH HISTORY

The health history is obtained at the first visit and reviewed at subsequent visits. The importance of the health history should be explained to all patients because they often omit information that they do not relate to their dental problems. This history aids the clinician in (1) *the evaluation of oral manifestations of systemic disease*, (2) *the detection of systemic conditions that may be affecting the periodontal tissue response*, and (3) *the detection of systemic conditions that require special precautions and modifications in treatment procedures.* Adequate information is imperative for the correct diagnosis and treatment plan by the dentist, and in order to provide safe, appropriate care for each individual.

For specific questions to be asked, the reader is referred to any one of several adequate health history forms available on the market. Also, the American Dental Associa-

127

tion has carefully devised both a short and a long form addressing pertinent diseases and conditions.

DENTAL HISTORY

Questions should be asked about each of the patient's chief complaints. Frequently, individuals with gingival or periodontal disease will describe "bleeding gums," "loose teeth," "spreading of the teeth with the appearance of spaces where none existed before," "foul taste in the mouth," or "itchy feeling in the gums, relieved by digging with a toothpick." There may also be pain of varied types and duration, such as "constant dull gnawing pain," "dull pain after eating," "deep radiating pains in the jaws," "acute throbbing pain," "sensitivity to percussion," "sensitivity to heat and cold," "burning sensation in the gums," and "extreme sensitivity to inhaled air." This information helps the clinician to address the individual's perceived problem, thus aiding in reassurance and motivation of the patient. Also, the existence of emergency problems can be evaluated and the patient referred for appropriate treatment.

ORAL EXAMINATION

Intraoral and Extraoral Examination

The entire oral cavity should be carefully examined. The examination should include the lips, floor of the mouth, tongue, palate, oropharyngeal region, the quality and quantity of saliva, and the cervical lymph nodes. Although these findings may not be related to the periodontal problem, it is the clinician's responsibility to detect any pathology present in the mouth. Textbooks on oral medicine and oral diagnosis cover this topic in detail.

Oral Hygiene

The "cleanliness" of the oral cavity is appraised in terms of the extent of accumulated food debris, plaque, materia alba, and tooth surface stains. Disclosing solution should be used routinely to detect plaque that would otherwise be unnoticed.

Mouth Odors

Halitosis, also called "fetor ex ore" or "fetor oris," is foul or offensive odor emanating from the oral cavity. Mouth odors may be of diagnostic significance, and their origin may be either (1) local or (2) remote (extraoral).

Local Sources. Local sources of mouth odors include the retention of odoriferous food particles on and between the teeth, coated tongue, acute necrotizing ulcerative gingivitis, dehydration states, caries, dentures, tobacco smoke, and healing wounds. The fetid odor characteristic of acute necrotizing ulcerative gingivitis is easily identified. Chronic periodontal disease with pocket formation may also cause unpleasant mouth odor from accumulated debris and the increased rate of putrefaction of the saliva.

Extraoral or Remote Sources. These may include adjacent structures involved with rhinitis, sinusitis, tonsillitis, or diseases of the lungs and bronchi. Odors are also emanated through the lungs from aromatic substances in the blood stream, such as alcohol, acetone in diabetics, and the uremic breath that accompanies kidney dysfunction.

DENTAL EXAMINATION

The teeth are examined for caries, developmental defects, anomalies of tooth form, wasting, hypersensitivity, and proximal contact relationships.

Wasting Disease of the Teeth

Wasting is defined as any gradual loss of tooth substance characterized by the formation of smooth, polished surfaces, without regard to the possible mechanism of this loss.

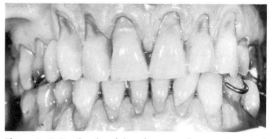

Figure 9–1. Erosion involving the enamel, cementum, and dentin.

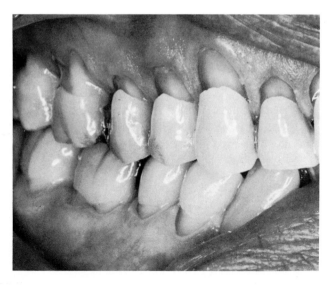

Figure 9–2. Abrasion attributed to aggressive toothbrushing. Involvement of the roots is followed by undermining of the enamel.

The forms of wasting are erosion, abrasion, and attrition.

Erosion is a sharply defined wedge-shaped depression in the cervical area of the facial tooth surface (Fig. 9–1). The long axis of the eroded area is perpendicular to the vertical axis of the tooth. The surfaces are smooth, hard, and polished. Erosion generally affects groups of teeth. In the early stages, it may be confined to the enamel, but it generally extends to involve the underlying dentin, as well as the cementum and dentin of the root. The etiology of erosion is not known. Decalcification by acid beverages or citrus fruits[18] and the combined effect of acid salivary secretion and friction[20] are suggested causes.

Abrasion refers to the loss of tooth substance induced by mechanical wear other than that of mastication (Fig. 9–2). Abrasion results in saucer-shaped or wedge-shaped indentations with a smooth, shiny surface. Abrasion starts on exposed cementum surfaces rather than on the enamel and extends to involve the dentin of the root. Continued exposure to the abrasive agent, combined with decalcification of the enamel by locally formed acids, may result in a loss of the enamel, followed by loss of the dentin of the crown.

Toothbrushing with abrasive dentifrice or hard toothbrushes and the action of partial denture clasps are common causes of abrasion. The first is by far the more prevalent. The degree of tooth wear from toothbrushing depends upon the abrasive effect of the dentifrice and the angle of brushing.[17] Horizontal brushing at right angles to the vertical axis of the teeth results in the severest loss of tooth substance. Occasionally abrasion of the incisal edges occurs as a result of habits such as holding bobby pins or tacks between the teeth.

Attrition is the occlusal wear due to functional contacts with opposing teeth. It is described on page 119.

Dental Stains

Pigmented deposits on the tooth surface are called *stains*. They are primarily esthetic problems resulting from the pigmentation of ordinarily colorless developmental and acquired dental coatings by chromogenic bacteria, foods, and chemicals. They vary in color and composition and in the firmness with which they adhere to the tooth surface.

Brown Stain

Brown stain is a thin, translucent, acquired, usually bacteria-free, pigmented pellicle. It occurs in individuals who do not brush sufficiently or who use a dentifrice with inadequate cleansing action. It is found most commonly on the buccal surface of the maxillary molars and on the lingual surface of the mandibular incisors. The brown color is usually due to the presence of tannin from coffee or tea.

dark Br / Black

Tobacco Stain — *Pits, fissures, enamel dentin*

Tobacco produces tenacious dark brown or black surface deposits and brown discoloration of tooth substance. Staining results from coal tar combustion products and from penetration of pits and fissures, enamel, and dentin by tobacco juices. Staining is not necessarily proportional to the amount of tobacco consumed, but depends to a considerable degree upon preexistent acquired coatings that attach the tobacco products to the tooth surface.

Chromogenic Bacteria —

Black Stain *Gram + Actinomyces*
firmly attached — recur after rem.

Typical Picture

Black stain usually occurs as thin black lines on the facial and lingual surfaces of the teeth near the gingival margin and as diffuse patches on proximal surfaces. It is firmly attached, tends to recur after removal, is more common in women, and may occur in mouths with excellent hygiene. The black stain that occurs on human primary teeth is typically associated with a low incidence of caries in affected children.[31, 33] Chromogenic bacteria have been implicated. The microflora of black stain is dominated by gram-positive rods, primarily *Actinomyces* species, and evidence implicates these bacteria as a probable cause. Isolated *Actinomyces* species can produce black pigmentation, and other in vitro investigations have demonstrated black pigment formation caused by *Actinomyces* in the dentin.[31] The chromogenic bacterium *Bacteroides melaninogenicus* accounts for less than 1 per cent of isolated bacteria and is not considered an important cause of black stain.[31]

Yellowish green — Children

Green Stain *enamel cuticle*

This is a green or greenish-yellow stain, sometimes of considerable thickness, which is common in children. It is considered to be the stained remnants of the enamel cuticle, but this has not been substantiated.[2] The discoloration has been attributed to fluorescent bacteria and fungi such as *Penicillium* and *Aspergillus*.[3] Green stain usually occurs on the gingival half of the facial surfaces of maxillary anterior teeth, and usually appears more often in boys (65 per cent) than in girls (43 per cent).[11]

gingival 1/2 F Max ant

Boys —

Bacteria / Fungi — Penicillin aspergillus

Orange Stain

Orange stain is less common than green or brown stain. It may occur on both the facial and lingual surfaces of anterior teeth. *Serratia marcescens* and *Flavobacterium lutescens* have been suggested as the responsible chromogenic organisms.[4]

M/B Permanent   Copper — green   Iron Me

Metallic Stains *Iron — Brown (Black*

Metals and metallic salts may be introduced into the oral cavity in dust inhaled by industrial workers or through orally administered drugs. The metals combine with acquired dental coatings (usually pellicle), producing a surface stain, or they penetrate the tooth substance and cause permanent discoloration. Copper dust produces a green stain and iron dust a brown stain. Medicines containing iron cause a black iron sulfite deposit. Other occasionally occurring metallic stains are manganese (black), mercury (greenish black), nickel (green), and silver (black).

Tissue   Yellowish Brown to Brownish

Chlorhexidine Stain

Chlorhexidine was introduced as a general disinfectant with a broad antibacterial action against gram-positive and gram-negative bacteria and yeasts.[8, 15] In countries where its use is permitted, it is commonly used in mouthwashes and toothpastes to control plaque accumulation. The continued use of chlorhexidine solution promotes discoloration in the mouth.[8, 15, 21] Chlorhexidine is retained in the human oral cavity[8] because of its affinity for sulfate and acidic groups such as those found in plaque constituents, carious lesions, pellicle, and bacterial cell walls.[8, 10, 21] The retention of chlorhexidine is concentration- and time-dependent. It is not influenced by the temperature or pH of the rinsing solution.

Chlorhexidine stain imparts a yellowish-brown to brownish color to the tissues of the oral cavity.[8] The staining appears in the cervical and interproximal regions of the teeth, on restorations, in plaque, and on the surface of the tongue.[8, 15, 21] It appears that the presence of aldehydes and ketones, which are normally intermediates of both mammalian and microbial metabolism, are essential for formation of discoloration by chlorhexidine.[21]

Cervical / Interprox — teeth
restorations, plaque
tongue & tissues

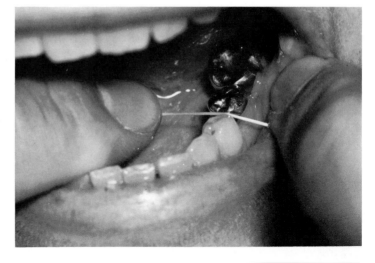

Figure 9–3. Tightness of contact points checked with dental floss.

No permanent staining of the enamel or dentin is observed clinically, since tooth-brushing with a dentifrice or professional prophylaxis can remove the accumulated stain.[21] Similar staining occurs with the use of alexidine.

Dentinal Sensitivity

Root surfaces exposed by gingival recession may be sensitive to thermal changes or tactile stimulation. Patients often point out the sensitive areas; others may be located by gentle exploration with a probe or cold air.

Proximal Contact Relations

Slightly open contacts permit food impaction. The tightness of contacts should be checked by clinical observation, radiographic observation, and with dental floss (Fig. 9–3).

Tooth Mobility

All teeth have a slight degree of physiologic mobility, which varies in different teeth (highest in the central and lateral incisors) and at different times of the day.[22] It is highest upon arising in the morning and progressively decreases. The increased mobility in the morning is attributed to slight extrusion of the teeth because of limited occlusal contact during sleep. During the waking hours mobility is reduced by chewing and swallowing forces, which intrude the teeth in the sockets. Tooth mobility that occurs beyond the physiologic range is termed pathologic or abnormal mobility.

As a general rule, mobility is graded clinically by a simple method. The tooth is held firmly between the handles of two metal instruments or with one metal instrument and one finger, and effort is made to move it in all directions (Fig. 9–4). Abnormal mobility most often occurs in the faciolingual direction. Mobility is graded according to the

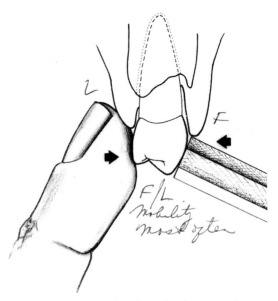

Figure 9–4. Tooth mobility checked with one metal instrument and one finger.

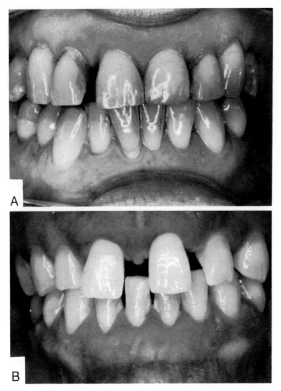

Figure 9–5. Stages in pathologic migration. *A,* Migration of right maxillary lateral incisor. *B,* Migration and extrusion of maxillary and mandibular incisors.

ease and extent of tooth movement, according to simple criteria:

Physiologic mobility, Grade 0.

Pathologic mobility, Grade 1—slightly more than physiologic.

Pathologic mobility, Grade 2—moderately more than physiologic.

Pathologic mobility, Grade 3—severe mobility faciolingually and/or mesiodistally combined with vertical displacement.

Causes of Pathologic Mobility

Mobility is pathologic in the sense that it exceeds the limits of normal mobility values, rather than that the periodontium is necessarily diseased at the time of examination. Pathologic mobility is caused by one or more of several factors:

1. *Loss of tooth support (bone loss).* The amount of mobility depends upon the severity and distribution of the bone loss on individual root surfaces, the length and shape of the roots, and the root size compared to the crown.

2. *Trauma from occlusion.* Injury produced by excessive occlusal forces or incurred because of abnormal occlusal habits such as bruxing and clenching is a common cause of tooth mobility (see Chapter 8).

3. *The extension of inflammation from the gingiva into the periodontal ligament results in degenerative changes that increase mobility.* The changes usually occur in periodontal disease that has advanced beyond the early stages, but tooth mobility is sometimes observed in severe gingivitis. The spread of inflammation from an acute periapical abscess produces a temporary increase in tooth mobility in the absence of periodontal disease. *Mobility is also temporarily increased for a short period after periodontal surgery.*

4. *Tooth mobility is increased in pregnancy and is sometimes associated with the menstrual cycle or the use of hormonal contraceptives.* It occurs in patients with or without periodontal disease, presumably because of physicochemical changes in the periodontal tissues.

Mobility can also result from jaw processes that destroy the alveolar bone and/or the roots of the teeth. Osteomyelitis and tumors of the jaws are examples.

Pathologic Migration of Teeth

Pathologic migration (Fig. 9–5) refers to tooth displacement that results when the balance among the factors which maintain physiologic tooth position is disturbed by periodontal disease. Pathologic migration is relatively common and may be an early sign of disease, or it may occur in association with gingival inflammation and pocket formation as the disease progresses.

Pathologic migration occurs most frequently in the anterior region, but posterior teeth may also be affected. The teeth may move in any direction, and the migration is usually accompanied by mobility and rotation. Pathologic migration in the occlusal or incisal direction is termed extrusion or elongation. All degrees of pathologic migration are encountered, and one or more teeth may be affected.

Causes of Pathologic Migration

1. Weakened periodontal support renders the teeth unable to maintain normal positions in the arch and they will move

away from occlusal forces, unless restrained by proximal contact. The abnormality in pathologic migration rests with the weakened periodontium. The force itself need not be abnormal.

2. Changes in magnitude, direction, or frequency of the forces exerted upon the teeth can induce pathologic migration of one or more teeth. These forces need not be abnormal if the periodontium is sufficiently weakened. Changes in the forces may occur for the following reasons:

    a. *Unreplaced missing teeth* allow drifting of teeth into the spaces created. Drifting does not result from destruction of the periodontal tissues, however, it usually creates conditions that lead to periodontal disease. Drifting generally occurs in a mesial direction, combined with tilting or extrusion beyond the occlusal plane. The premolars often drift distally. Although drifting is a common sequel when missing teeth are not replaced, it does not always occur.

    b. *Failure to replace first molars* causes a pattern resulting in many changes. The second and third molars tilt, the premolars move distally, and the mandibular incisors tilt or drift lingually. The mandibular premolars, while drifting distally, lose their intercuspating relationship with the maxillary teeth and may tilt distally. Anterior overbite is increased, the mandibular incisors strike the maxillary incisors near the gingiva and may traumatize it. The maxillary incisors are pushed labially and laterally and the anterior teeth extrude because the incisal apposition has largely disappeared. Diastemata are often created by the separation of the anterior teeth.

    The disturbed proximal contact relationships lead to food impaction, gingival inflammation, and pocket formation, followed by bone loss and tooth mobility. Occlusal disharmonies created by the altered tooth positions traumatize the supporting tissues of the periodontium and aggravate the destruction caused by the inflammation. Reduction in periodontal support leads to further migration of the teeth and mutilation of the occlusion.

3. Trauma from occlusion may cause a shift in tooth position either by itself or in combination with inflammatory periodontal disease. The direction of movement depends upon the occlusal force.

4. Pressure from the tongue may cause drifting of the teeth in the absence of periodontal disease or contribute to pathologic migration of teeth with reduced periodontal support.

PERIODONTAL EXAMINATION

It is important to look for the earliest signs of gingival and periodontal disease. The examination should be systematic, starting in the molar area in either the maxilla or the mandible and proceeding around the arch. This will avoid overemphasis on spectacular findings at the expense of other conditions which, though less striking, may be very important.

Plaque and Calculus

There are many methods of assessing plaque and calculus accumulation.[7] For the detection of *subgingival calculus* each tooth surface is carefully checked to the level of the gingival attachment with a sharp explorer (Fig. 9–6). Gentle blasts of air may be used to deflect the gingiva and aid in visualization of the calculus. The presence of supragingival calculus can be directly observed, and the amount easily estimated. Radiographs reveal heavy calculus deposits interproximally (Fig. 9–7) and sometimes on the facial and lingual surfaces of teeth, but *cannot be relied upon for the thorough detection of calculus.*

Gingiva

Observations of gingiva should be made after slight air drying because light reflection from moisture obscures detail. Visual examination, exploration with instruments, and firm but gentle palpation should be used for detecting pathologic alterations in normal resilience, as well as locating areas of pus formation.

Each of the following features of the gingiva should be considered: *color, size, contour,*

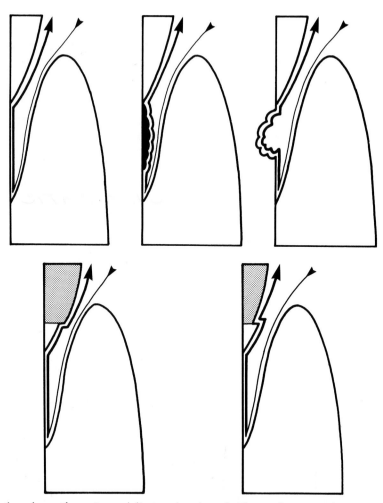

Figure 9–6. Detection of smoothness *(upper left)* **or various irregularities on the root surface** with outward motion of probe or explorer. *Upper center,* Calculus. *Upper right,* Caries. *Lower left and right,* Irregular margins of restorations.

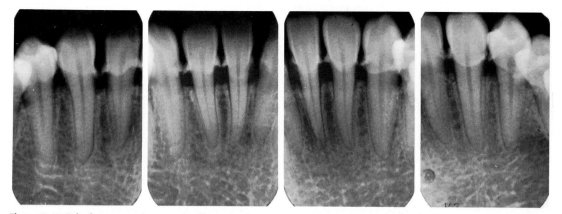

Figure 9–7. Calculus appears interproximally as angular spurs. The radiopaque image of calculus on the facial and lingual surface is superimposed on teeth.

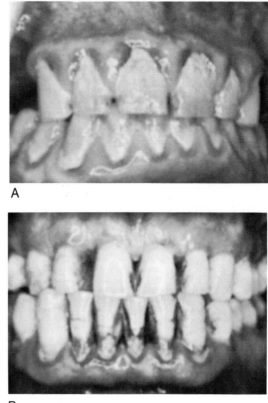

Figure 9–8. Types of gingival inflammation. *A,* **Edematous type.** Note loss of stippling, increase in size, abundant plaque and materia alba, and change in color. *B,* **Fibrotic type.** Note the abundant calculus and the gingival recession. The patient has pockets of moderate to severe depth in the mandibular anterior teeth and shallower pockets in the maxillary teeth.

consistency, surface texture, position, ease of bleeding, and *pain* (see Chapter 2). No deviation from the normal should be overlooked. The distribution of gingival disease and its acuteness or chronicity should also be noted.

Gingival inflammation can produce two basic types of tissue response: *edematous* and *fibrotic* (Fig. 9–8). Edematous tissue is characterized by a smooth, glossy, soft gingiva. Fibrotic gingiva has some normal characteristics; the gingiva is firm, stippled, and opaque, but is usually thicker than normal gingiva and the margin appears rounded.

The position of the gingiva warrants special mention. For accurate appraisal of recession, attention should be given to difference between the *apparent position* and the *actual position* of the gingival attachment on each tooth surface (see Chapter 2).

Periodontal Pockets

Examination of periodontal pockets should include the presence and distribution on each tooth surface, probing depth, and levels of epithelial attachment on the roots.

The only accurate method of detecting and evaluating periodontal pockets is careful exploration with a periodontal probe. Pockets are not reliably detected or measured by radiographic examination. Periodontal pockets are soft tissue changes. Radiographs indicate areas of bone loss where pockets may occur but do not show whether pockets are present and do not reveal pocket depth.

Pocket Probing

There are two different pocket depths: the biologic or histologic depth, and the clinical or probing depth[12] (Fig. 9–9) (see Chapter 1).

The *biologic* or *histologic depth* is the distance between the gingival margin and the bottom of the pocket (the coronal end of the junctional epithelium). This can be measured only in carefully prepared histologic sections.

The *clinical* or *probing depth* is the distance to which a periodontal probe penetrates into the pocket. The depth of penetration depends on factors such as the size of the probe, the force with which it is introduced, the direction of penetration, the resistance of the tissues, and the convexity of the crown.

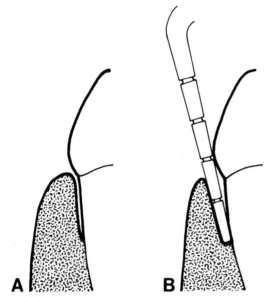

Figure 9–9. A, **Biologic pocket depth.** B, **Probing or clinical pocket depth.**

Several studies have evaluated the depth of penetration of a probe in a sulcus or pocket. Armitage et al.[1] evaluated the penetration of a probe in beagle dogs, using a standardized force of 25 ponds. (One pond

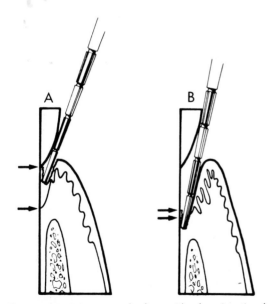

Figure 9–10. A, In a **normal sulcus,** with a long junctional epithelium (between arrows), probe penetrates about one third to one half the length of the junctional epithelium. B, In a **periodontal pocket,** with a short junctional epithelium (between arrows), the probe penetrates beyond the apical end of the junctional epithelium.

is equal to 1 gram of absolute force.) They reported that in healthy specimens the probe penetrated the epithelium to about two thirds of its length, in gingivitis specimens it stopped 0.1 mm short of the apical end of the epithelial attachment, and in periodontitis specimens the probe tip consistently went past the most apical cells of the junctional epithelium (Fig. 9–10).

The depth of penetration of the probe in the connective tissue apical to the junctional epithelium in periodontal pockets is about 0.3 mm.[14, 32] This is important in evaluating differences in probing depth before and after treatment, as the decreased penetrability of the tissues may play a significant role in probing depth changes.[12, 16]

Probing Technique. The probe should be inserted in line with the vertical axis of the tooth and "walked" circumferentially around each surface of each tooth to detect the areas of deepest probe penetration (Fig. 9–11). In addition, special attention should be directed to detecting the presence of interdental craters and furcation involvements. To detect an *interdental crater* the probe should be placed obliquely from both the facial and lingual surfaces so as to explore the deepest portion of the pocket located beneath the contact point (Fig. 9–12). Definitive evaluation of possible *furcation involvements* is made by clinical examination with specially de-

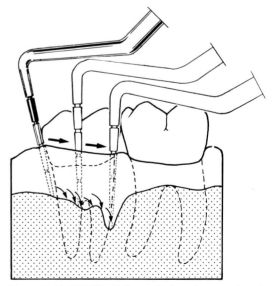

Figure 9–11. "Walking" the probe in order to explore the pocket in all its extent.

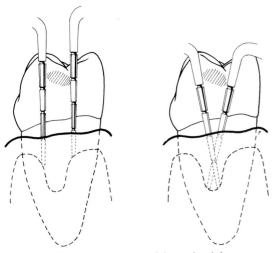

Figure 9–12. Vertical insertion of the probe *(left)* may not detect **interdental craters;** oblique positioning of the probe *(right)* reaches the depth of the crater.

signed probes (Fig. 9–13). Instruments like the Nabers probe may reveal lesions undetected with regular probes.

Level of Attachment Versus Probing Depth. *The level of attachment of the epithelium at the base of the pocket to the tooth surface is of greater diagnostic significance than the probing depth of the pocket.* Probing depth is simply the distance between the base of the pocket and the gingival margin. It can vary in untreated periodontal disease from causes like mechanical irritation, which can result in shrinkage of the pocket wall and some reduction in pocket depth. The level of attachment of the base of the pocket on the tooth

surface affords a better indication of the severity of periodontal disease. *Shallow pockets attached at the level of the apical third of the roots connote more severe destruction than deep pockets attached in the coronal third of the roots* (see Chapter 10).

The level of attachment of the base of a periodontal pocket may vary on different surfaces of the same tooth and even in different areas of the same surface. Inserting the probe on all surfaces and in more than one area on individual surfaces reveals the depth and conformation of the pocket. The level of attachment is determined in a gingival pocket by subtracting from the total depth the distance from the gingival margin to the cemento-enamel junction (Figs. 9–14 and 9–15). When the gingival margin coincides with the cemento-enamel junction, the level of attachment and the pocket depth are equal; when the gingival margin is located apical to the cemento-enamel junction, the loss of attachment will be greater than the pocket depth. Drawing the gingival margin on the chart and denoting probing depths will clarify the evaluation of attachment loss.

Suppuration. To determine whether purulent exudate (pus) is present in a periodontal pocket, the ball of the index finger is applied along the lateral aspect of the marginal gingiva and pressure is applied in a rolling motion toward the crown (Fig. 9–16). The pus is formed on the inner pocket wall leaving the external appearance of the pocket unchanged so that visual examination without digital pressure is not adequate. Pus

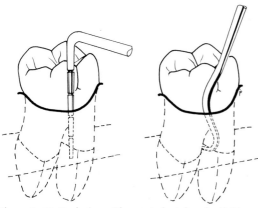

Figure 9–13. Exploring with a periodontal probe *(left)* **may not detect furcation involvement.** Specially designed instruments (Nabers probe) *(right)* can enter the furcation area.

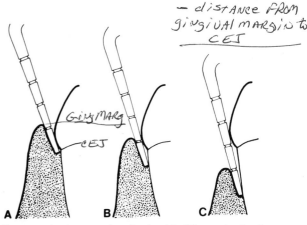

TOTAL DEPTH — distance from gingival margin to CEJ

Ging Marg
CEJ

A   B   C

Figure 9–14. Same pocket depth with different levels of attachment.

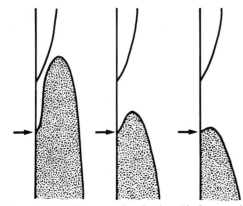

Figure 9–15. Different pocket depths with the same level of attachment. Bottom of pocket is indicated by *arrow*.

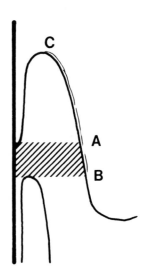

Figure 9–17. The shaded area shows the **attached gingiva**, which extends between the projection on the external surface of the bottom of the pocket (A) and the mucogingival junction (B). The keratinized gingiva may extend from the mucogingival junction (B) to the gingival margin (C).

formation does not occur in all periodontal pockets, but it is often found in pockets where it is not suspected.

Amount of Attached Gingiva. The width of the attached gingiva is the distance between the mucogingival junction and the projection on the external surface of the bottom of the gingival sulcus or the periodontal pocket. It should not be confused with the width of the keratinized gingiva, since this includes the marginal gingiva (Fig. 9–17).

The width of the attached gingiva is determined by subtracting the sulcus or pocket depth from the total width of the keratinized gingiva (from the

gingival margin to the mucogingival junction). This is done by stretching the lip or cheek in order to demarcate the mucogingival line while the pocket is probed (Fig. 9–18). It is generally considered that the amount of attached gingiva is insufficient when stretching the lip or cheek induces movement of the free gingival margin.

Alveolar Bone Loss. Alveolar bone levels are evaluated by clinical and radiographic examination. Probing is helpful for determining the height and contour of the facial and lingual bone obscured on the radiograph by the dense roots and for determining the architecture of the interdental bone.

TRAUMA FROM OCCLUSION

Trauma from occlusion refers to *tissue injury* produced by occlusal forces—not to the occlusal forces themselves. Trauma from occlusion is suspected because of the condition of the periodontal tissues.

Periodontal findings that suggest the presence of trauma from occlusion are the following: excessive tooth mobility, particularly in teeth showing radiographic evidence of a widened periodontal space; vertical or angular bone destruction; infrabony pockets; and pathologic migration, especially of the anterior teeth.

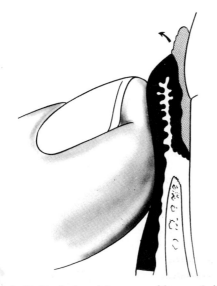

Figure 9–16. Purulent exudate expressed from periodontal pocket by digital pressure.

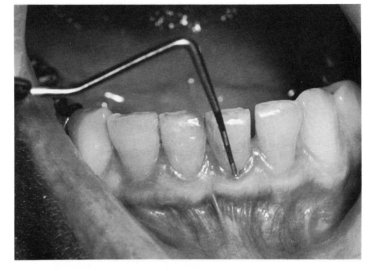

Figure 9–18. To determine the width of the attached gingiva, the pocket is probed at the same time that the lip (or cheek) is extended to demarcate the mucogingival line.

Additional findings that suggest the presence of abnormal occlusal relationships are neuromuscular disturbances such as impaired function of the masticatory musculature, which in severe cases results in muscle spasm and temporomandibular joint disorders.

Special notice should be made of *pathologic migration of the anterior teeth* as a sign of trauma from occlusion. Premature tooth contacts in the posterior region that deflect the mandible anteriorly contribute to destruction of the periodontium of the maxillary anterior teeth and to pathologic migration.

ACTIVITY OF PERIODONTAL LESIONS

The determination of the depth of the pocket or the level of connective tissue attachment does not provide information on the activity of periodontal lesions. Although there is no positively identified method at present, several indicators are useful: bleeding, gingival fluid measurements, and microbial analysis of plaque.[9]

Inactive lesions may show little or no bleeding upon probing and minimal amounts of fluid; the bacterial flora, as revealed by darkfield microscopy, consists mostly of coccoid cells.

Active lesions bleed more readily upon probing and have large amounts of fluid and exudate; their bacterial flora show greater numbers of spirochetes and motile bacteria.[13]

RADIOGRAPHIC EXAMINATION

Radiographs are valuable aids for evaluating periodontal disease and the outcomes of treatment. *They are an adjunct to the clinical examination, not a substitute for it.*

The radiographic image results from the superimposition of tooth, bone, and soft tissues in the pathway between the cone of the machine and the film. The radiograph reveals alterations in calcified tissue, which are not the result of current cellular activity but the effects of past cellular experience upon the bone and roots. Showing changes in the soft tissues of the periodontium requires special techniques that are not yet in routine clinical use.

Normal Interdental Septa

Because the facial and lingual bony plates are obscured by the relatively dense root structure, radiographic evaluation of bone changes in periodontal disease is based mainly upon the appearance of the interdental septa (Fig. 9–19). The septum normally presents a thin radiopaque border, adjacent to the periodontal ligament and at the crest, referred to as the *lamina dura*. This appears radiographically as a continuous white line, but it is perforated by numerous small foramina, containing blood vessels, lymphatics, and nerves, which pass between the periodontal ligament and the bone. *Since the*

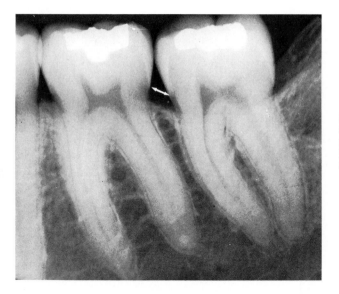

Figure 9–19. Crest of interdental septum is normally parallel to a line drawn between the cemento-enamel junctions of adjacent teeth *(arrow)*. Note also the radiopaque lamina dura around the roots and interdental septum.

lamina dura represents the bone surface lining the tooth socket, the shape and position of the root, changes in the angulation of the x-ray beam, and altered exposure times produce considerable variations in its appearance.[19]

The width and shape of the interdental septum and the angle of the crest normally vary according to the convexity of the proximal tooth surfaces and the level of the cemento-enamel junction of the approximating teeth.[28] The interdental space and the interdental septum between teeth with prominently convex proximal surfaces are wider anteroposteriorly than are those between teeth with relatively flat proximal surfaces. The faciolingual diameter of the bone is related to the width of the proximal root surface. *The angulation of the crest of the interdental septum is generally parallel to a line between the cemento-enamel junctions of the approximating teeth* (see Fig. 9–19). When there is a difference in the levels of the cemento-enamel junctions, the crest of the interdental bone is angulated rather than horizontal.

In order to rely on radiographs of pre- and post-treatment comparisons, standardized, reproducible techniques are required to obtain reliable radiographs.[23, 25, 29]

Bone Destruction in Periodontal Disease

Because radiographs do not reveal minor destructive changes in bone,[5, 6, 26] periodontal disease that produces even slight radiographic changes has progressed beyond the earliest stages. The radiographic image tends to show less severe bone loss than is actually present.[34] The difference between the alveolar crest height and the radiographic appearance ranges from 0 to 1.6 mm,[27] mostly due to x-ray angulation.

The amount and distribution of radiographic bone loss suggest the location of destructive local factors in different areas of the mouth and around different surfaces of the teeth.

The Pattern of Bone Destruction

In periodontal disease, the interdental septa undergo changes that affect the lamina dura, the crestal radiodensity, the size and shape of the medullary spaces, and the height and contour of the bone. The interdental septa may be reduced in height, with the crest perpendicular to the long axis of the adjacent teeth, termed *horizontal bone loss* (Fig. 9–20), or they may present angular or arcuate defects, called *angular or vertical bone loss* (Fig. 9–21).

For several reasons, radiographs do not indicate the internal morphology or depth of the crater-like interdental defects that appear as angular or vertical defects, nor do they reveal the extent of involvement on the facial and lingual surfaces. Facial and lingual surface bone destruction is obscured by the

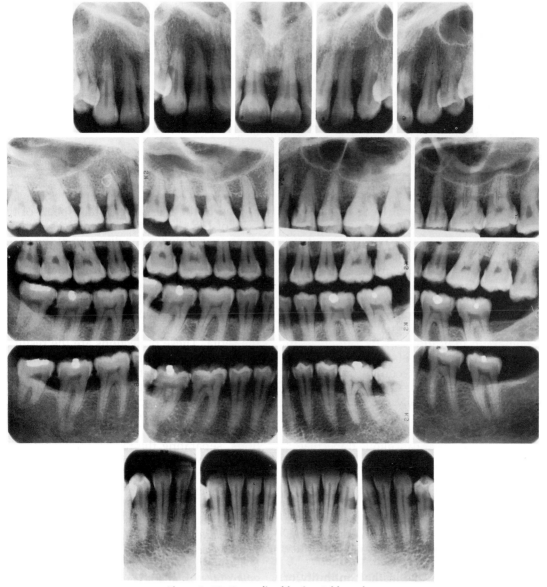

Figure 9–20. Generalized horizontal bone loss.

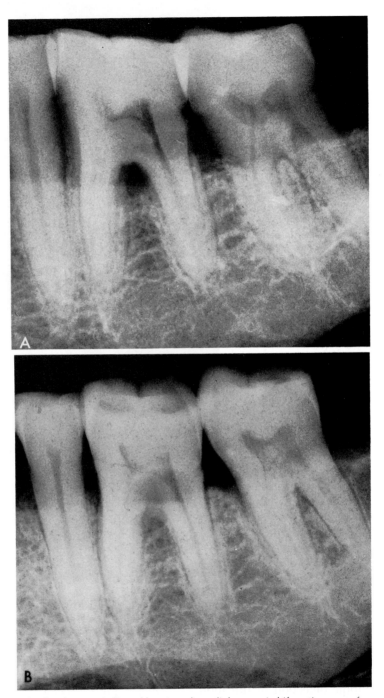

Figure 9–23. *A,* **Bifurcation involvement** indicated by triangular radiolucence in bifurcation area of mandibular first molar. The second molar presents only a slight thickening of the periodontal space in the bifurcation area. *B,* **Same area, different angulation.** The triangular radiolucence in the bifurcation of the first molar is obliterated, and involvement of the second molar bifurcation is apparent.

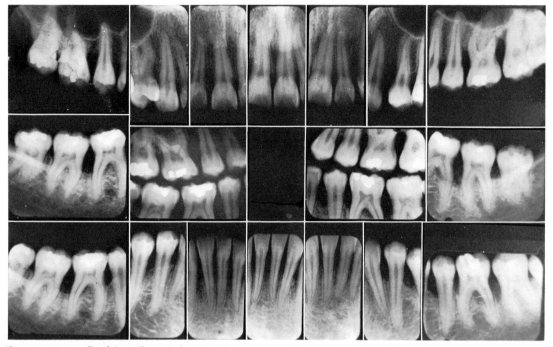

Figure 9–24. Localized juvenile periodontitis. The accentuated bone destruction in the anterior and first molar areas is considered characteristic of this disease, formerly called "periodontosis."

of alveolar bone is localized in the early stages to a single tooth or group of teeth and tends to become generalized as the disease progresses. The bone loss occurs initially in the maxillary and mandibular incisor and first molar areas, usually bilaterally. The interdental septa present vertical, arc-like, or angular destructive patterns. When the bone loss is generalized, it is least pronounced in the mandibular premolar areas (Fig. 9–24).

Generalized alteration in the trabecular pattern of the alveolar bone consists of less clearly defined trabecular markings and of increases in the size of the cancellous spaces.

EXFOLIATIVE CYTOLOGY

Exfoliative cytology is not used for periodontal diagnosis, but the hygienist may be called upon to obtain material for the evaluation by the pathologist to rule out the suspicion of oral cancer.

Exfoliative cytology is a diagnostic procedure consisting of the microscopic examination of cells obtained by scraping the surface of the suspected area or by rinsing the oral cavity. The former is preferred. Its reliability for the diagnosis of cancer is 86 per cent, as compared with the close to 100 per cent reliability of the oral biopsy procedure.[30] Exfoliative cytology is not a substitute for bi-

opsy, but it is valuable if a biopsy cannot be done for some reason. It is helpful in screening large groups of people for the presence of malignancy, provided it is used in conjunction with a careful oral examination, and in the diagnosis of bullous and vesicular oral lesions.

To obtain a specimen, the entire surface of the abnormal mucosa is firmly scraped with the edge of a wooden tongue depressor. The material thus removed is spread directly on a glass slide, immediately fixed in 95 per cent alcohol, and submitted for microscopic diagnosis.

NUTRITIONAL STATUS

If, when examining a patient, it is the clinician's impression that a nutritional deficiency exists, this suspicion must be corroborated by a medical evaluation of the patient's nutritional status. Nutritional therapy in the treatment of periodontal disturbances must be based on a demonstrated need, which is best determined by a nutritionist.

Nutrition refers to the complex relationship between the individual's total health status and the intake, digestion, and utilization of nutrients. *Nutritional deficiency connotes an inadequacy in the nutritional status of the tissue.* Malnutrition or poor nutrition may result from excessive food intake and improper nutrient balance as well as from an insufficiency of nutrients.

Nutritional deficiencies may be (1) *primary*, resulting from overt insufficiency of nutrients; or (2) *secondary (conditioned)*, resulting from bodily conditions that interfere with the ingestion, transport, cellular uptake, or utilization of essential nutrients in the presence of adequate food intake. Nutritional deficiencies usually develop in the following stages: (1) *depletion of the tissue nutrient reserve*, (2) *biochemical tissue lesions*, (3) *morphologic and functional abnormalities that are expressed as* (4) *clinical signs and symptoms*, and finally (5) *tissue death*.

A diagnosis of nutritional deficiency is based on four sequential routes of inquiry: (1) medical, social, and dietary history; (2) clinical examination; (3) laboratory tests; and (4) therapeutic trial. A nutrition text will provide detailed discussion of these procedures. Clinical findings identified with specific nutritional deficiencies and their oral manifestations are described in Chapter 11.

References

1. Armitage, G. C., Svanberg, G. K., and Löe, H.: Microscopic evaluation of clinical measurements of connective tissue attachment levels. J. Clin. Periodontol., 4:173, 1977.
2. Ayers, P.: Green stains. J. Am. Dent. Assoc., 26:3, 1939.
3. Badanes, B. B.: The role of fungi in deposits upon the teeth. Dent. Cosmos, 75:1154, 1933.
4. Bartels, H. A.: A note on chromogenic microorganisms from an organic colored deposit of the teeth. Int. J. Orthod., 25:795, 1939.
5. Bender, I. B., and Seltzer, S.: Roentgenographic and direct observation of experimental lesions in bone. J. Am. Dent. Assoc., 62:152, 1961.
6. Bender, I. B., and Seltzer, S.: Roentgenographic and direct observations of experimental lesions in bone. II. J. Am. Dent. Assoc., 62:708, 1961.
7. Fischman, S. L., and Picozzi, A.: Review of the literature: the methodology of clinical calculus evaluation. J. Periodontol., 40:607, 1969.
8. Gjermo, P.: Chlorhexidine in dental practice. J. Clin. Periodontol., 1:143, 1974.
9. Hancock, E. B.: Determination of periodontal disease activity. J. Periodontol., 52:492, 1981.
10. Heyden, G.: Relation between locally high concentrations of chlorhexidine and staining as seen in the clinic. J. Periodont. Res., 8(Suppl.):76, 1973.
11. Leung, S. W.: Naturally occurring stains on the teeth of children. J. Am. Dent. Assoc., 41:191, 1950.
12. Listgarten, M. A.: Periodontal probing: what does it mean? J. Clin. Periodontol., 7:165, 1980.
13. Listgarten, M. A., and Hellden, L.: Relative distribution of bacteria at clinically healthy and periodontally diseased sites in humans. J. Clin. Periodontol., 5:115, 1978.
14. Listgarten, M. A., Mao, R., and Robinson, P. J.: Periodontal probing: the relationship of the probe tip to periodontal tissues. J. Periodontol., 47:511, 1976.
15. Löe, H., and Schiott, C.: The effect of mouth rinses and topical application of chlorhexidine on the development of dental plaque and gingivitis in man. J. Periodont. Res., 5:79, 1970.
16. Magnusson, I., and Listgarten, M. A.: Histological evaluation of probing depth following periodontal treatment. J. Clin. Periodontol., 7:26, 1980.
17. Manly, R. S.: Factors influencing tests on the abrasion of dentin by brushing with dentifrices. J. Dent. Res., 23:59, 1944.
18. Mannerberg, F.: Saliva factors in cases of erosion. Odont. Revy, 14:156, 1963.
19. Manson, J. D.: The lamina dura. Oral Surg., 16:432, 1963.
20. Miller, W. D.: Experiments and observations on the wasting of tooth tissue variously designated as erosion, abrasion, chemical abrasion, denudation, etc. Dent. Cosmos, 49:1, 1907.
21. Nordno, H.: Discoloration of human teeth by a combination of chlorhexidine and aldehydes or ketones in vitro. Scand. J. Dent. Res., 79:356, 1971.
22. O'Leary, T. J.: Tooth mobility. Dent. Clin. North Am., 3:567, 1969.
23. Patur, B., and Glickman, I.: Roentgenographic evaluation of alveolar bone changes in periodontal disease. Dent. Clin. North Am., 4:47, 1960.
24. Pauls, V., and Trott, J. R.: A radiological study of experimentally produced lesions in bone. Dent. Pract., 16:254, 1966.
25. Puckett, J.: A device for comparing roentgenograms of the same mouth. J. Periodontol., 39:38, 1968.
26. Ramadan, A. B. E., and Mitchell, D. F.: A roentgenographic study of experimental bone destruction. Oral Surg., 15:934, 1962.
27. Regan, J. E., and Mitchell, D. F.: Roentgenographic and dissection measurements of alveolar crest height. J. Am. Dent. Assoc., 66:356, 1963.
28. Ritchey, B., and Orban, B.: The crests of the interdental septa. J. Periodontol., 24:75, 1953.
29. Rosling, B., Hollender, L., Nyman, S., and Olsson, G.: A radiographic method for assessing changes in alveolar bone height following periodontal therapy. J. Clin. Periodontol., 2:211, 1975.
30. Shklar, G., Cataldo, E., and Meyer, I.: Reliability of cytologic smear in diagnosis of oral cancer. A controlled study. Arch. Otolaryngol., 91:158, 1970.
31. Slots, J.: The microflora of black stain on human primary teeth. Scand. J. Dent. Res., 82:484, 1974.
32. Spray, J. R., et al.: Microscopic demonstration of the position of periodontal probes. J. Periodontol., 49:148, 1978.
33. Sutcliffe, P.: Extrinsic tooth stains in children. Dent. Pract., 17:175, 1967.
34. Theilade, J.: An evaluation of the reliability of radiographs in the measurement of bone loss in periodontal disease. J. Periodontol., 31:143, 1960.

Chapter 10

Rationale, Prognosis, and Treatment

RATIONALE FOR PERIODONTAL THERAPY

The effectiveness of periodontal therapy is made possible by the remarkable healing capacity of the periodontal tissues. Periodontal therapy allows chronically inflamed gingiva to become clinically and structurally identical to gingiva that has never been exposed to excessive plaque accumulation.[15]

Properly performed, periodontal treatment can be relied upon to eliminate pain, eliminate gingival inflammation[27] and gingival bleeding, reduce periodontal pockets and eliminate infection, stop pus formation, arrest the destruction of soft tissue and bone,[28] reduce abnormal tooth mobility,[10] establish optimal occlusal function, reestablish the physiologic gingival contour necessary for the preservation of periodontal health, prevent the recurrence of disease, reduce tooth loss,[23] and sometimes restore tissue destroyed by disease.

The removal of plaque and of all the factors that favor its accumulation is essential to restore gingival health.

HEALING AFTER PERIODONTAL THERAPY

The basic healing process consists of the removal of degenerated tissue debris and the replacement of tissues destroyed by disease. *Regeneration, repair,* and *reattachment* are aspects of periodontal healing that have significant effects on the results of periodontal treatment.

Regeneration

Regeneration is the growth and differentiation of new cells and intercellular substances to form new tissues or parts. It consists of fibroplasia, endothelial proliferation, the deposition of interstitial ground substance and collagen, epithelial hyperplasia, and the maturation of connective tissue.

Regeneration takes place by growth of the same tissues that had been destroyed or by differentiation from their precursors. Gingival epithelium is replaced by epithelium, and the underlying connective tissue and periodontal ligament are derived from connective tissue. Bone and cementum are not replaced by existing bone or cementum but by connective tissue, which is the precursor of both. Undifferentiated connective tissue cells develop into osteoblasts and cementoblasts, which form bone and cementum.

Regeneration of the periodontium is a continuous physiologic process. Under normal conditions new cells and tissues are constantly being formed to replace those that mature and die; this is called "wear and tear repair."

147

Mitotic activity in the gingival epithelium and the connective tissue of the periodontal ligament, bone formation, and continuous deposition of cementum are normal findings in the healthy periodontium.

Regeneration also occurs during active periodontal disease. Most gingival and periodontal diseases are chronic inflammatory processes that are healing lesions exhibiting tissue regeneration. Plaque accumulation is injurious to the regenerating tissues and prevents complete healing.

By removing bacterial plaque and creating the conditions to prevent its formation, periodontal treatment enhances regeneration. There is a brief spurt in regenerative activity immediately following periodontal treatment, but there are no local treatment procedures that promote or accelerate regeneration.

Repair

Repair is a microscopic activity that is not the same as restoration of destroyed periodontal tissues. In most instances, repair simply restores the continuity of the diseased marginal gingiva and reestablishes a normal gingival sulcus at the same level on the root as the base of the preexistent periodontal pocket (Fig. 10–1). This process, also called "healing by scar"[26] arrests bone destruction without necessarily increasing bone height. Restoration of the destroyed periodontium to a degree which is clinically and/or radiographically detectable occurs less frequently and is dependent upon reattachment.

Reattachment

Reattachment is the embedding of new periodontal ligament fibers into new cementum and the attachment of the gingival epithelium to a tooth surface previously denuded by disease (Fig. 10–2). Attachment of the gingiva or the periodontal ligament to areas of the tooth from which they may be removed in the course of treatment or during the preparation of teeth for restorations represents *simple healing* of the periodontium, not reattachment. *Reattachment* refers specifically to the restoration of the marginal periodontium, and not to repair of other areas of the root, such as that following traumatic cemental tears, tooth fractures, or the treatment of periapical lesions. Since new fibers are formed and attach to new cementum, there is a tendency to use the term *new attachment* rather than *reattachment*. The terms may be used interchangeably.

Epithelial adaptation is the close apposition of the gingival epithelium to the tooth surface without complete obliteration of the pocket. The pocket space does not permit passage of a probe. Although this may be a tenuous situation because bacteria can still penetrate the pocket, several clinical studies have shown that with adequate maintenance ther-

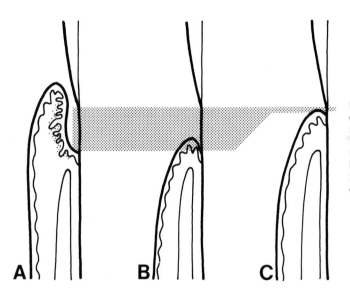

Figure 10–1. Two possible outcomes of pocket elimination. *A*, Periodontal pocket before treatment. *B*, Normal sulcus re-established at the level of the base of the pocket. *C*, Periodontium restored on the root surface previously denuded by disease. The latter is called reattachment. Shaded areas show denudation caused by periodontal disease.

A   B   C

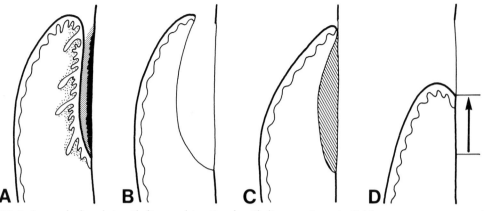

Figure 10–2. Removal of pocket epithelium and junctional epithelium creates potential for post-treatment reattachment. A, Periodontal pocket. B, After scaling, root planing, and curettage. C, Blood clot formed between instrumented pocket wall and cementum surface. D, Reattachment has increased the height of gingival attachment.

apy these deep sulci lined by long, thin epithelium may be acceptable. The absence of bleeding or secretion upon probing, the absence of clinically visible inflammation, and the absence of stainable plaque on the root surface when the pocket wall is deflected from the tooth may indicate that the "deep sulcus" persists in an inactive state, causing no further loss of attachment.[4, 42] A post-therapy depth of 4 or 5 mm may be acceptable in these cases.

Opinions differ regarding the extent and conditions under which reattachment is attainable after periodontal treatment. It occurs more often following the treatment of infrabony pockets[24, 38] than suprabony pockets,[33, 37] except in patients with one-wall vertical defects (see Chapter 3). It has been demonstrated histologically following the treatment of infrabony pockets,[32] but with suprabony pockets both positive and negative microscopic findings[19] have been reported. Reattachment has been observed histologically in experimental animals following the healing of artificially created pockets[16, 17, 25] and following the surgical removal of inflamed gingiva. However, the likelihood of obtaining reattachment is increased by the elimination of infection and the correction of excessive tooth mobility. Several other factors are important to consider.

Removal of Junctional Epithelium

The posttreatment location of the junctional epithelium limits the height to which

periodontal fibers become attached to the tooth. The level of attachment of the periodontal ligament in turn determines the maximum posttreatment height that the bone can attain. *Removal of the junctional epithelium creates conditions in which connective tissue fibers could reattach to the tooth surface coronal to the pretreatment level and creates the potential for increased bone height and the repair of vertical defects.*

In the treatment of periodontal pockets, complete removal of the junctional epithelium cannot be determined by clinical examination. Some investigators report complete removal of the junctional epithelium,[22] the lateral epithelium,[1, 20] and some underlying inflamed connective tissue following gingival curettage, whereas others observed remnants of both tissues.[35, 37,]

Preparation of the Root Surface

Changes in the tooth surface wall of periodontal pockets, such as the degeneration of Sharpey's fibers, accumulation of bacteria and their products, and disintegration of the cementum and dentin, interfere with reattachment. *These obstacles to reattachment can be eliminated by thorough root planing.*[13]

Several substances have been used in attempts to better condition the root surface for the attachment of new connective tissue fibers. The *citric acid* demineralization of root surfaces has been extensively investigated in animals and humans. Several mechanisms for its action have been postulated[11]: accel-

erated cementogenesis, widened dentinal tubules to allow for connective tissue ingress,
exposed root dentinal collagen fibers, extraction of endotoxin and other toxic plaque
products, and induction of mesenchymal cell
differentiation to osteoblasts or possibly cementoblasts. Studies in experimental animals
have given encouraging results,[29, 30] especially for the treatment of furcation lesions,[6]
but the results of studies in humans have
been contradictory.[5, 28, 31, 34]

Fibronectin is the glycoprotein that fibroblasts require in order to attach to root surfaces. The addition of fibronectin to the root
surface may promote reattachment.[9, 36] Clinical studies are not yet available.

*Sodium deoxycholate and human plasma frac-
tion Cohn IV* can dissociate endotoxin into
subunits and might render diseased root surfaces detoxified. The human plasma fraction
possibly contains fibronectin. Animal experiments using these agents have shown increased connective tissue attachment.[39, 40]

Granulation Tissue

This tissue, adjacent to the pocket wall, is
removed to provide better visibility of and
accessibility to the root surface. Its removal
does not represent a sacrifice of tissue because it is replaced in the healing process.

The Clot

The clot forms the initial protective covering of the treated area. It is replaced by
granulation tissue, which may extend up to
the clot surface. The vascularity and bulk of
the granulation tissue are reduced as it
undergoes maturation to connective tissue.
The height of the granulation tissue may
affect the level at which the epithelium becomes attached to the root, because the proliferating epithelium is guided by the connective tissue surface along which it moves.

Other Factors

*Trauma from occlusion impairs posttreatment
healing of the supporting periodontal tissues and
reduces the likelihood of reattachment.* Widened
periodontal spaces, angular bone defects,
and tooth mobility often result when trauma
persists during healing.

*Reattachment is more likely to occur when the
destructive process has been rapid.* This may be
seen following the treatment of pockets complicated by acute periodontal abscesses or
the treatment of acute necrotizing ulcerative
gingivitis.

The formation of new cementum and the
embedding of periodontal ligament fibers can
occur on the cementum and dentin of vital
teeth; in nonvital teeth it can occur on cementum but is not likely to occur on exposed
dentin.[20]

PROGNOSIS

*The prognosis is the prediction of the duration,
course, and termination of a disease and the
likelihood of its response to treatment.* It must be
determined before the treatment is planned.
The prognosis of gingival and periodontal
disease is critically dependent upon the patient—his attitude, his desire to retain his
natural teeth, and his willingness and ability
to maintain good oral hygiene. Without
these, treatment will not succeed.

Gingival Disease

If inflammation is the only pathologic
change, the prognosis is favorable provided
all local irritants are eliminated, gingival contours conducive to the preservation of health
are attained, and the patient cooperates by
maintaining good oral hygiene.

When inflammation is superimposed upon
systemically caused tissue changes (such as
in gingival enlargement associated with
phenytoin therapy or in patients with nutritional, hematologic, or hormonal disorders),
gingival health may be improved temporarily
by local therapy alone, but the long term
prognosis depends upon the control or correction of the contributing systemic factors.

Periodontal Disease

The prognosis in patients with periodontal
disease is dependent upon two considerations: *the overall prognosis* and *the prognosis of
individual teeth.*

The Overall Prognosis

The overall prognosis is concerned with
the dentition as a whole. It is an evaluation

of the likelihood of success of treatment. Several considerations are required for this determination to be made.

Assessment of Past Bone Response. The past response of the alveolar bone to local factors is a useful guide for predicting the bone response to treatment and the likelihood of arresting the bone-destructive process. Assessment of the past bone response entails consideration of the severity and distribution of the periodontal bone loss in terms of the following: the patient's age; the distribution, severity, and duration of local irritants such as plaque, calculus, and food impaction; occlusal abnormalities; and habits. If the amount of bone loss can be accounted for by the local factors, local treatment can be expected to arrest the bone destruction, and the overall prognosis for the dentition is good. If the bone loss is more severe than one would ordinarily expect at the patient's age in the presence of local factors of comparable severity and duration, factors other than those in the oral cavity are contributing to the bone destruction, and the overall prognosis is generally poor.

Height of Remaining Bone. When bone loss is severe and generalized, the remaining bone may be insufficient for proper tooth support, even if the bone destruction is stopped. Generally, bone height alone is insufficient for determining overall prognosis because individuals exhibit varying degrees of bone loss.

Patient's Age. *All other factors being equal, the prognosis is better in the older of two patients with comparable levels of remaining alveolar bone.* This is because the younger patient has suffered a more rapid bone destruction than the older patient.

Periodontal Pockets. The location of the base of the periodontal pocket is more important than probing depth in deciding the overall prognosis. Because pocket depth and the severity of bone loss are not necessarily related, a patient with deep pockets and little bone loss has a better prognosis than a patient with shallow pockets and severe bone destruction.

Malocclusion. Irregularly aligned teeth, malformation of the jaws, and abnormal occlusal relationships may be important factors in the etiology of periodontal disease because they may interfere with plaque control or produce occlusal interferences. In these cases, correction by orthodontic or prosthetic means is essential if periodontal treatment is to succeed. *The overall prognosis is poorer in patients with occlusal deformities that cannot be corrected than in those without.*

Individual Teeth

The prognosis of individual teeth is separate from the overall prognosis. It is common to have patients with good overall prognoses and poor prognoses of individual teeth. Also, many times, most of the teeth are lost but a few can be retained to support prostheses. Pocketing, mobility, and tooth morphology are important factors in determining these prognoses.

Mobility. The principal causes of tooth mobility are loss of alveolar bone, inflammatory changes in the periodontal ligament, and trauma from occlusion. Tooth mobility caused by inflammation and trauma from occlusion is correctable.[21] Tooth mobility resulting from loss of alveolar bone alone is not likely to be corrected. *The likelihood of restoring tooth stability is inversely proportional to the extent to which it is caused by loss of alveolar bone.*

Periodontal Pockets. In suprabony pockets the location of the base of the pocket affects the prognosis of individual teeth more than the probing depth. *Proximity to frenum attachments and to the mucogingival line jeopardizes the prognosis unless corrective procedures are included in the treatment.* The prognosis is adversely affected if the base of the pocket is close to the root apex, even if there is no evidence of apical disease. The incidence of degenerative pulp changes is increased in teeth affected by periodontal disease, usually without clinical symptoms or pulp necrosis. In these cases the prognosis is generally poor. However, striking apical and lateral bone repair is sometimes obtained by combining endodontic and periodontal therapy.

Tooth Morphology. Treatment prognosis is poor in teeth with short, tapered roots and relatively large crowns. Because of the disproportionate crown-root ratio and the reduced root surface available for periodontal support,[14] the periodontium is also more susceptible to injury by occlusal forces.

The *morphology of the tooth root* is a very important consideration in therapy.[12] Scaling and planing the root surface by the clinician

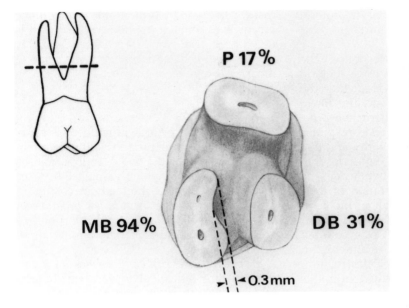

Figure 10–3. Root concavities in maxillary first molars sectioned 2 mm apical to the furca. (Data from Bower, R. C.: J. Periodontol., 50:366, 1979). The furcal aspect of the root is concave in 94 per cent of the mesiobuccal (MB) roots, 31 per cent of the distobuccal (DB) roots, and 17 per cent of the palatal (P) roots. The deepest concavity is found in the furcal aspects of the mesiobuccal root (mean concavity, 0.3 mm). The furcal aspect of the buccal roots diverges toward the palate in 97 per cent of the teeth (mean divergence, 22°).

and oral hygiene by the patient can be made very difficult by complex root morphology. Recognition of the presence of root anomalies plays an essential role in treatment planning and prognosis determination. Anomalies offer no problem as long as they are apical to the epithelial attachment, not exposed to the lumen of the pocket. As soon as the disease progresses to uncover these areas, the problems appear.

Root concavities and the morphology of the furcation areas are features that can in-

hibit plaque removal. *Concavities* can vary from shallow flutings to deep depressions present in the proximal surfaces. They increase the attachment area and produce a root shape that is more resistant to torquing forces (Fig. 10–3 and 10–4). Concavities appear more marked in the maxillary first premolars, in the mesiobuccal root of the maxillary first molar, in both roots of the mandibular first molars, and in the mandibular incisors.[2, 3] Access to the *furcation area* is sometimes very difficult to obtain. In 58 per

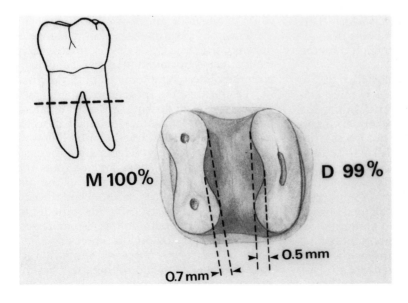

Figure 10–4. Root concavities in mandibular first molars sectioned 2 mm apical to the furca. (Data from Bower, R. C.: J. Periodontol., 50:366, 1979). Concavity of the furcal aspect was found in 100 per cent of mesial (M) roots and 99 per cent of distal (D) roots. Deeper concavity was found in the mesial roots (mean concavity, 0.7 mm).

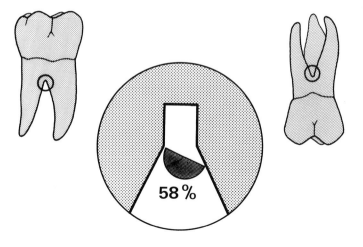

Figure 10–5. The furcation entrance is narrower than a standard curette in 58 per cent of first molars. (Data from Bower, R. C.: J. Periodontol., 50:366, 1979.)

58%

cent of upper and lower first molars, the furcation entrance diameter is narrower than the width of commonly used periodontal curettes[2] (Fig. 10–5).

Other anatomic structures inhibit plaque control. The presence of *developmental grooves*, which sometimes appear in the maxillary lateral incisors (palatogingival grooves) or in the lower incisors, also creates accessibility problems[7, 12] and worsens the prognosis.[41] Enamel projections extend into the furcation of 28.6 per cent of mandibular molars and 17 per cent of maxillary molars.[18] An intermediate bifurcation ridge has been described in 73 per cent of mandibular first molars, crossing from the mesial to the distal root at the midpoint of the bifurcation.[8]

Furcation Involvement. The presence of bifurcation or trifurcation involvement does not indicate a hopeless prognosis. However, when a lesion reaches the furcation it causes two additional important problems: (1) the difficulty of access to the area for scaling and root planing, and (2) inaccessibility of the area to plaque control by the patient. If both of these problems can be resolved, the prognosis will be similar to that of single-rooted teeth with similar degrees of bone loss.

SEQUENCE OF TREATMENT

After the evaluation and prognosis have been determined, the treatment is planned.

The treatment plan is the blueprint for case management. The dental treatment plan includes all procedures required for the establishment and maintenance of oral health, including which teeth are to be extracted, the need for surgical procedures, occlusal correction, and types of restorations to be placed. Periodontal treatment requires long-range planning. *Its value to the patient is measured in years of healthful functioning of the entire dentition, not by the number of teeth retained at the time of treatment.* It is directed to establishing and maintaining the health of the periodontium throughout the mouth rather than to spectacular efforts to "tighten loose teeth."

Phases of Therapeutic Procedures

Periodontal therapy is an inseparable part of dental therapy. The sequence of procedures presented here includes all dental procedures. Those that are part of periodontal therapy, whether performed by the dentist or the dental hygienist, are preceded by an asterisk (*).

Preliminary Phase

Treatment of emergencies
  Dental or periapical
  *Periodontal
  Other

Extraction of hopeless teeth and provisional replacement if needed (may be postponed to a more convenient time)

Phase I Therapy (Etiotropic Phase)

*Plaque control

*Diet control (in patients with rampant caries)

*Removal of calculus and root planing

Correction of restorative and prosthetic irritational factors

Excavation of caries and restoration (temporary or final, depending on whether a definitive prognosis for the tooth has been determined.

Occlusal therapy

Minor orthodontic movement

*Provisional splinting

Evaluation of Response to Phase I

Rechecking

*Pocket depth and gingival inflammation

*Plaque, calculus, and caries

Phase II Therapy (Surgical Phase)

*Periodontal surgery

Root canal therapy

Phase III Therapy (Restorative Phase)

Final restorations

Fixed and removable prosthodontics

Evaluation of Periodontal Response to Restorative Procedures

Phase IV Therapy (Maintenance Phase)

*Periodic recalls and evaluation of:

Plaque and calculus

Gingival condition (pockets, inflammation)

Caries

Occlusion, tooth mobility

Other pathology

ANSWERING PATIENT'S QUESTIONS

Patients frequently ask questions regarding periodontal treatment. Several suggestions.

are presented to help explain the treatment plan.

Be specific. Assuming that a definitive diagnosis has been made, tell patients: "You have gingivitis" or "You have periodontitis." Then, explain exactly what these conditions are, how they are treated, and what is likely to happen in the future after treatment. *Avoid vague statements* such as: "You have trouble with your gums" or "Something should be done about your gums." It is not easy to understand the significance of such statements and they are often disregarded.

Start your discussion on a positive note. Talk about the teeth that can be retained and the long-term service they can be expected to render. Do not begin with statements like "The following teeth have to be extracted." This creates a negative impression which may add to the hopeless attitude many patients have about their teeth.

Make it clear that every effort will be made to retain as many teeth as possible, *but do not dwell on the patient's loose teeth.* Emphasize the fact that one important purpose of the treatment is to prevent the other teeth from becoming as severely diseased as the loose teeth.

Avoid creating the impression that treatment consists of separate procedures, some or all of which may be selected by the patient. *Make it clear that dental restorations and prostheses contribute as much to the health of the gums as does the elimination of inflammation and periodontal pockets.* Do not speak in terms of "having the gums treated" and "then taking care of the necessary restorations later" as if these were unrelated treatments.

Patients frequently ask: Are my teeth worth treating?" "Would you have them treated if you were I?" "Why don't I just go along the way I am until the teeth really bother me, and then have them all extracted?" *Respond by making it clear that the best results are obtained by prompt treatment. If the condition is not treatable, the teeth should be extracted. Explain that "doing nothing" or holding onto hopelessly diseased teeth as long as possible is inadvisable* because it impairs proper mastication of food. This can lead to "bolting" food or nutritional imbalances from eating only soft foods. Exudate from periodontal pockets may also spoil the taste of food. In addition, the incorporation of purulent material into the food may irritate the mucosa of the stomach and lead to gastritis. Infection in the periodontal area is also a potential source of bacteremia. Also important is the fact that it is not feasible to place restorations on periodontally unsound teeth, which potentially causes both impaired function and appearance.

Failure to eliminate periodontal disease not only results in the loss of teeth already hopelessly involved but also shortens the life span of other teeth that, with proper treatment, could serve as the foundation for a healthy, functioning dentition. It is the dental clinician's responsibility to inform and motivate patients about proper periodontal care as well as other dental needs.

References

1. Blass, J. L., and Lite, T.: Gingival healing following surgical curettage: a histopathologic study. N.Y. Dent. J., 25:127, 1959.
2. Bower, R. C.: Furcation morphology relative to periodontal treatment—furcation entrance architecture. J. Periodontol., 50:23, 1979.
3. Bower, R. C.: Furcation morphology relative to periodontal treatment—furcation root surface anatomy. J. Periodontol., 50:366, 1979.
4. Caffesse, R. G., Ramfjord, S. P., and Nasjleti, C. E.: Reverse bevel periodontal flaps in monkeys. J. Periodontol., 39:219, 1968.
5. Cole, R., Nilveus, R., Ainamo, J., Bogle, G., Crigger, M., and Egelberg, J.: Pilot clinical studies on the effect of topical citric acid application on healing after replaced flap surgery. J. Periodont. Res., 16:117, 1981.
6. Crigger, M., Bogle, G., Nilveus, R., Egelberg, J., and Selvig, K.: Effect of topical citric acid application on the healing of experimental furcation defects in dogs. J. Periodont. Res., 13:538, 1978.
7. Everett, F. G., and Kramer, G. N.: The distolingual groove in the maxillary lateral incisor, a periodontal hazard. J. Periodontol., 43:352, 1972.
8. Everett, F. G., Jump, E. B., Holder, T. D., and Williams, G. C.: The intermediate bifurcational ridge: a study of the morphology of the bifurcation of the lower first molar. J. Dent. Res., 37:162, 1958.
9. Fernyhough, W., and Page, R. C.: Attachment, growth and synthesis of human gingival fibroblasts on demineralized or fibronectin-treated normal and diseased tooth roots. J. Peridontol., 54:133, 1983.
10. Ferris, R. T.: Quantitative evaluation of tooth mobility following initial periodontal therapy. J. Periodontol., 37:190, 1966.
11. Fialkoff, B., and Fry, H. R.: Acid demineralization in periodontal therapy: a review of the literature. J. Western Soc. Periodontol., 30:52, 1982.
12. Gher, M. E., and Vernino, A. R.: Root morphology—clinical significance in pathogenesis and treatment of periodontal disease. J. Am. Dent. Assoc., 101:627, 1980.
13. Jones, W. A., and O'Leary, T. J.: The effectiveness of "in vivo" root planing in removing bacterial endotoxin from the roots of periodontally involved teeth. J. Periodontol., 49:337, 1978.
14. Kay, S., Forscher, B. K., and Sackett, L. M.: Tooth root length-volume relationships. An aid to periodontal prognosis. I. Anterior teeth. Oral Surg., 7:735, 1954.
15. Lindhe, J., Parodi, R., Liljenberg, B., and Fornell, J.: Clinical and structural alterations characterizing healing gingiva. J. Periodont. Res., 13:410, 1978.
16. Linghorne, W. J.: Studies in the reattachment and regeneration of the supporting structures of the teeth. IV. Regeneration in epithelialized pockets following the organization of a blood clot. J. Dent. Res., 36:4, 1957.
17. Linghorne, W. J., and O'Connell, D. C.: Studies in the reattachment and regeneration of the supporting structures of the teeth. II. Regeneration in epithelialized pockets. J. Dent. Res., 34:164, 1955.
18. Master, D. H., and Hoskins, S. W. P.: Projection of cervical enamel into molar furcations. J. Periodontol., 35:49, 1964.
19. Morris, M. L.: Healing of naturally occurring periodontal pockets about vital human teeth. J. Periodontol., 26:285, 1955.
20. Morris, M. L.: Healing of human periodontal tissues following surgical detachment and extirpation of vital pulps. J. Periodontol., 31:23, 1960.
21. Morris, M. L.: The diagnosis, prognosis and treatment of the loose tooth. Oral Surg., 6:1037, 1953.
22. Morris, M. L.: The removal of pocket and attachment epithelium in humans: a histological study. J. Periodontol., 25:57, 1954.
23. Oliver, R. C.: Tooth loss with and without periodontal therapy. Periodont. Abstracts, 17:8, 1969.
24. Prichard, J.: The infrabony technique as a predictable procedure. J. Periodontol., 28:202, 1957.
25. Ramfjord, S. P.: Experimental periodontal reattachment in Rhesus monkeys. J. Periodontol., 22:67, 1951.
26. Ratcliff, P. A.: An analysis of repair systems in periodontal therapy. Periodont. Abstracts, 14:57, 1966.
27. Rateitschak, K.: The therapeutic effect of local treatment on periodontal disease assessed upon evaluation of different diagnostic criteria. 2. Changes in gingival inflammation. J. Periodontol., 35:155, 1964.
28. Rateitschak, K., Engleberger, A., and Marthaler, T. M.: The therapeutic effect of local treatment on periodontal disease assessed upon evaluation of different dignostic criteria. 3. Radiographic changes in appearance of bone. J. Periodontol. 35:263, 1964.
29. Register, A. A., and Burdick, F. A.: Accelerated reattachment with cementogenesis to dentin, demineralized in situ. 1. Optimum range. J. Periodontol., 46:646, 1975.
30. Register, A. A., and Burdick, F. A.: Accelerated reattachment with cementogenesis to dentin, demineralized in situ. 2. Defect repair. J. Periodontol., 47:497, 1976.
31. Renvert, S., and Egelberg, J.: Healing after treatment of periodontal intraosseous defects. II. Effect of citric acid conditioning of the root surface. J. Clin. Periodontol., 8:459, 1981.
32. Schaffer, E. M., and Zander, H.: Histological evidence of reattachment of periodontal pockets. Paradentologie, 7:101, 1953.

33. Shapiro, M.: Reattachment in periodontal disease. J. Periodontol., *24*:26, 1953.

34. Stahl, S., and Froum, S.: Human clinical and histologic repair responses following the use of citric acid in periodontal therapy. J. Periodontol., *48*:261, 1977.

35. Stone, S., Ramfjord, S., and Waldron, J.: Scaling and gingival curettage. A radioautographic study. J. Periodontol., *37*:415, 1966.

36. Terranova, V. P., and Martin, G. R.: Molecular factors determining gingival tissue interaction with tooth structure. J. Periodont. Res., *17*:530, 1982.

37. Waerhaug, J.: Microscopic demonstration of tissue reaction incident to removal of subgingival calculus. J. Periodontol., *26*:26, 1955.

38. Williams, C. H. M.: Rationalization of periodontal pocket therapy. J. Periodontol., *14*:67, 1943.

39. Wirthlin, M. R., and Hancock, E. B.: Biologic preparation of diseased root surfaces. J. Periodontol., *51*:291, 1980.

40. Wirthlin, M. R., Hancock, E. B., and Gangler, R. W.: Regeneration and repair after biologic treatment of root surfaces in monkeys. I. Facial surfaces, maxillary incisors. J. Periodontol., *52*:729, 1981.

41. Withers, J. A., et al.: The relationship of palatogingival grooves to localized periodontal disease. J. Periodontol., *52*:41, 1981.

42. Yukna, R. A.: A clinical and histologic study of healing following the excisional new attachment procedure in Rhesus monkeys. J. Periodontol., *47*:701, 1976.

Chapter 11

Systemic Factors Influencing Periodontal Disease and Its Treatment

SYSTEMIC INFLUENCES ON PERIODONTAL DISEASE

Nutritional Influences

There are a number of oral manifestations of nutritional disease. These include alterations of the lips, oral mucosa, bone, and the periodontal tissues. Nutritional deficiencies do not cause gingivitis or periodontal disease, but they affect the condition of all tissues and can aggravate the injurious effects of local irritants.

Theoretically, there may exist a "border zone" in which local irritants of insufficient severity could cause gingival and periodontal disorders if their effects were potentiated by nutritional deficiency. On this theoretic basis, some clinicians enthusiastically adhere to the theory that nutritional deficiencies or imbalances play a key role in the etiology of periodontal diseases. Although research conducted up to this time does not in general support this view, it has been pointed out that numerous problems in experimental design and data interpretation may render current findings incomplete.[1]

Numerous experiments in animals have shown that the *physical character of the diet* may play some role in the accumulation of plaque and the development of gingivitis. Soft diets, although nutritionally adequate, lead to plaque and calculus formation.[6, 21] Hard, fibrous foods provide surface cleansing action and stimulation, which result in less plaque accumulation in animals[7] even if the diet is nutritionally inadequate. However, studies in humans have not demonstrated reduced plaque formation when hard foods are consumed.[21, 52] This difference may be related to variation in tooth anatomy or the fact that experimental animals can be fed exclusively on hard-consistency diets, while human subjects eat combinations of foods. The presence of high sucrose content in human diets also leads to the production of thick plaques.

The *effect of vitamin C on the periodontium* is considered separately here because of the traditional association of this vitamin with gingival pathology. Severe vitamin C deficiency in humans results in scurvy, a disease characterized by hemorrhagic diathesis, retardation of wound healing, and increased susceptibility to infection.

Scurvy results in defective formation and

157

maintenance of collagen, mucopolysaccharide ground substance, and intercellular cement substance in mesenchymal tissues. Its effect on bone is marked by retardation or cessation of osteoid formation, impaired osteoblastic function, and osteoporosis.[53] Vitamin C deficiency is also characterized by increased capillary permeability and susceptibility to traumatic hemorrhages.

Several studies in large populations that have analyzed the relation between periodontal status and ascorbic acid levels have failed to establish a causal relationship between levels of vitamin C and the prevalence or severity of periodontal disease.[40] Gingivitis, with enlarged, hemorrhagic, bluish-red gingiva, is described as one of the classic signs of vitamin C deficiency, but it is caused by bacterial plaque. Vitamin C deficiency may aggravate the gingival response to plaque and worsen the edema, enlargement, and bleeding.[14] However, although the severity of the condition may be reduced by correcting the deficiency, gingivitis will remain as long as bacterial irritation is present. Vitamin C deficiency does not produce periodontal pockets. However, when pocket formation occurs in individuals with vitamin C deficiency, pockets are of greater depth than would be produced in normal patients with comparable local irritants.

Analysis of the literature[54] reveals that microscopic signs of vitamin C deficiency are quite different from those found in plaque-induced human periodontal disease. Individuals with acute or chronic vitamin C deficient states and no plaque accumulation show minimal signs, if any, of changes in their periodontal health.

Hormonal Influences

Hormones are organic substances produced by the endocrine glands. They are secreted directly into the blood stream and exert an important physiologic influence on the functions of human cells and organ systems. Some hormone-related conditions that have oral manifestations of clinical interest will be described.

Hyperparathyroidism

Parathyroid hypersecretion produces generalized demineralization of the skeleton, the formation of bone cysts and giant cell tumors, increased osteoclasis, occasional osteoid formation, and proliferation of the connective tissue in the marrow spaces and the haversian canals. The proportion of patients with hyperparathyroidism who present with oral changes ranges from 25 per cent[44] to 45[36] to 50 per cent.[46] Oral changes include malocclusion, tooth mobility, and radiographic evidence of alveolar osteoporosis characterized by closely meshed trabeculae, widening of the periodontal ligament space, absence of the lamina dura, and radiolucent cyst-like spaces. Giant cell tumors in the jaws and loss of the lamina dura are late signs of the relatively uncommon hyperparathyroid bone disease. The periodontal changes in hyperparathyroidism are a typical example of the effects of a systemic disease on the periodontal tissues, totally unrelated to the presence or absence of plaque-induced periodontitis.

Diabetes

Diabetes is a metabolic disease characterized by hypofunction or lack of function of the beta cells of the islets of Langerhans in the pancreas, leading to high blood glucose levels and excretion of sugar in the urine. It is a complicated biochemical disease; the metabolic regulation of carbohydrates involves not only beta cells, which secrete the insulin that reduces glycemia, but also the alpha cells of the pancreas which secrete glucagon, the corticoadrenal hormones, and the anterior pituitary hormones, all of which increase glycemia.

Two basic types of diabetes have been described, insulin dependent and non–insulin dependent. *Insulin dependent diabetes* is also known as juvenile diabetes or juvenile-onset diabetes, although it may appear at older ages. This type of disease is very unstable, is difficult to control, has a marked tendency toward ketosis and coma, is not preceded by obesity, and requires insulin therapy. The disease presents the symptoms traditionally associated with diabetes, such as polyphagia, polydipsia, polyuria, predisposition to infections, and anorexia. *Non–insulin dependent diabetes* is the adult type, with onset usually after age 45. It generally occurs in obese individuals and can often be controlled by diet or by oral hypoglycemic agents. The development of ketosis and coma

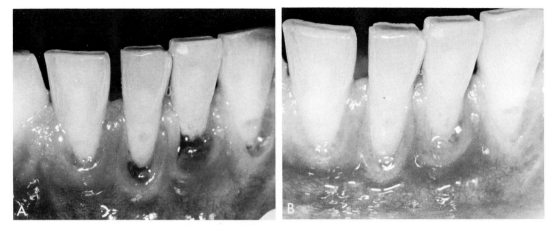

Figure 11–1. Adult diabetic patient. *A,* Blood glucose level 400 mg per 100 ml. Note gingival inflammation, spontaneous bleeding, and edema. *B,* After 4 days of insulin therapy (glucose level less than 100 mg per 100 ml) the clinical periodontal picture has improved in the absence of local therapy. (Courtesy of Dr. Joan Otomo.)

is not common. Adult-onset diabetes has the same symptoms as juvenile diabetes but is less severe.

Diabetes and the Periodontium. The most significant periodontal findings in uncontrolled diabetics are the reduction in defense mechanisms and the increased susceptibility to infections that may lead to destructive periodontal disease. Controlled diabetics exhibit normal tissue response and normal defense against infections. However, the possibility that the control of the disease may be inadequate makes it important to exercise special care in the periodontal treatment of all diabetics.

A variety of periodontal changes have been described in diabetic patients, such as the tendency toward abscess formation, enlarged gingiva, polypoid gingival proliferations, and loosened teeth (Fig. 11–1).[38]

In general, the rate of periodontal destruction appears to be similar for diabetics and nondiabetics up to the age of 30 years[13, 48]; after age 30 there is a greater degree of destruction in diabetics. Patients showing overt diabetes over a period of more than 10 years have greater loss of periodontal structures than those with shorter histories of diabetes.[13] The extensive literature on the subject and the overall impressions of clinicians indicate that periodontal disease in diabetics follows no consistent pattern. Very severe gingival inflammation, deep periodontal pockets, and frequent periodontal abscesses often occur in diabetics with poor oral hygiene. In juvenile diabetics, there is

often extensive periodontal destruction. However, in many other diabetic patients, both juvenile-onset and adult-onset, gingival changes and bone loss are not found. *The distribution and severity of local irritants affect the severity of periodontal disease in diabetics.* Diabetes does not cause gingivitis or periodontal pocketing, but alterations in tissue response to local irritants hastens bone loss in periodontal disease and retards healing after periodontal treatment. Frequent periodontal abscesses appear to be an important manifestation of periodontal disease in diabetics.

Puberty

Sex hormones complicate the tissue response to local irritation in adolescents at puberty, resulting in exaggerated gingival inflammation. Pronounced inflammation, bluish-red discoloration, edema, and enlargement result from plaque accumulation that would ordinarily elicit mild responses (Fig. 11–2). Excessive anterior overbite aggravates these symptoms because of the complicating effects of food impaction and injury to the gingiva on the labial aspects of the mandibular teeth and the palatal aspects of the maxillary teeth. The response diminishes as adulthood is approached, but complete return to normal requires the removal of local irritants. Puberty-associated gingivitis is not a universal occurrence and with proper preventive measures can be avoided.

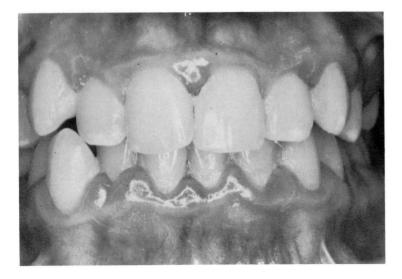

Figure 11–2. Gingivitis in puberty, with edema, discoloration, and enlargement.

Menstrual Cycle

As a general rule, the menstrual cycle is not accompanied by notable gingival changes, but occasional changes have been reported. During the menstrual period the prevalence of gingivitis increases. Patients may complain of bleeding gums or a bloated, tense feeling in the gums in the days preceding menstrual flow. Horizontal tooth mobility does not change significantly.[12] The salivary bacterial count is increased during menstruation and at ovulation, 10 to 14 days earlier.[34] The exudate from inflamed gingiva is increased during menstruation, suggesting that existent gingivitis is aggravated, but the cre-vicular fluid flow of normal gingiva is unaffected.[15]

Pregnancy

Gingivitis in pregnancy is caused by local irritants. Hormonal changes in pregnancy accentuate the gingival response and produce a clinical picture different from that seen in nonpregnant women. No notable changes occur in the gingiva during pregnancy in the absence of local irritants.

The severity of gingivitis in pregnancy increases from the second or third month. Women with slight, chronic gingivitis that was unnoticed before pregnancy become

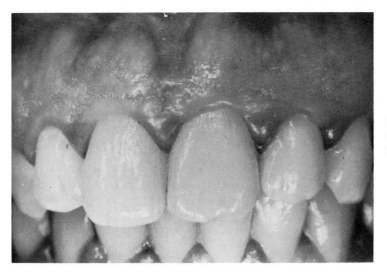

Figure 11–3. Gingivitis in pregnancy. Early changes in the interdental papillae.

aware of gingival areas that are enlarged, edematous, and discolored (Fig. 11–3). Increased gingival bleeding is also noticed. The gingivitis becomes more severe by the eighth month and decreases during the ninth; plaque accumulation follows a similar pattern.[24] The greatest severity has been reported in the second and third trimesters. The correlation between gingivitis and the quantity of plaque is higher after parturition than during pregnancy.

Clinical Features of Pregnancy Gingivitis. Pronounced vascularity is the most striking clinical feature of pregnancy gingivitis. The gingiva becomes inflamed and varies in color from bright red to bluish-red. The marginal and interdental gingivae are edematous, pit on pressure, appear smooth and shiny, are soft and friable, and sometimes present a raspberry-like appearance. The extreme redness results from marked vascularity, and there is an increased tendency to bleed. The changes are usually painless unless complicated by acute infection. In some cases the inflamed gingiva forms discrete tumor-like masses called "pregnancy tumors." There is partial reduction of symptoms by two months postpartum; however, as long as local irritants are present, the gingiva does not return to normal.

There is a marked increase in estrogen and progesterone during pregnancy and a reduction after parturition. The severity of gingivitis is related to these hormone levels.[16] The gingival response has been principally attributed to progesterone, which produces dilatation and proliferation of the microvasculature, circulatory stasis, and increased susceptibility to mechanical irritation—all of which favor leakage of fluid into the perivascular tissues.[27, 31]

Hormonal Contraceptives

Hormonal contraceptives aggravate the gingival response to local irritants in a manner similar to pregnancy. When taken for long periods of time (longer than 1.5 years), increased periodontal destruction has been reported.[20] Although some brands of oral contraceptives produce more dramatic changes than others,[33] no correlation has been found between gingival response and progesterone or estrogen content in various brands. Cumulative exposure to oral contraceptives apparently has no effect on gingival inflammation or oral debris index scores.[17]

Hematologic Diseases

Oral changes are often the earliest indication of hematologic disturbances, but they cannot be relied upon for diagnosis of the hematologic disorder. Oral findings may suggest blood disturbances, but specific diagnoses require complete physical examination and hematologic studies. Comparable oral changes occur in more than one form of blood dyscrasia, and secondary inflammatory changes produce wide variations in oral findings.

Leukemia

The leukemias are "malignant neoplasias of white blood cell precursors, characterized by (1) diffuse replacement of the bone marrow with proliferating leukemic cells; (2) abnormal numbers and forms of immature white cells in the circulating blood; and (3) widespread infiltrates in the liver, spleen, lymph nodes and other sites throughout the body."[36] According to the type of white blood cell involved, leukemias can be lymphocytic, myelogenous, or monocytic. These forms can be acute, which is rapidly fatal; subacute; or chronic. The replacement of the bone marrow elements by leukemic cells reduces normal white blood cell and platelet production, leading to anemia and bleeding disorders.

Oral manifestations occur with the greatest frequency in acute and subacute monocytic leukemia, less frequently in acute and subacute lymphatic and myelogenous leukemia, and seldom in chronic leukemia. Periodontal changes in leukemia can be (1) primary changes, those directly attributable to the hematologic disturbance; and 2) secondary changes, those superimposed upon the oral tissues by the omnipresent local factors, which induce a wide range of inflammatory changes.

Changes that may occur in acute and subacute leukemia include diffuse, cyanotic, bluish-red discoloration of the entire gingival mucosa; diffuse, edematous enlargement obliterating details of the normal gingival surface; rounding and tenseness of the gingival margin; blunting of the interdental papillae;

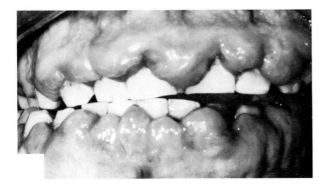

Figure 11–4. Acute myelocytic leukemia. Frontal view of gingival enlargement. (Courtesy of Dr. Spencer Woolfe.)

and varying degrees of gingival inflammation with ulceration, necrosis, and pseudomembrane formation (Fig. 11–4).

Microscopically, the gingiva presents a dense, diffuse infiltration of predominantly immature leukocytes in the attached as well as the marginal gingiva. The normal connective tissue components are displaced by the leukemic cells; the nature of the cells seen depends on the type of leukemia. The periodontal ligament and the alveolar bone may also be infiltrated with mature and immature leukocytes.

The inflamed gingiva of leukemic patients is extremely susceptible to infection so that plaque can cause severe necrosis and pseudomembrane formation in acute and subacute leukemias. These oral changes can cause great difficulty for patients and can result in systemic toxic effects, loss of appetite, nausea, blood loss from gingival bleeding, and constant pain.

Hemophilia

Hemophilia is an inherited sex-linked disease affecting only males and transmitted by females. The defect is passed to the female offspring, who exhibit no symptoms of the disease but pass it to male children. Hemophilia is characterized by prolonged hemorrhage from even slight wounds and also by spontaneous bleeding into the tissues. Spontaneous bleeding from mucous membranes is not a feature of the disease, but chronic marginal gingivitis in hemophiliac patients can constitute a serious complication because of the bleeding problem.

The clotting time in hemophilia is markedly prolonged, but the bleeding time remains normal. The prolonged clotting time

is due to a deficiency of serum protein antihemophilic globulin (AHG; Factor VIII), which presumably results in platelet resistance to disintegration. The normal bleeding time may be explained because capillary contraction is normal, causing cessation of bleeding. When the capillaries later expand, however, there is no clot present to plug the defect, and bleeding resumes.

Focal Infection

According to the concept of focal infection, a primary site of infection in one part of the body may serve as the focus (the Latin word for *hearth*) from which the infection emanates to other parts of the body. Interest in focal infection has fluctuated considerably from the initial enthusiasm stimulated by the original investigation of Rosenow in 1917. In the early days of the focal infection concept, the oral cavity attracted attention because it harbored teeth with chronic apical disease. Interest has since shifted from the periapical areas to the periodontal pockets.[45] Within the limitations that govern the concept of focal infection, *the periodontal pocket represents a greater potential menace than periapical disease* because (1) infection is always present, (2) there is a greater variety of organisms and they penetrate the soft tissue walls, (3) mechanical stimulation from mastication is a constant potential source of bacteremia, and (4) periodontal pockets are more prevalent in the population than is periapical disease.

The potential role of periodontal pathogens in anaerobic infections elsewhere in the body has been recently emphasized. Organisms associated with periodontal diseases have been found in infected wounds, lung abscesses, subacute bacterial endocarditis, and other infections.

Bacteremia

The literature consistently points to disease of the gingiva as a source of bacteremia following mechanical manipulation of the teeth. Murray and Moosnick[29] found positive blood cultures in 55 per cent of persons with varying degrees of dental caries and periodontal disease who chewed paraffin cubes for 30 minutes. Positive blood cultures were also reported after tooth extractions in nine patients with periodontal disease.[10] Okell and Elliott[30] reported 72 positive blood cultures following extraction in 100 patients with gingival disease. A significantly lower incidence of bacteremia was found in patients with no clinical periodontal disease. In addition, when marked gingival disease was present, rocking of the teeth alone sufficed to produce bacteremia in 86 per cent of the patients.[8] Bacteremia occurred more frequently in association with deep periodontal pockets. The penetration of bacteria into the epithelium and connective tissue of the pocket wall may favor bacteremia.[41] Burket and Burn[5] painted a nonpathogen, *Serratia marcescens*, into the gingival sulcus prior to extraction and recovered it in postextraction blood cultures in 18 of 90 cases. This information emphasizes the *necessity* of premedication precautions for patients with certain systemic conditions.

PERIODONTAL TREATMENT FOR PATIENTS WITH SYSTEMIC CONDITIONS

Many medical problems require special management in the dental setting. Several common conditions are presented here with the appropriate precautions to be taken so that the clinician can render safe, responsible periodontal treatment. If there is any question of safety for the patient or the operator, it is proper to consult the patient's physician prior to treatment.

Cardiovascular Diseases

Several cardiovascular conditions warrant modification of the periodontal treatment plan; history of angina pectoris, myocardial infarction, cerebrovascular accident, transient ischemic attacks, cardiac bypass surgery, and congestive heart failure are some of the most common. In most cases the patient's cardiologist should be consulted, and the following precautions should be taken to avoid stress: (1) schedule morning appointments, (2) maintain an open, concerned atmosphere during treatment, and 3) keep appointments short.

Angina Pectoris

Patients with histories of unstable angina pectoris (angina that occurs irregularly or on multiple occasions without predisposing factors) should be treated for emergencies only. Patients with stable angina (that which occurs infrequently, is associated with exertion or stress, and is easily controlled with medication and rest) can undergo elective dental procedures if the following precautions are taken:

1. Premedicate as needed with diazepam, nitrous oxide–oxygen, or short-acting barbiturates such as pentobarbital (30 to 60 mg) or secobarbital (60 to 100 mg).[4, 42]

2. Adequate anesthesia is required. Recommended procedure is to aspirate frequently and inject slowly.

3. If the patient feels stressed, sublingual nitroglycerin premedication (1/200 grain) 5 minutes prior to the procedure is suggested.

The patient's medication (generally nitroglycerin) should be readily accessible on the dental tray. Check the expiration date of the patient's nitroglycerin as well as that of the office's emergency medical kit, because the drug rapidly loses potency. If the patient becomes fatigued or has a sudden change in heart rhythm or rate, the dental procedure should be discontinued as soon as possible.

A patient who has an anginal episode in the dental chair requires the following emergency medical treatment:

1. Discontinue the procedure.
2. Administer one tablet (0.3 to 0.6 mg) of nitroglycerin sublingually.
3. Reassure the patient.
4. Loosen restrictive garments.
5. Administer oxygen with the patient in a reclining position.
6. If the signs and symptoms cease within 3 minutes, complete the procedure if

dental procedures poor dental hygiene or other dental diseases such as periodontal or periapical infections may induce bacteremia."[18] *The report recommended antibiotic prophylaxis for all dental procedures that are likely to cause gingival bleeding.* This includes almost all periodontal treatment procedures. In order to provide adequate preventive measures for BE, the major concern should be to reduce the microbial population in the oral cavity so as to minimize soft tissue inflammation and bacteremia. Studies have confirmed that patients with periodontal disease have greater and more frequent bacteremia than those without periodontal disease.

Preventive measures in the dental setting *must* include the following:

1. Careful health histories must be taken to identify susceptible individuals.
2. Oral hygiene instruction should begin with gentle toothbrushing with a soft brush and oral rinses. No antibiotic coverage for this procedure is necessary. The bacteremia caused by oral hygiene procedures is dependent upon the degree of periodontal tissue inflammation. As gingival health improves, more aggressive oral hygiene may be performed. Dental irrigation devices have been implicated in association with BE; therefore their use should be discouraged.[50]
3. *Currently recommended prophylactic antibiotic regimens should be practiced for all susceptible patients.*[2] These are listed in Table 11–1. If patients have been receiving continuous oral penicillin for secondary prevention of rheumatic fever, penicillin-resistant alpha-hemolytic streptococci are occasionally found in the oral cavity. It is recommended that regimen A with erythromycin (see Table 11–1) be followed in these cases.
4. Treatment should be designed to ac-

TABLE 11–1. PROPHYLAXIS OF INFECTIVE ENDOCARDITIS: ANTIBIOTIC REGIMENS FOR DENTAL PROCEDURES

Regimen for patients with valvular heart disease, prosthetic heart valves, most forms of congenital heart disease, idiopathic hypertrophic subaortic stenosis, and mitral valve prolapse.

Note: 1. Oral regimens are safer and preferred for most patients.
2. Parenteral regimens have a greater effectivity and are recommended for patients with prosthetic valves, patients who have had previous bouts with endocarditis, or patients who are on continuous oral penicillin for rheumatic fever prophylaxis.

ORAL ROUTE

Adult Dosage: 2.0 gm penicillin V 1 hr before dental procedure and 1.0 gm 6 hr later.

Child Dosage: If child weighs more than 27 kg (60 lb), administer adult dose; if child weighs less than 27 kg (60 lb), administer one half the adult dosage before procedure and repeat 6 hr later.

Penicillin Allergy

Adult Dosage: 1.0 gm erythromycin 1 hr before and 500 mg 6 hr after procedure.

Child Dosage: 20 mg/kg erythromycin 1 hr before procedure and 10 mg/kg 6 hr later.

PARENTERAL ROUTE

Adult Dosage: 1 gm ampicillin IM or IV 30 min to 1 hr before procedure and repeat 8 hr later;

or

two million units of aqueous penicillin G IM or IV 30 min to 1 hr before procedure and repeat 8 hr later *plus* 1.5 mg/kg gentamicin IM or IV 30 min to 1 hr before procedure and repeat 8 hr later.

Child Dosage: 50 mg/kg ampicillin IM or IV 30 min to 1 hr before procedure and repeat 8 hr later;

or

50,000 units/kg aqueous penicillin G IM or IV 30 min before procedure and repeat 8 hr later *plus* 2.0 mg/kg gentamicin IM or IV 30 min to 1 hr before procedure and repeat 8 hr later.

Penicillin Allergy

Adult Dosage: 1 gm vancomycin IV infused over 1 hr beginning 1 hr before procedure and repeat 8 hr later.

Child Dosage: 20 mg/kg vancomycin IV infused over 1 hr beginning 1 hr before procedure and repeat 8 hr later.

*From American Heart Association recommendations, revised 1985. (Courtesy of Dr. F. M. Lucatorto.)

commodate the susceptible patient's particular degree of periodontal involvement. When faced with long-term therapy, multiple visits, and procedures that easily induce bleeding, the following guidelines are recommended:

a. All periodontal treatment procedures, including probing, should be performed only with antibiotic coverage. Gentle oral hygiene procedures are excluded.

b. It is prudent to provide additional antibiotic doses in cases of delayed healing. Also, suture removal can be performed more safely by utilizing antibiotic coverage on the day of suture removal or by placing resorbable sutures.

c. Prolonged impingement of the gingival tissues with ligatures or tissue retractors should be avoided.

d. For multiple appointments 10 to 14 days should elapse before starting new coverage.[22] Alternatively, antibiotics can be rotated to minimize the emergence of resistant organisms.

e. Prior to surgical procedures, the gingival tissues should be disinfected with antiseptics such as 1 to 5 per cent topical iodine.[3]

f. Regular recall appointments emphasizing oral hygiene and periodontal maintenance are extremely important for these individuals.

g. *If there is any question about the need for antibiotic coverage for the prophylaxis of subacute bacterial endocarditis, it is better to err on the side of safety.*[51]

Radiotherapy

Postirradiation morbidity manifested as osteoradionecrosis occurs in 5 to 10 per cent of patients irradiated for head or neck carcinoma.[35] Osseous healing may progress slowly or not at all. A decreased vascular supply, along with damaged and diminished numbers of osteocytes and osteoblasts, contribute to this painful, debilitating, pathologic response. Any trauma or infection may lead to osteoradionecrosis including extractions or periodontal disease that exacerbates into abscesses. The teeth also become somewhat brittle after full-course radiation therapy to the head or neck.[11, 43] For these reasons, *postirradiation periodontal care should be limited to routine scaling and root planing, oral hygiene reinforcement, and fluoride treatments.* Ultrasonic instrumentation is not recommended. Periodontal surgical procedures that could expose osseous structures should *not* be performed, especially on the mandible. *Periodontal care should remain conservative for the duration of the patient's life because radiation effects are cumulative.*

Diabetes

Diabetic patients require special precautions prior to periodontal therapy. The following is an outline of periodontal therapy for diabetics with respect to the amount of glucose intolerance and the degree of disease control.

Periodontal treatment in the uncontrolled diabetic is contraindicated.

If a patient is suspected to be diabetic, the following procedures should be performed:

1. Physician consultation.

2. Analysis of laboratory tests for fasting blood glucose, postprandial blood glucose, glucose tolerance test, and urinary glucose.

3. Rule out the possibility of acute orofacial infection, or severe dental infection because insulin and glucose requirements are altered in these cases. Only antibiotic and analgesic care should be administered until a complete physical examination is performed and diabetic control is attained. If emergency periodontal treatment is required, antibiotic coverage is required prior to incision and drainage of abscesses. The physician should monitor insulin requirements.

If the patient is a "brittle" diabetic, one whose disease is difficult to control, treatment of periodontal disease may reduce insulin requirements; therefore optimal periodontal health is a necessity. Glucose levels should be monitored, and periodontal treatment should be performed only when the patient is in a well-controlled state. Prophylactic antibiotics, started 2 days preoperatively and continued through the immediate postoperative therapy, should be administered. Penicillin is the drug of choice. Periodontal recall maintenance appointments at frequent intervals are important for periodontitis and diabetes stabilization. The clinician must also be able to recognize the signs of an oncoming diabetic coma or insulin reaction.

The well-controlled diabetic may be treated as an ordinary patient.[23] *However, there are guidelines that should be followed to ensure diabetes control:*

1. Phase I therapy: Make certain that prescribed insulin and meals have been taken. Morning appointments after breakfast usually provide optimal insulin levels.
2. Phase II therapy:
   a. There is no agreement on medical management before and after periodontal therapy. Individual physician consultation is a prerequisite. If general anesthesia, intravenous, or surgical procedures are performed that alter the patient's ability to maintain a normal caloric intake, postoperative insulin doses must be altered.
   b. Tissues should be handled atraumatically and appointments should be short.
   c. Endogenous epinephrine may increase insulin requirements; therefore, anxious patients may require preoperative sedation. The anesthetic should contain epinephrine in doses no greater than 1:100,000.
   d. Schedule morning appointments.
   e. Diet recommendations that enable the patient to maintain a proper glucose balance should be given.
   f. There remains a controversy regarding antibiotic prophylaxis for the prevention of infection. If therapy is extensive, antibiotic coverage is recommended.
3. Maintenance therapy: Frequent recall appointments and fastidious oral home care are required. Studies indicate that controlled diabetics and patients without diabetes have similar therapeutic responses.

Pregnancy

The aim of periodontal therapy for the pregnant woman is to minimize the potentially exaggerated inflammatory response related to hormonal alterations. *Meticulous plaque control, scaling, root planing, and polishing should be the only nonemergency periodontal procedures performed.*

The second trimester is the safest time in which treatment may be performed. However, long, stressful appointments and periodontal surgery should be waived until postpartum.

Because of "supine hypotensive syndrome" that occurs during the third trimester, decreased blood pressure, syncope, and loss of consciousness may occur as a result of uterine pressure upon the inferior vena cava. Appointments should be short, and the patient should be allowed to change positions frequently. Fully reclined positions should be avoided. Other precautions during pregnancy relate to the potential toxic or teratogenic effects of therapy on the fetus. No medications should be prescribed or radiographs taken unless there is an emergency situation.

Bleeding Disorders

Patients with a history of bleeding problems caused by disease or drugs should be managed to minimize risks. Coagulation disorders, including those related to aspirin therapy, and leukemia and agranulocytosis will be described.

Coagulation Disorders

Periodontal care for patients on anticoagulation therapy should be altered, depending on the medication utilized to reduce intravascular clotting. Drugs that perform this function include heparin, bishydroxycoumarin (dicumarol), sodium warfarin (Coumadin), phenindione derivatives, cyclocumarol, ethyl biscoumacetate, and aspirin.

Periodontal treatment should be altered as follows:

1. Physician consultation to determine the nature of the underlying medical problem and the degree of required anticoagulation (the general therapeutic range is a prothrombin time between 1.5 and 3.0 times normal).
2. Periodontal scaling, surgery, and extractions require a prothrombin time <1.5 times normal (25 to 30 per cent of normal).

a. The physician should be consulted about discontinuing or reducing the anticoagulant dosage to achieve the desired prothrombin time.

b. Changes in prothrombin time are not apparent until 2 to 3 days after changing dosages.

c. A prothrombin time measurement is required on the day of the procedure. If it is >1.5 times normal, cancel the procedure and reschedule it for 1 to 3 days later. Prothrombin time should be remeasured on the day of treatment.

3. After scaling and curettage, the patient should not be dismissed until bleeding has stopped.

4. It is preferable to perform periodontal surgery in a hospital, but small segments of the mouth may be treated in the dental office if adequate precautions are taken.

5. Do not perform scaling or periodontal surgery if the patient has an acute infection.

6. The patient should return in 3 to 5 days to determine whether healing is normal; if so, the physician should resume the patient's anticoagulation therapy.

Aspirin Therapy. Individuals on aspirin therapy should be screened for bleeding time and partial thromboplastin time. Salicylates have been known to exert a Coumadin-like effect and interfere with normal platelet function in patients on long-term and high-dose therapy. Aspirin should not be prescribed for patients who are known to be receiving anticoagulation therapy or who are known to have bleeding tendencies.

Leukemia

The alterations in periodontal treatment for leukemic patients are based on their enhanced susceptibility to infection, bleeding tendency, and the effects of chemotherapy. Close cooperation with the physician is imperative in these cases.

Agranulocytosis

Patients with agranulocytosis (cyclic neutropenia and granulocytopenia) are more susceptible to infection than unaffected subjects. There is a reduction in the total white blood cell count and a reduction or elimination of granular leukocytes. The periodontal response to inflammation is exaggerated. Treatment should be performed only during remission of the disease and should be conservative. Scaling, root planing, and oral hygiene instruction should be carefully performed under antibiotic prophylaxis.

Infectious Diseases

Rarely does one contract or transfer an infectious disease if necessary precautions are taken. It is the undiagnosed, untreated patient who provides an incomplete medical history who is a potential hazard to the doctor, the staff, and other patients. This section covers several infectious diseases of interest to dental practitioners.

Hepatitis

Hepatitis presents three clinically similar diseases (A; B; and non-A, non-B), that differ in virology, epidemiology, and precautions to be taken. Because up to 75 per cent of individuals infected with hepatitis are undiagnosed, the clinician must be able to screen for and recognize the signs and symptoms of hepatitis. High-risk patients are renal dialysis patients, hospital personnel, blood bank personnel, mortuary workers, homosexuals, obstetrics and gynecology personnel, immunosuppressed patients, drug users, and institutionalized patients. Because 10 to 15 per cent of hepatitis B patients may have chronic forms of the disease, patients who report past histories of hepatitis should be carefully screened.

The framework for treating patients with hepatitis follows:

I. Diagnosis of history of hepatitis or active hepatitis.

A. If the disease is active, only emergency care should be provided.

B. Past history of hepatitis.

1. Type A. Only emergency procedures should be performed if the disease is active. If the patient has recovered, treatment is routine.

2. Type B.

a. Only emergency treatment should be performed if the disease is active and acute.

b. If the patient has recovered, consult with the physician and ascertain hepatitis B antigen (HB_sAg) and hepatitis B antibody (anti-HB_s) determinations.

(1) If HB_sAg-, the patient may be treated routinely.

(2) If the tests are negative but you are highly suspicious that HB virus is present, order another anti-HB_s determination.

(3) If HB_sAg+, the patient is probably infective; the degree of infectivity is measured by an HB_eAg determination.

(4) If anti-HB_s+, the patient may be treated routinely.

II. Disinfection and sterilization procedures.

A. All personnel in clinical contact with the patient should wear masks, gloves, and glasses (or goggles); for surgical situations, disposable gowns should be worn. All should practice aseptic technique.

B. All instruments should be placed on sheets of aluminum foil.

C. All disposable items (gauzes, floss, saliva ejectors, masks, gowns, gloves, and aluminum foil) should be placed in one lined wastebasket.

D. Minimize aerosol production by not using ultrasonic scalers, air syringes, or high-speed handpieces. Saliva is a distillate of the virus.

E. When the procedure is completed, all equipment, including handpieces, should be scrubbed and sterilized.

F. The dental chair and unit should be wiped down with dilute hypochlorite.

G. Use as many disposable covers as possible; aluminum foil may be used for covering light handles, drawer handles, and bracket trays. Headrest covers should also be used.

H. All disposable items should be gathered, bagged in plastic, tied, labeled, and removed for proper disposal.

If you are exposed to a known HB_sAg+ patient, the currently available method of secondary prevention is immune globulin. Hepatitis B immune globulin (0.05 to 0.07 ml/kg of body weight) is administered within 7 days of exposure, and a second dose is given 25 to 30 days later. Immune serum globulin is effective in preventing hepatitis A if given within 2 weeks of exposure. A vaccine of hepatitis B surface antigen is available for immunization in three doses over a 6-month span. It is felt to be effective for 5 years and is indicated for the high-risk population.

Sexually Transmitted Diseases

The Public Health Service has categorized three groups of sexually transmitted diseases: syphilis, gonorrhea, and herpes. Those with active disease should receive emergency care only. Prophylactic measures as listed under hepatitis should be followed. Remember that oral lesions of primary and secondary syphilis, gonorrhea, and herpes are *infectious*. Patients found to be free of disease may receive routine periodontal therapy. If one finds lesions or symptomatology suggestive of syphilis or gonorrhea, the patient should be referred for medical evaluation. The patient with herpetic lesions may receive treatment when the lesions resolve. One should, however, take precautionary measures if a history of recurrent lesions is given.

Currently there is great concern about treating patients with acquired immune deficiency syndrome (AIDS). At this time there are no accepted standards for treating these patients. Because this syndrome is transmitted through blood serum and is highly infectious, dental clinicians should seek the most recent information about treatment precautions. The local Public Health Service, the U.S. Center for Disease Control in Atlanta, Georgia, and the local Dental Society are the best sources of current information.

References

1. Alfano, M. C.: Controversies, perspectives and clinical implications of nutrition in periodontal disease. Dent. Clin. North Am., 20:519, 1976.
2. American Heart Association Committee Report: prevention of bacterial endocarditis. Circulation, 56:139A, 1977.
3. Brown, A. A.: Prevention of bacterial endocarditis. Ontario Dent., 54:14, 1977.
4. Burkett, L. W.: Oral Medicine. 6th ed. Philadelphia, J. B. Lippincott Company, 1971.
5. Burket, L. W., and Burn, G. G.: Bacteremia following dental extraction. Demonstration of source of bacteria by means of a nonpathogen. J. Dent. Res., 16:521, 1937.
6. Burwasser, P., and Hill, T. J.: The effect of hard and soft diets on the gingival tissues of dogs. J. Dent. Res., 18:389, 1939.
7. Egelberg, J.: Local effect of diet on plaque formation and development of gingivitis in dogs. I. Effect of hard and soft diets. Odont. Revy, 16:31, 1965.
8. Elliott, S. D.: Bacteremia and oral sepsis. Proc. R. Soc. Med., 32:747, 1939.

9. Falace, D. A., and Ferguson, T. W.: Bacterial endocarditis: survey of patients treated between 1963 and 1975. Oral Surg., *42*:189, 1976.
10. Fish, E. W., and MacLean, L.: Distribution of oral streptococci in the tissues. Br. Dent. J., *61*:336, 1936.
11. Frank, R. M., Herdly, J., and Philippe, E.: Acquired dental defects and salivary gland lesions after irradiation for carcinoma. J. Am. Dent. Assoc., *70*:868, 1965.
12. Friedman, L. A.: Horizontal tooth mobility and the menstrual cycle. J. Periodont. Res., *7*:125, 1972.
13. Glavind, L., Lund, B., and Löe, H.: The relationship between periodontal state and diabetes duration, insulin dosage and retinal changes. J. Periodontol., *39*:341, 1968.
14. Hodges, R. E., Baker, E. M., Hood, J., et al.: Experimental scurvy in man. Am. J. Clin. Nutr., *22*:535, 1969.
15. Holm-Pederson, P., and Löe, H.: Flow of gingival exudate as related to menstruation and pregnancy. J. Periodont. Res., *2*:13, 1967.
16. Hugoson, A.: Gingival inflammation and female sex hormones. A clinical investigation of pregnant women and experimental studies in dogs. J. Periodontol. Res., *5*(Suppl.), 1970.
17. Kalkwarf, K. L.: Effect of oral contraceptive therapy on gingival inflammation in humans. J. Periodontol., *49*:560, 1978.
18. Kaplan, E. L., and Taranta, A. V. (eds.): Infective Endocarditis: An American Heart Association Symposium. Dallas, Am. Heart Assoc. Monograph Series, 52, 1977.
19. Kimura, T.: An epidemiological study of hypertension. Clin. Sci. Mol. Med., *43*:103, 1974.
20. Knight, G. M., and Wade, A. B.: The effects of hormonal contraceptives on the human periodontium. J. Periodont. Res., *9*:18, 1974.
21. Lindhe, J., and Wicen, P. O.: The effects on the gingivae of chewing fibrous foods. J. Periodont. Res., *4*:193, 1969.
22. Little, J. W.: Management of the patient with a history of rheumatic fever in dental practice. J. Oral Med., *33*:47, 1978.
23. Little, J. W., and Falace, D. A.: Dental Management of the Medically Compromised Patient. St. Louis, C. V. Mosby Company, 1980.
24. Löe, H.: Periodontal changes in pregnancy. J. Periodontol. *36*:209, 1965.
25. Malamed, S. F.: Medical Emergencies in the Dental Office. St. Louis, C. V. Mosby Company, 1978.
26. McCarthy, T. M.: Emergencies in Dental Practice. 3rd ed. Philadelphia, W. B. Saunders Company, 1979.
27. Mohamed, A. H., Waterhouse, J. P., and Friederici, H. H.: The microvasculature of the rat gingiva as affected by progesterone: an ultrastructural study. J. Periodontol., *45*:50, 1974.
28. Moser, M., et al.: Report of the Joint National Committee on Detection, Evaluation, and Treatment of High Blood Pressure. J.A.M.A., *237*:255, 1977.
29. Murray, M., and Moosnick, F.: Incidence of bacteremia in patients with dental disease. J. Lab. Clin. Med., *26*:801, 1941.
30. Okell, C. C., and Elliott, S. D.: Bacteremia and oral sepsis. Lancet, *2*:869, 1935.
31. Nyman, S.: Studies on the influence of estradiol and progesterone on granulation tissue. J. Periodont. Res., *7*(suppl.), 1971.
32. Peart, W. S.: Arterial Hypertension. *In* Beeson, P. B., and McDermott, W. (eds.): Textbook of Medicine. 14th ed. Philadelphia, W. B. Saunders Company, 1975, pp. 981–992.
33. Perry, D. A.: Oral contraceptives and periodontal health. J. Western Soc. Periodontol., *29*:72, 1981.
34. Prout, R. E. S., and Hopps, R. M.: A relationship between human oral bacteria and the menstrual cycle. J. Periodontol., *41*:98, 1970.
35. Rankow, R. M., and Weissman, B.: Osteoradionecrosis of the mandible. Ann. Otol. Rhinol. Laryngol., *80*:603, 1971.
36. Robbins, S. L., Cotran, R. S., Kumar, V.: Pathologic Basis of Disease, 3rd ed. Philadelphia, W. B. Saunders Co., 1984.
37. Rosenberg, E. H., and Guralnick, W. C.: Hyperparathyroidism. Oral Surg., *15*(Suppl. 2):84, 1962.
38. Rudy, A., and Cohen, M. M.: The oral aspects of diabetes mellitus. N. Engl. J. Med., *219*:503, 1938.
39. Russel, R. P.: Systemic hypertension. *In* Harvey, A. (ed.): Osler's Principles and Practice of Medicine. 19th ed. New York, Appleton-Century-Crofts, 1976, pp. 370–392.
40. Russell, A. L.: International nutrition surveys: a summary of preliminary dental findings. J. Dent. Res., *42*:233, 1963.
41. Saglie, R., Newman, M. S., Carranza, F. A., Jr., and Pattison, G. L.: Bacterial invasion of gingival tissue in advanced periodontitis in humans. J. Periodontol., *53*:217, 1982.
42. Scopp, I. W.: An overview of the heart patient in dental practice. N.Y. J. Dent., *49*:48, 1979.
43. Shannon, I. L., Westcott, W. B., Starcke, E. N., and Mira, J.: Laboratory study of cobalt-60 irradiated human dental enamel. J. Oral Med., *33*:23, 1978.
44. Silverman, S., Gordan, G., Grant, T., Steinbach, H., Eisenberg, E., and Manson, R.: The dental structures in primary hyperparathyroidism. Oral Surg., *15*:426, 1962.
45. Stortebecker, T. P.: Dental infectious foci and diseases of the nervous system. Acta Psychiatr. Neurol. Scand., *36*(Suppl. 157), 1961.
46. Strock, M. S.: The mouth in hyperparathyroidism. N. Engl. J. Med. *224*:1019, 1945.
47. Sylvan, S. L., et al.: Bacterial endocarditis—changing concepts in dental management. J. Hosp. Dent., *12*:138, 1978.
48. Sznajder, N., Carraro, J. J., Rugna, S., and Sereday, M.: Periodontal findings in diabetic and nondiabetic patients. J. Periodontol., *49*:445, 1978.
49. Thalen, H. J., and Meere, C. C. (eds.): Fundamentals of Cardiac Pacing. Boston, Nyhoff Publishers, 1979.
50. Therapeutics Advisory Committee: Prevention of infective endocarditis associated with dental treatment and dental disease: report of the committee. Aust. Dent. J., *25*:51, 1980.
51. Trefez, B. R.: SBE prophylaxis reconsidered: rationale, questions, answers. Dent. Rev., *18*:7, 1978.
52. Wilcox, C. E., and Everett, F.: Friction on the teeth and the gingiva during mastication. J. Am. Dent. Assoc., *66*:5, 1963.
53. Wolbach, S. B., and Bessey, O. A.: Tissue changes in vitamin deficiencies. Physiol. Rev., *22*:233, 1942.
54. Woolfe, S. N., Hume, W. R., and Kenney, E. B.: Ascorbic acid and periodontal disease: a review of the literature. J. Western Soc. Periodontol., *28*:44, 1980.

Chapter 12

Periodontal Emergencies

The treatment of acute gingival disease entails the alleviation of the acute symptoms and the elimination of all other periodontal disease, chronic as well as acute, throughout the oral cavity. *Treatment is not complete so long as periodontal pathology or factors capable of causing it are still present.*

ACUTE NECROTIZING ULCERATIVE GINGIVITIS

Acute necrotizing ulcerative gingivitis can occur in mouths free of gingival involvement or superimposed on underlying chronic gingival disease. *The simplest part of clinical treatment is the alleviation of the acute symptoms; correction of the underlying chronic gingival disease requires more comprehensive procedures.*

At the *first visit* the clinician should obtain a general impression of the patient's background, including information regarding recent illness, living conditions, dietary background, type of employment, hours of rest, and mental stress. Observe the patient's general appearance, apparent nutritional status, and responsiveness or lassitude, and *take the patient's temperature.* Palpate the submaxillary and submental areas to detect enlarged lymph glands.

Examine the oral cavity for the "characteristic lesions" of acute necrotizing ulcerative gingivitis, their distribution, and the possible involvement of the oropharyngeal region.

Evaluate the patient's oral hygiene; check for the presence of pericoronal flaps, periodontal pockets, and local irritants.

Question the patient regarding the history of previous occurrences of the acute disease and its onset and duration. Determine if the recurrences were associated with specific factors such as menstruation, particular foods, exhaustion, or mental stress. Inquire about treatment received and the patient's impression of its effectiveness.

After the diagnosis has been established, the patient is treated as either "nonambulatory" or "ambulatory," based upon the following criteria:

Nonambulatory patients are those with symptoms of generalized toxicity, high fever, malaise, and lassitude. Bed rest may be necessary, and extensive office treatment should be postponed until the systemic symptoms subside.

Ambulatory patients may have localized adenopathy and slightly elevated temperatures but there should be no serious systemic complications.

Treatment for Nonambulatory Patients

Day One

On the first day, local treatment is limited to gently removing the necrotic pseudomembrane with a pellet of cotton saturated with hydrogen peroxide. The patient should be

173

advised to rest in bed and to rinse the mouth every 2 hours with a glassful of an equal mixture of warm water and 3 per cent hydrogen peroxide. If systemic antibiotics are needed, penicillin is usually administered. Erythromycin or metronidazole, which is extensively used in Europe, may also be used. The patient should return to the office after 24 hours.

Day Two

If the patient's condition has improved, proceed to the treatment for ambulatory patients. If there is no improvement at the end of 24 hours, the oral condition, the possibility of oropharyngeal involvement, and the patient's temperature should be checked. Swab the involved gingiva again with hydrogen peroxide, and repeat the previous instructions. Have the patient return after 24 hours.

Day Three

In most instances, the patient is improved by this time and is started on the treatment for ambulatory patients. If not, the patient's physician should be consulted (Fig. 12–1).

Treatment for Ambulatory Patients

Day One

Treatment is confined to the acutely involved areas, which are isolated with cotton rolls and dried. A topical anesthetic is applied, and after 2 or 3 minutes the areas are gently swabbed with cotton pellets to remove the pseudomembrane and nonattached surface debris. Each cotton pellet is used in a small area and is then discarded; sweeping motions over large areas with a single pellet are not recommended. Cleanse the area with warm water and remove the superficial calculus if the procedure can be tolerated. *Ultrasonic scalers are very useful for this purpose.*

Deep scaling and curettage are contraindicated at this time because of the possibility of extending the infection into deeper tissues and also of causing a bacteremia. Unless an emergency exists, procedures such as extractions or periodontal surgery should be postponed until the patient has been symptom-free for a period of 4 weeks, in order to minimize the likelihood of exacerbation of the acute symptoms.

The patient should be advised of the extent of the total treatment the condition requires and warned that treatment is not complete when the pain stops. He or she should be informed of the presence of chronic gingival and periodontal disease which must be eliminated in order to prevent recurrence of the acute symptoms.

The patient should be told to avoid alcohol, tobacco, and condiments, and to return in 24 hours. Heat and the products of tobacco are particularly irritating to the inflamed tissue and also retard healing.

Rinsing with an equal mixture of 3 per cent

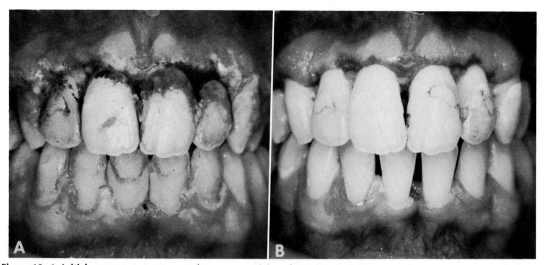

Figure 12–1. Initial response to treatment of acute necrotizing ulcerative gingivitis. *A,* Severe acute necrotizing ulcerative gingivitis. *B,* Third day. There is still some erythema, but the condition is markedly improved.

hydrogen peroxide and warm water every 2 hours is recommended. Usual physical activities may be pursued, but excessive physical exertion and prolonged exposure to the sun should be avoided. Toothbrushing should be confined to the removal of surface debris with a bland dentifrice; zealous brushing will be painful. Dental floss, interdental cleaners, and water irrigation under medium pressure are also suggested. These patients are easily dehydrated so consumption of copious amounts of fluids should be encouraged.

Day Two

The patient's condition has usually improved after one day; the pain is diminished or no longer present. The gingival margins of the involved areas are erythematous, but without a superficial pseudomembrane.

The procedures performed on Day One are repeated. Shrinkage of the gingiva may expose previously covered calculus, which may be removed by gentle scaling of the teeth. The instructions to the patient are the same as on Day One. If there have been undesirable effects from the hydrogen peroxide, warm water alone should be used for rinsing.

Day Three

The patient should be essentially symptom-free. There is still some erythema in the involved areas, and the gingiva may be slightly painful on tactile stimulation. Scaling and curettage are repeated. The patient is instructed in plaque control procedures that are essential for the success of the treatment and the maintenance of periodontal health. The hydrogen peroxide rinses are discontinued.

Day Four

Tooth surfaces in the involved areas are scaled and smoothed, and plaque control by the patient is checked and corrected.

Day Five

Unfortunately, treatment is often stopped at this time because the acute condition has subsided, but this is when comprehensive treatment of the patient's chronic periodontal problem should start. Appointments should be scheduled for the treatment of chronic gingivitis, periodontal pockets, *pericoronal flaps, and for the elimination of all forms of local irritation, plus necessary occlusal adjustment.*

Patients without gingival disease other than the treated acute involvement are dismissed for 1 week. If the condition is satisfactory following that period of time, the patient should be recalled in 1 month, examined, treated if necessary, and the schedule for subsequent recall visits determined.

Drug Treatment

A large variety of drugs have been used topically in the treatment of acute necrotizing ulcerative gingivitis.[2] *Topical drug therapy is only an adjunctive measure in the treatment of this disease; no drug, when used alone, can be considered complete therapy.*

Escharotic drugs such as phenol, silver nitrate, and chromic acid should not be used. They are necrotizing agents that alleviate the painful symptoms by destroying the nerve endings in the gingiva. They also destroy the young cells necessary for repair and delay healing. Their repeated use results in the loss of gingival tissue, which cannot be restored when the disease subsides.[3]

Antibiotics are administered systemically in patients with toxic systemic complications or local adenopathy but are not recommended for topical use because of the risk of sensitization. Phenoxymethylpenicillin (penicillin V) or metronidazole are the drugs of choice.

In addition to systemic antibiotics, supportive treatment consists of copious fluid consumption and analgesics for relief of pain. Bed rest is necessary for patients with toxic systemic complications such as high fever, malaise, anorexia, and general debility.

Gingival Changes with Healing

The characteristic lesions of acute necrotizing ulcerative gingivitis undergo the following changes in the course of healing in response to treatment:

1. Removal of the surface pseudomembrane exposes the underlying red, hemorrhagic, crater-like depressions in the gingiva.

2. Subsequently, the bulk and redness of the crater margins are reduced, but the surface remains shiny.

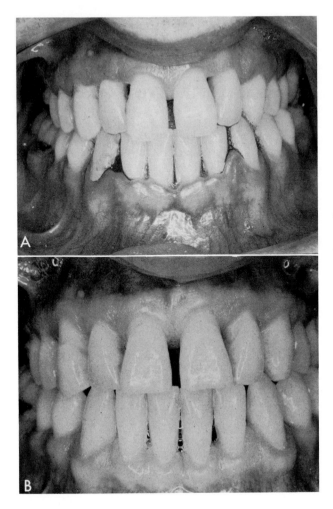

Figure 12–2. Physiologic contour and reattachment of gingiva following treatment of acute necrotizing ulcerative gingivitis. *A,* Acute necrotizing ulcerative gingivitis showing the characteristic punched-out eroded gingival margin with surface pseudomembrane. *B,* After treatment. Note the restoration of physiologic gingival contour and reattachment of the gingiva to the surfaces of the mandibular teeth, which had been exposed by the disease.

3. This is followed by the early signs of the restoration of normal gingival contour and color.

4. In the final stage, the normal gingival color, consistency, surface texture, and contour are restored. Portions of the root exposed by the acute disease are covered by healthy gingiva (Fig. 12–2).

When the *menstrual period* occurs in the course of treatment, there is a tendency toward exacerbation of the acute signs and symptoms, giving the appearance of a relapse. Female patients should be informed of this possibility and spared any unnecessary anxiety regarding this oral condition.

Even in cases of severe gingival necrosis, healing ordinarily leads to restoration of the normal gingival contour. However, shelf-like gingival margins that favor the retention of food and the recurrence of gingival inflam-

mation sometimes result. This can be corrected by surgical reshaping of the gingiva.

Sequelae of Treatment

Persistent or "Nonresponsive" Cases

If it has been necessary to change from drug to drug in an effort to relieve a "stubborn" case of acute necrotizing ulcerative gingivitis, something is wrong with the overall treatment regimen, which is not likely to be corrected by changing drugs. *When this problem occurs the following measures should be taken:*

1. *All local drug therapy should be discontinued so that the condition may be studied in an uncomplicated state.*

2. Careful differential diagnosis should be

made to rule out diseases that resemble acute necrotizing ulcerative gingivitis.

3. A search should be made for contributing local and systemic etiologic factors that may have been overlooked.

4. Special attention must be given to instructing the patient in plaque control before undertaking comprehensive local treatment.

Recurrent Disease

The following factors should be explored in patients with recurrent acute necrotizing ulcerative gingivitis:

Inadequate Local Therapy. Too often treatment is discontinued when the symptoms have subsided, without eliminating the chronic gingival disease and periodontal pockets which remain after the superficial acute condition is relieved. Persistent chronic inflammation causes degenerative changes that predispose the gingiva to recurrence of acute involvement.

Pericoronal Flap. Recurrent acute involvement in the mandibular anterior area is often associated with persistent pericoronal inflammation arising from difficult eruption of third molars. The anterior involvement is less likely to recur after the third molar situation is corrected.

Anterior Overbite. Marked overbite is often a contributing factor in the recurrence of disease in the anterior region. When the incisal edges of the maxillary teeth impinge upon the labial gingiva or the mandibular teeth strike the palatal gingiva, the resultant tissue injury predisposes the gingiva to recurrent acute disease. Less severe overbite produces food impaction and gingival trauma. Correction of the overbite is necessary for the complete treatment of acute necrotizing ulcerative gingivitis.

Inadequate Plaque Control and Heavy Use of Tobacco. These are common causes of recurrent disease.

ACUTE PERICORONITIS

Pericoronitis is the acute and painful inflammation of flaps of gingiva over partially erupted teeth, usually the third molars.[1]

Treatment

The treatment of pericoronitis depends on the severity of the inflammation, the systemic complications, and the advisability of retaining the involved tooth. All pericoronal flaps should be viewed with suspicion. *Persistent symptom-free pericoronal flaps should be removed as a preventive measure against subsequent acute involvement.* If a patient presents with painful, severely involved acute pericoronitis, the following treatment is recommended.

Day One

The extent and severity of the involvement of adjacent structures and toxic systemic complications should be determined. The area should be gently flushed with warm water to remove superficial debris and surface exudate, and a topical anesthetic should be applied. The flap should be gently elevated from the tooth with a scaler, the underlying debris removed, and the area flushed with warm water. Extensive curettage or surgical procedures are contraindicated at the initial visit. Instructions to the patient should include hourly rinses with warm saline solution, rest, and copious fluid intake. Systemic antibiotics should be administered if fever or other general symptoms are present. The patient should return in 24 hours.

Day Two

After 24 hours, the patient's condition is usually markedly improved. The flap should be gently separated from the tooth and the area flushed with warm water. The patient should continue with the instructions of the previous day and to return in 24 hours.

Day Three

At this time it is necessary to determine whether the tooth is to be retained or extracted, or if the pericoronal flap should be removed (Fig. 12–3). If the decision is to remove the flap, *it is necessary to remove the tissue distal to the tooth as well as the flap on the occlusal surface.* Incising only the occlusal portion of the flap will leave a deep distal pocket that invites recurrence of acute pericoronal involvement.

ACUTE HERPETIC GINGIVOSTOMATITIS

Acute herpetic gingivostomatitis is the initial reaction of the oral tissues to inoculation

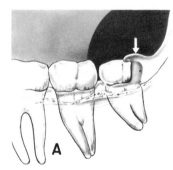

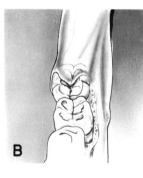

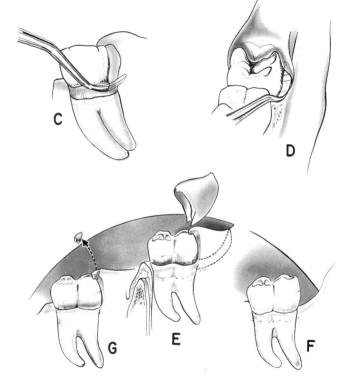

Figure 12–3. Treatment of acute periocoronitis. *A,* Inflamed periocoronal flap *(arrow)* in relation to the mandibular third molar. *B,* Anterior view of third molar and flap. *C,* Lateral view with scaler in position to gently remove debris under flap. *D,* Anterior view of scaler in position. *E,* Removal of section of the gingiva distal to the third molar, after the acute symptoms subside. The line of incision is indicated by the broken line. *F,* Appearance of the healed area. *G,* Incorrect removal of the tip of the flap, permitting deep pocket to remain distal to the molar.

with herpes type 1 virus. The treatment of acute herpetic gingivostomatitis consists of palliative measures to make the patient comfortable until the disease has run its course in 7 to 10 days.

Plaque, food debris, and superficial calculus should be removed to reduce gingival inflammation, which can complicate the acute herpetic involvement. Extensive periodontal therapy should be postponed until the acute symptoms subside in order to avoid the possibility of exacerbation of the patient or inoculation of the clinician. Painful her-

petic infection of clinicians' fingers have been reported.[4]

Relief of pain to enable the patient to eat comfortably is obtained with dyclonine hydrochloride (Dyclone), a topical anesthetic mouthwash, which is available in a 0.5 per cent solution that may be diluted 1:1 with water. It is held in the mouth for 1 or 2 minutes and swished around to produce an anesthetic effect that lasts for 40 minutes. It is helpful when used before meals but may be used more often without toxic effects.

Supportive measures include copious fluid

intake and systemic antibiotic therapy if toxic systemic complications arise. For pain relief, 10 grains of aspirin every 3 hours may be recommended for adults, with smaller doses for children.

PERIODONTAL ABSCESSES

Periodontal abscesses may be acute or chronic. Acute abscesses are painful, edematous, red, shiny ovoid elevations of the gingival margin and/or attached gingiva. After their purulent content is partially exuded, they become chronic. Chronic abscesses may produce dull pain and may undergo acute exacerbation.

Acute Abscesses

The purpose of treatment of an acute abscess is *to alleviate the pain, to control the spread of infection, and to establish drainage.* The patient's general systemic response should be evaluated and the temperature taken. Drainage is established through the pocket or by means of an incision from the outer surface. The former method is preferable.

Drainage Through the Pocket

After application of a topical or local anesthetic, a flat instrument or a probe is carefully introduced into the pocket in an attempt to distend the pocket wall. A curette can then be used gently to penetrate the tissue and establish drainage. When drainage cannot be easily established via the pocket or when the abscess can be seen pointing through the gingiva, an external incision is indicated.

Drainage Through External Incision

The abscess should be isolated with gauze sponges and dried and swabbed with an antiseptic solution, followed by a topical or local anesthetic. Wait 2 or 3 minutes for the anesthetic to become effective; then the abscess is palpated gently to locate the most fluctuant area. A vertical incision is made with a scalpel blade through that part of the lesion, extending from the mucogingival fold to the gingival margin. If the swelling is on the lingual surface, the incision is started just apical to the swelling and extended through the gingival margin. The blade should penetrate to firm tissue to be sure of reaching deep purulent areas. After the initial extravasation of blood and pus, irrigate the area with warm water and gently spread the incision to facilitate draining (Fig. 12–4).

If the tooth is extruded, the occlusion should be adjusted slightly to avoid contact with antagonists. Stabilize the tooth with the index finger to reduce vibration and discomfort. It is often preferable to adjust teeth in the opposing jaw to avoid discomfort.

After the drainage stops, the area should be dried and painted with an antiseptic. Patients without systemic complications should be instructed to rinse hourly with saline solution and to return the next day. Penicillin or other antibiotics are prescribed for patients with elevated temperatures. The patient should be instructed to avoid exertion and to consume copious fluids; and analgesics may be prescribed for pain.

The next day, the swelling will generally be markedly reduced or absent, and the symptoms should have subsided. If acute symptoms persist, the patient should continue the regimen prescribed the previous day and to return in 24 hours. The symptoms invariably disappear by then, and the lesion is ready for surgical correction.

Chronic Abscesses

Chronic abscesses are treated by gingivectomy or flap surgery techniques (see Chapter 15).

Differential Diagnosis Between Types of Abscesses

The following are useful guides in the differential diagnosis between *periodontal* and *periapical* abscesses:

If the tooth is nonvital, the lesion is most likely periapical. Generally, periodontal abscesses do not cause devitalization of teeth. In severe cases the periodontal abscess may extend to the apex and cause pulpal involvement and necrosis.

When the apex and lateral surface of a root are involved by a single lesion that can be probed directly from the gingival margin, it

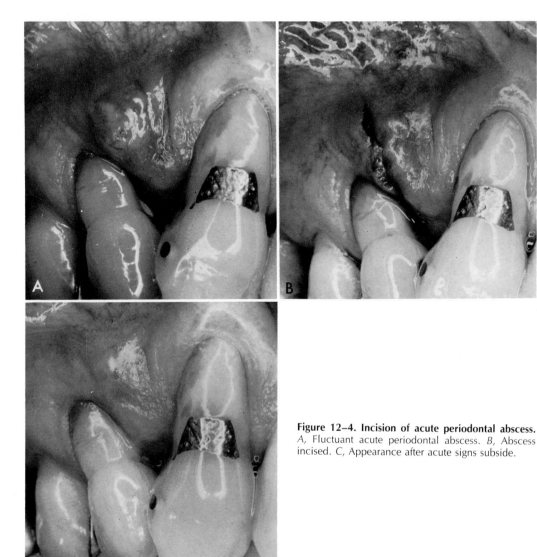

Figure 12–4. Incision of acute periodontal abscess.
A, Fluctuant acute periodontal abscess. B, Abscess incised. C, Appearance after acute signs subside.

is likely to be a periodontal abscess. Rarely will an apical abscess spread along the lateral aspect of the root to the gingiva.

Radiographs are of limited use in differentiating between early periodontal and early periapical abscesses because frequently no radiographic changes are seen. A radiolucency present along the lateral surface of the root suggests the presence of a periodontal abscess, whereas apical rarefaction suggests a periapical abscess. Clinical findings, such as the presence of extensive caries, pocket formation, tooth vitality, and the existence of continuity between the gingival margin and

the abscess area are often of greater diagnostic value than radiographs.

The presence of a fistula on the lateral aspect of the root suggests periodontal rather than apical involvement; a sinus and fistula from a periapical lesion is more likely to be located farther apically. However, sinus and fistula location is not conclusive because in many instances, particularly with children, the sinus from a periapical lesion drains on the side of the root rather than at the apex.

The *periodontal abscess* must also be differentiated from the *gingival abscess*. The principal differences between the two are identified through knowledge of the location and history of the lesions. The gingival abscess is confined to the gingival margin, and it often occurs in previously disease-free mouths. It is usually an acute inflammatory response to foreign material forced into the gingiva. In rare instances it results from infection of an epithelium-lined gingival cyst. The periodontal abscess involves the supporting periodontal tissues and generally occurs in the course of chronic destructive periodontal disease.

References

1. Ash, M. M., Jr., Costich, E. R., and Hayward, J. R.: A study of periodontal hazards of third molars. J. Periodontol., 33:209, 1962.
2. Burket, L. W.: Oral Medicine. 3rd ed. Philadelphia, J. B. Lippincott Company, 1946, p. 53.
3. Glickman, I., and Johannessen, L. B.: The effect of a 6 per cent solution of chromic acid on the gingiva of the albino rata: correlated gross, biomicroscopic, and histologic study. J. Am. Dent. Assoc., 41:674, 1950.
4. Snyder, M. L., Church, D. H., and Rickles, N. H.: Primary herpes infection of right second finger. Oral Surg., 27:598, 1969.

Chapter 13

Phase I Therapy

The first phase of periodontal therapy, commonly called Phase I therapy or initial therapy, is directed at (1) removing all local irritants that may cause gingival inflammation and (2) instructing and motivating the patient in plaque control. In some cases, particularly uncomplicated gingivitis, Phase I therapy is all that is required (Fig. 13–1).

It is a common error to perform this phase of therapy, followed by needed surgical treatment and restorative procedures, and only then to place the patient in the maintenance phase. *The initial phase of therapy should be followed immediately by the maintenance phase; recall appointments should be scheduled and patient maintenance checked at regular intervals.* Periodontal surgical and restorative procedures should be performed while the patient is on a maintenance schedule for the entire mouth.

INITIAL TREATMENT FOR PERIODONTAL DISEASE

Rationale

Initial therapy or *Phase I therapy* is the first therapeutic step in the chronologic sequence of procedures that constitute periodontal treatment. The objective of initial therapy is the reduction or elimination of gingival inflammation; this is achieved by the complete removal of calculus, correction of defective restorations, removal or temporization of carious lesions, and comprehensive plaque control instruction (Fig. 13–2). Phase I therapy also provides the opportunity to evaluate tissue response and patient attitudes toward periodontal care, both of which are crucial to the prognosis of periodontal conditions.

The purpose of Phase I therapy is (1) to reduce

183

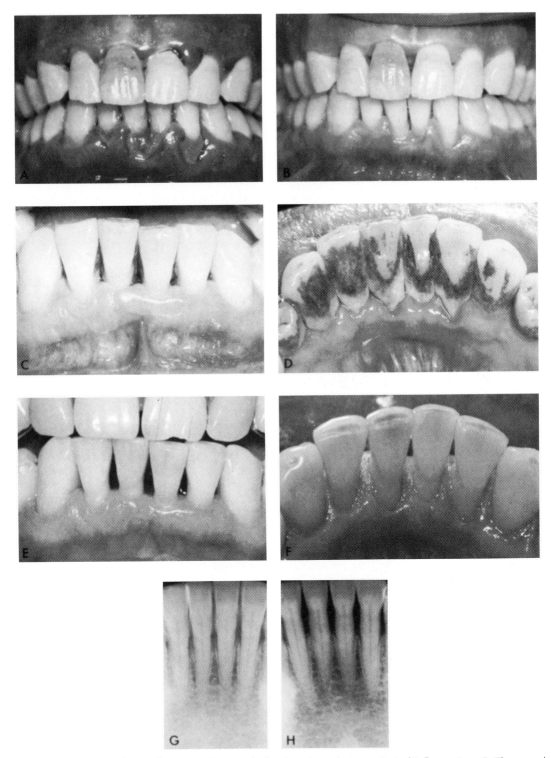

Figure 13–1. Results of Phase I therapy. *A,* Heavy calculus deposits and severe gingival inflammation. *B,* Three weeks after elimination of irritants, gingival healing has resulted. *C–H,* One case before and 1½ years after Phase I therapy. (Courtesy of Dr. Steven Levine.) *C,* and *D,* clinical preoperative view. Note edematous gingival enlargement and abundant calculus. *E* and *F,* Clinical postoperative views after Phase I therapy and maintenance visits. Note excellent gingival contour and color. *G* and *H,* Radiographs taken before and 1½ years after treatment. Note presence of calculus in the preoperative radiograph and the clean root surface seen after treatment. Bone height remained unchanged.

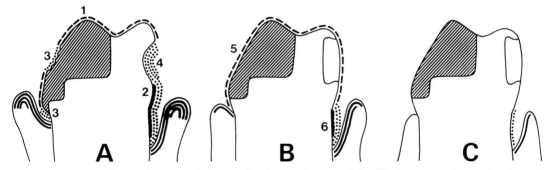

Figure 13–2. Steps in Phase I therapy. *A,* Before starting therapy. Interrupted line (1) shows areas that can be cleaned by the patient. Dotted lines are areas that have to be prepared by the dentist before the patient can clean them; 2, calculus; 3, rough surfaces and overhanging margins of restorations; 4, caries. Parallel lines in the gingiva denote presence and degree of inflammation. *B,* After removal of supragingival calculus, correction of restoration, and removal and obturation of caries, the area that the patient can clean (interrupted line, 5) has been considerably extended. Inflammation (parallel lines in gingiva) is reduced. 6, subgingival calculus still not removed. *C,* After removal of subgingival calculus. Pocket persists and plaque accumulated in it cannot be removed by patient. Surgical pocket elimination may be indicated.

or eliminate gingival inflammation, (2) to eliminate periodontal pockets produced by the edematous enlargement of inflamed gingiva, and (3) to achieve surgical manageability of the gingiva, firm consistency and minimal bleeding.

The specific aim of Phase I therapy is to facilitate daily plaque removal by eliminating rough and irregular contours from the tooth surfaces and establishing suitable plaque control regimens. Phase I therapy is primarily concerned with establishing smooth and regular tooth surfaces as a prerequisite for achieving the goal of effective plaque control. Adequate plaque removal by the patient can be expected only if the tooth surfaces are free of rough deposits or irregular contours and readily accessible for oral hygiene aids.

After careful analysis of a case, the number of appointments needed to complete this phase of treatment is estimated. Patients with only slight amounts of calculus and relatively healthy tissues can be treated completely in one appointment. Many patients will require several appointments. The estimated number of appointments is based on the number of teeth in the mouth, the amount and location of plaque and calculus, and the depth of pockets.

Treatment Planning

Frequently, supragingival and subgingival calculus removal, root planing, comprehensive plaque control instruction, and overhang recontouring are performed in combination

in a series of appointments. In these cases treatment is completed in quadrant or sextant segments, allowing the operator multiple appointments to reinforce or augment oral hygiene instructions and reevaluate areas treated at previous appointments. In these cases, the most severely involved areas should be treated first. At other times, deposits of plaque and calculus are so heavy that the first appointment requires a full mouth scaling and debridement, followed by a series of appointments for more definitive therapy.

Within 3 to 4 weeks substantial reduction or elimination of gingival inflammation usually occurs following removal of calculus, elimination of necrotic cementum, recontouring or planing of irregular tooth surfaces, and institution of plaque control. This healing process is frequently accompanied by transient root sensitivity as well as by marked recession of the gingival margin that may be unesthetic. The patient must be informed in advance of these therapeutic sequelae so as to prevent potential distrust or loss of motivation regarding periodontal therapy. In the following sections, the sequence of treatment is described.

Plaque Control Instruction

Introducing an oral hygiene program to the patient is of high priority in every periodontal treatment plan. Plaque control instructions should begin at the first therapeutic appointment. The patient is taught how to clean all surfaces of the teeth; however, calculus, defective restorations, carious lesions, or necrotic cementum may prevent sufficient access for oral hygiene aids. Patients should not be expected to remove plaque adequately from these areas.

An appropriate toothbrushing technique should be taught at this stage of therapy. Patients should be taught to use dental floss on proximal tooth surfaces even though flossing around sharp edges and coarse surfaces of calculus or overhanging restorations may be somewhat difficult. As Phase I therapy progresses, oral hygiene instruction can be reinforced and additional aids introduced as needed. Chapter 14 is devoted to this topic.

Removal of Calculus and Root Planing

Calculus provides a highly retentive surface for the oral microflora and thus promotes the accumulation of dental plaque (see Chapter 6). Since adequate removal of plaque from calculus surfaces is not feasible with current oral hygiene techniques, calculus must be eliminated entirely in order to facilitate effective plaque control.

In the presence of inflamed, friable gingiva adjacent to deep periodontal pockets, calculus is first dislodged from all supragingival tooth surfaces. Complete interproximal access for scaling instruments is often difficult, especially between incisor teeth with narrow embrasures. In those areas, sharp-pointed sickle scalers rather than round-ended curettes should be used to reach close to the contact zones. Crowding of anterior teeth frequently results in very long, tight contacts and extremely narrow embrasures. This makes access difficult even for sickle scalers.

Subgingival calculus removal, elimination of necrotic cementum, and root planing is then initiated.

Subgingival calculus is removed with curettes (Fig. 13–3). Since these accumulations are much harder and more tenacious than supragingival calculus, subgingival scaling requires considerable force and good control of the working instrument (Fig. 13–4). Inadvertent curettage of the soft periodontal tissues adjacent to the root surface being treated is not uncommon.

It is not enough to eliminate the calculus from the root surface. After subgingival calculus has been completely removed, there may be areas in which the roots feel rough because the cementum has undergone necrotic changes or because heavy instrumentation has produced grooves and scratches in the surfaces. *The root must be planed until it is smooth. Smoothness of the root surface is essential for optimal plaque control and is one of the most reliable clinical signs for diagnosing the absence of calculus or necrotic cementum.*

It is not an objective of this book to present

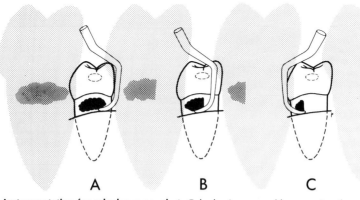

Figure 13–3. Instrumentation for calculus removal. *A,* Calculus is removed by engaging the apical border of deposits with the cutting edge of the scaler; a vertical movement of the instrument will remove the fragment of calculus engaged by the instrument, as seen in the shaded drawing. *B,* The instrument is moved laterally and again engages the apical border of calculus, overlapping to some extent the previous stroke; the shaded drawing shows further removal. *C,* The final portion of the calculus is engaged and removed. Note how in an interdental space the operation is done entering facially and lingually.

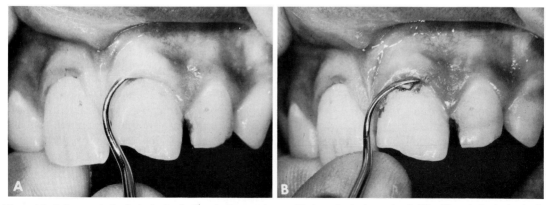

Figure 13–4. Removal of subgingival calculus. *A,* Currette inserted below gingival margin. *B,* Flint-like subgingival calculus removed.

a detailed discussion and analysis of instrumentation procedures. For this the reader is directed to the excellent text by Pattison and Pattison, *Periodontal Instrumentation.*[29]

Manual scaling and root planing are strenuous procedures. Because of this, the applicability of power-driven instruments to these tasks has gained attention. Comparative studies indicate that ultrasonic and rotary scalers can be used safely and effectively in the debridement and planing of periodontally diseased root surfaces, although there is a high risk of tissue damage if they are used improperly.[10, 35]

Scaling invariably leaves the treated tooth, especially the cementum and dentin, with a rough and scratched surface that favors the quick reestablishment of plaque and calculus. Therefore, following calculus removal, the tooth roots must be planed and exposed surfaces polished with abrasive paste. Smooth, polished tooth surfaces are highly conducive to effective plaque control and resist calculus formation considerably better than rough surfaces.[37]

Recontouring of Defective Restorations and Treatment of Carious Lesions

Rough, overcontoured, overhanging, or smooth but subgingivally located restorations and orthodontic appliances are associated with pronounced accumulations of plaque, periodontal inflammation, and loss of alveolar bone and periodontal attachment. Like calculus, these restorations or appliances in-

terfere with efficient plaque control and must be corrected or removed to allow the reduction or elimination of gingival inflammation. Correction of existing restorations is as important as the removal of calculus and should be accomplished during Phase I therapy. *Adequate plaque control by patients on restored teeth is feasible only if the restorations are well contoured and their surfaces are smooth.*

Defective restorations, especially overhanging margins, are detected clinically by moving a fine explorer tip continuously back and forth across the margins. In the presence of overhangs, clicking sounds are produced and definite catches may be felt. Bitewing radiographs may be a helpful in determining the approximate dimensions of proximal overhangs.

Overhanging margins should be eliminated either by replacing the restorations or by correcting the contours of the existing restorations. Recontouring, although often only a temporary measure, can improve the immediate results of Phase I therapy.

Overhanging portions of *amalgam* or *resin* restorations may be removed with scalers, finishing burs, or diamond-coated files mounted on special handpiece attachments that generate reciprocating strokes of high frequency. Scalers are efficient for the gross removal of overhangs from accessible areas, but they leave a relatively rough surface on the restoration that needs to be smoothed with abrasive discs or finishing strips.

Caries in the vicinity of the gingiva interferes with gingival health, even in the absence of adjacent calculus or defective restorations, because it acts as a large reservoir for microorganisms. Definitive or provisional treatment of carious lesions is an integral part of Phase I therapy. Complete removal of the lesions and permanent closure of the cavities are desirable whenever possible, however, temporary restorations are acceptable. The dentist should place them in cases when permanent restorative care is not immediately available to the patient or when the prognosis of the decayed teeth depends upon the result of periodontal therapy.

Tissue Reevaluation

The periodontal tissues must be reexamined by the dentist after 3 or 4 weeks to determine the need for further therapy. Pockets are reprobed and tissue condition reevaluated. Further improvement of the patient's periodontal condition following surgery can be expected only if Phase I therapy has been successfully completed. Therefore, surgical reduction or elimination of periodontal pockets should be attempted only if a patient is exercising effective plaque control and if the periodontal tissues are free of overt inflammation.

TREATMENT OF UNCOMPLICATED GINGIVITIS

Uncomplicated chronic gingivitis is the most common disease of the gingiva. It affects the interdental and marginal gingivae. *It should be detected in its earliest stages and treated as soon as detected* (Fig. 13–5). Usually painless, it is the most common cause of gingival bleeding. Failure to treat it invites destruction of the underlying periodontal tissues and premature tooth loss.

Chronic gingivitis is always caused by local irritation. Systemic conditions may aggravate the inflammation caused by local irritants and should be appropriately managed, but no systemic conditions, by themselves, cause chronic gingivitis.

Treatment

The first step in the treatment of uncomplicated gingivitis is explaining the importance of plaque control and teaching the patient all procedures necessary to achieve it. *This gives the patient a realistic perspective regarding the treatment of gingivitis; it includes something he must do for himself, as well as something the dental clinician does for him.* It also provides an opportunity to demonstrate that plaque control really benefits the gums.

Ideally, at a second appointment the condition of the gums is reviewed with the patient, and improvement is pointed out. The teeth should be stained with disclosing solution and plaque control reinforced. The teeth should be scaled to remove all deposits, and all tooth surfaces polished with an abrasive paste. *Polishing is an important preventive measure against the recurrence of gingivitis because plaque, the most important cause of gingivitis and the initial stage in the formation of calculus, tends to form more readily on rough surfaces.*

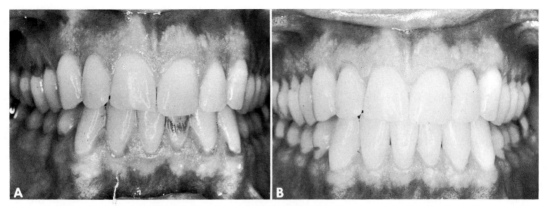

Figure 13–5. Uncomplicated chronic marginal gingivitis. *A,* Before treatment. *B,* After treatment.

Other sources of local irritation, such as overhanging margins, should be identified and eliminated.

At subsequent appointments, the gingivae must be evaluated and plaque control reviewed. Special attention should be given to areas of persistent inflammation; this usually entails rescaling and emphasizing oral hygiene technique in these difficult areas. The patient is then placed on maintenance schedule *with a careful explanation of the reasons for periodic visits and the importance of the care given the mouth in the intervening periods.*

Causes of Failure

The treatment of chronic gingivitis should present no problem. However, if disease persists, there are several likely causes:

1. Failure to adequately remove calculus, often found just beneath the cemento-enamel junction.
2. Failure to polish the tooth surfaces after deposits were removed.
3. Failure to eliminate sources of irritation other than deposits on the teeth, such as food impaction areas.
4. Inadequate plaque control because of insufficient patient instruction or lack of patient cooperation.
5. The tendency to seek a remote systemic etiology for persistent gingivitis caused by overlooked local irritants.
6. Dependence upon vitamins, mouthrinses, and topical application of drugs. *Except for topical anesthetics, drugs serve only as adjuncts in the treatment of chronic gingivitis.*

ANTIMICROBIAL AGENTS IN PERIODONTAL THERAPY

Antimicrobial agents have been used in periodontal therapy since early times.[19, 20, 42] In the last two decades, reports that systemically administered antibiotics were excreted via the saliva and/or the gingival fluid have triggered great interest in the subject.[1, 2] It has been shown in experimental animals that the systemic administration of antibiotics results in changes in the plaque flora, reduces gingivitis, and slows bone loss.[18, 24, 38] In humans, however, the use of antibiotics may present problems, such as the development

of resistant strains of organisms and allergic manifestations.[12]

Antimicrobial agents can be used in patients with periodontitis for the following purposes:

1. In the treatment of systemic complications of the acute periodontal abscess or acute necrotizing ulcerative gingivitis. These topics are covered in Chapter 12.
2. For antibiotic coverage of patients with medical problems in order to prevent systemic complications. This topic is covered in Chapter 11.
3. As a mouthrinse used for plaque control and the prevention of gingivitis. This is discussed in Chapter 14.
4. As an adjunct in the treatment of periodontal disease (to be explained in detail in this chapter).

Uses of Antimicrobial Agents

In conjunction with the pocket treatment, antimicrobial agents may be of importance in the following ways:

1. *Antimicrobials may be used as adjuncts to nonsurgical therapy.* These agents may reach and kill bacteria that cannot be removed by scaling and curettage, such as bacteria that have penetrated into the tissues in advanced periodontitis[31] and localized juvenile periodontitis,[4] and bacteria located on the root surface in inaccessible areas of tortuous furcations or very deep pockets. The use of antimicrobials in conjunction with nonsurgical therapy may reduce or eliminate the indications for periodontal surgery. Antimicrobials may also be useful in increasing the interval between recall maintenance visits. Once bacteria have been removed from the pocket, it takes several weeks before a mature, aggressive plaque can repopulate.[28] The use of antimicrobials during the initial scaling visit or subsequently by the patient may prolong this interval.

2. *Antimicrobials may enhance the success of new attachment and bone regenerating procedures.* The reinfection of the pocket area is probably one of the major factors working against reattachment.[3] The maintenance of a sterile area may favor the new attachment of the tissues and is also likely to improve the chances for success of osseous and nonosseous grafts.

The rationale for the use of antibiotics in the treatment of periodontal disease should be the same as for any infection. The causative microorganism(s) should be identified and the most effective agent selected. Although this appears simple, the difficulty lies primarily in the identification of the *specific etiologic microorganism(s)* rather than those simply *associated* with various periodontal disorders.[6]

According to Gibson,[12] an *ideal* antibiotic for use in the prevention and treatment of periodontal disease should (1) act specifically on periodontal pathogens, (2) not be allergenic or toxic, (3) maintain activity in the oral environment or tissue for long periods, (4) not be in general use for treatment of other diseases, and (5) not be prohibitively expensive.

Antibiotics have been evaluated both systemically and topically as plaque-reducing agents. With some antibiotics the topical approach may be dangerous, since this is more likely to result in the development of hypersensitivity. The systemic route of administration provides bacteriostatic or bactericidal levels of some antibiotics in body fluids, including saliva and crevicular fluid.

The potential usefulness of antimicrobial agents in relation to pocket therapy requires considerably more investigation and development before specific clinical recommendations can be made.

Systemic Administration of Antibiotics

Several systemically administered antibiotics have been investigated for their effects in treating periodontal diseases.

Tetracyclines

Numerous studies have been made of the effect of tetracyclines on clinical and bacteriologic parameters of periodontal disease because these drugs reach a concentration in the gingival fluid 2 to 10 times that in the blood.[14]

Systemic tetracycline reduces plaque and gingival inflammation in dogs[24] and reduces bone loss in dogs[40] and rats.[38] Studies in humans have shown that the use of tetracycline as an *adjunct* to scaling and root planing enhances healing[24, 33] but does not result in an important gain of attachment.[24]

It has been reported that the tetracycline derivative *minocycline* reduced total bacterial counts and completely eliminated spirochetes for periods of up to 2 months and resulted in improved clinical parameters after administration of 200 mg per day for 1 week.[7] In the United States, the tetracyclines currently appear to be the antibiotic most likely to be of value for the treatment of periodontitis.

Metronidazole

This drug is active against anaerobic organisms and has been used successfully in England in the treatment of acute necrotizing ulcerative gingivitis.[9, 25, 32] Administered systemically (800 to 1000 mg per day for 2 weeks), this drug suppresses the growth of anaerobic flora, including spirochetes, and results in the disappearance of the clinical and histopathologic signs of periodontitis.[21, 23] Long-term studies are needed to explore the effect of discontinuing the use of metronidazole.

Penicillin

Penicillin is the drug of choice for the treatment of serious infections in humans; it also induces allergic reactions and bacterial resistance. Its use in periodontal therapy does not appear justified.

Erythromycin

This antibiotic presents the drawbacks described for penicillin; therefore it is not indicated for periodontal therapy.

Spiramycin

Spiramycin is a macrolide antibiotic active against gram-positive organisms; it is excreted in high concentrations in saliva. It is used as an adjunct to periodontal treatment in Canada and Europe, but its use has not been approved in the United States. Several studies have shown promising results when spiramycin is prescribed in advanced periodontal disease, as measured by the Gingival Index, the Plaque Index, pocket depth, and crevicular fluid flow.[27] In addition, it is a safe, non-toxic drug with few and infrequent side effects; also, it is not in general use for medical problems.[12]

Local Administration of Antibiotics and Antimicrobials

Antibiotics

The local delivery of antibiotics within periodontal pockets is considered to have excellent potential as an adjunct to traditional periodontal therapy. The following local delivery systems have been tried for different agents: dentifrices, mouthrinses, and professional administration into the pocket by means of syringes, water irrigation devices, and fibers.

Mouthrinses and dentifrices are inefficient delivery systems because of the transient period of contact of the drug with the tissue and the lack of penetration into periodontal pockets. Direct irrigation using a syringe with a blunt needle has been tried by several investigators[3, 34] (Fig. 13–6). Penetration of solutions to the apical portions of pockets occurs if the needle tip is placed 3 mm within the pocket.[16] This method of administration appears to be an excellent way to enhance the results obtained with scaling and root planing residual pockets at recall visits.

Goodson and coworkers[13] have suggested that tetracycline-filled hollow fibers placed into the gingival sulcus would provide therapeutic effects with less than 1/1000 the amount of tetracycline used in systemic therapy. The use of tetracycline in this manner has resulted in conflicting reports relative to the elimination of spirochetes and other motile microorganisms. However, the concept of a local delivery system for antibiotics deserves further investigation.[8]

Fluorides

Several studies have demonstrated the bactericidal effects of fluorides against plaque bacteria.[30] Stannous fluoride has a greater bactericidal effect in vitro than neutral sodium fluoride or acidulated phosphate fluoride.[43] The antibacterial effect of fluoride mouthrinses in humans has been shown.[36, 44] The direct lavage of otherwise untreated pockets with 1.64% stannous fluoride in advanced periodontitis was found to be effective in reducing Bleeding Index scores and in delaying the repopulation of the pocket by spirochetes and motile bacteria.[26]

Other Antimicrobials

The use of daily subgingival irrigation with chlorhexidine after one scaling and root planing session was evaluated by Wieder et al.[39] They found that a reduction in periodontitis was still apparent 2 months after the cessation of irrigation; the treatment permitted extension of the interval between recall visits.

Keyes and colleagues[17] have described a method of periodontal therapy based on patient-applied hypertonic salts in an oxidative antiseptic solution for controlling plaque microorganisms. Several studies have been made to evaluate this treatment modality,[15, 41] but the results are as yet inconclusive.

Treatment of Juvenile Periodontitis

Discussion of the treatment of juvenile periodontitis is included in this chapter be-

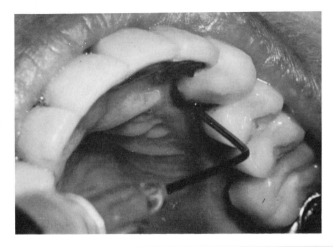

Figure 13–6. Placement of syringe into the pocket for irrigation after scaling and root planing.

cause of the importance of antibiotics in treatment.

The prognosis in cases of juvenile periodontitis depends on whether the disease is generalized or localized and on the degree of destruction present at the time of examination. The generalized forms, usually associated with some systemic disease, have a poorer prognosis than the localized forms. Juvenile periodontitis sometimes undergoes spontaneous remission.

Numerous treatments for localized juvenile periodontitis have been attempted, including extraction, transplantation, and conventional periodontal therapy. The general response to treatment has been poor.

In recent years several authors have reported greater success using antibiotics as adjuncts to therapy. Genco et al.[11] reported the treatment of localized juvenile periodontitis with scaling and root planing plus tetracycline (250 mg four times per day for 14 days) every 8 weeks. Measurements of vertical defects were made at intervals for up to 18 months after the initiation of therapy. Bone loss was stopped, and in one third of the defects there was an increase in bone level, whereas in the control group bone loss continued.

Liljenberg and Lindhe[22] treated localized juvenile periodontitis patients with tetracycline (250 mg four times per day for 2 weeks) and unrepositioned flaps and scheduled periodic recall visits (once a month for 6 months, then every 3 months). They reported that the lesions in patients with localized juvenile periodontitis healed more rapidly and more completely than similar lesions in other patients.

The lack of response of juvenile periodontitis to scaling and root planing may be due to the fact that *Actinobacillus actinomycetemcomitans*, the causative organism, is present in the tissues[4, 31] and remains after pocket therapy unless antibiotics are employed.[5]

Recommendations

At the present time antimicrobial agents appear to be indicated for the treatment of periodontal pockets in the following instances:

1. Tetracycline administration, 250 mg four times per day for 1 to 2 weeks, as an adjunct to the treatment of juvenile periodontitis and rapidly destructive, nonresponsive forms of advanced periodontitis.

2. Local irrigation of pockets with stannous fluoride (1.64 per cent) in order to delay the bacterial repopulation is indicated in deep pockets and furcation areas where access is difficult.

3. The value of systemic antibiotics in enhancing the success of new attachment and bone regeneration procedures is still uncertain.

References

1. Bader, H. I., and Goldhaber, P.: The passage of intravenously administered tetracycline into the gingival sulcus of dogs. J. Oral Therap. Pharmacol., 2:324, 1968.
2. Borzelleca, J., and Cherrick, H. M.: Excretion of drugs in saliva. J. Oral Therap. Pharmacol., 2:180, 1965.
3. Carranza, F. A., Sr.: Experiencias clinicas sobre reinsercion. Ensayos con penicilina. Rev. Asoc. Odontol. Argent., 39:55, 1951.
4. Carranza, F. A., Jr., Saglie, R., Newman, M. G., and Valentin, P.: Scanning and transmission electron microscopic study of tissue-invading microorganisms in localized juvenile periodontitis. J. Periodontol., 54:598, 1983.
5. Christersson, L. A., Albini, B., Zambon, J., Slots, J., and Genco, R. J.: Demonstration of *Actinobacillus actinomycetemcomitans* in gingiva of localized juvenile periodontitis lesions. J. Dent. Res., 62:198, 1983 (abstract).
6. Ciancio, S. G.: Use of antibiotics in periodontal therapy. *In* Newman, M. G., and Goodman, A. (eds.): Antibiotics in Dentistry. Chicago, Quintessence, 1983.
7. Ciancio, S. G., Slots, J., Reynolds, H., Zambon, J., and McKenna, J.: The effect of short-term administration of minocycline HCl on gingival inflammation and subgingival microflora. J. Periodontal., 53:557, 1982.
8. Coventry, J., and Newman, H. N.: Experimental use of a slow release device employing chlorhexidine gluconate in areas of acute periodontal inflammation. J. Clin. Periodontol., 9:129, 1982.
9. Duckworth, R., et al.: Acute ulcerative gingivitis. A double-blind controlled clinical trial of metronidazole. Br. Dent. J., 120:599, 1966.
10. Ellman, I. A.: Safe high-speed periodontal instrument. Dent. Survey, 36:759, 1960.
11. Genco, R. J., Ciancio, L. J., and Rosling, B.: Treatment of localized juvenile periodontitis. J. Dent. Res., 60:527, 1981 (abstract).
12. Gibson, W.: Antibiotics and periodontal disease: a selective review of the literature. J. Am. Dent. Assoc., 104:213, 1982.
13. Goodson, J. W., Haffajee, A., and Socransky, S. S.: Periodontal therapy by local delivery of tetracycline. J. Clin. Periodontol., 6:83, 1979.
14. Gordon, J. M., Walker, C. B., Murphy, J. C., Good-

son, J. M., and Socransky, S. S.: Concentration of tetracycline in human gingival fluid after single doses. J. Clin. Periodontol., 8:117, 1981.

15. Greenwell, H., Bissada, N. F., Maybury, J. E., and DeMarco, T. J.: Clinical and microbiological effectiveness of Keyes' method of oral hygiene on human periodontitis with and without surgery. J. Am. Dent. Assoc., 106:457, 1983.

16. Hardy, J. H., Newman, H. N., and Strahan, J. D.: Direct irrigation and subgingival plaque. J. Clin. Periodontol., 9:57, 1982.

17. Keyes, P. H., Wright, W. E., and Howard, S. A.: The use of phase-contrast microscopy and chemotherapy in the diagnosis and treatment of periodontal lesions. An initial report. I and II. Quintessence Internat., 9:51, 1978, 9:69, 1978.

18. Kornman, K. S., Caffesse, R. G., and Nasjleti, C. E.: The effects of intensive antibacterial therapy on the sulcular environment in monkeys. Changes in the bacteriology of the gingival sulcus. J. Periodontol., 51:34, 1980.

19. Kritchevsky, B., and Seguin, P.: The pathogenesis and treatment of pyorrhea alveolaris. Dent. Cosmos, 60:781, 1918. (Translated from La Presse Medicale, Paris, May 13, 1918.)

20. Krogh, H. W.: Reduction of the gingival flora preceding operation. J. Am. Dent. Assoc., 19:659, 1932.

21. Lekovic, V., Kenney, E. B., Carranza, F. A., Jr., and Endres, B.: Effect of metronidazole on human periodontal disease. A clinical and microbiologic study. J. Periodontol., 54:476, 1983.

22. Liljenberg, B., and Lindhe, J.: Juvenile periodontitis. Some microbiological, histopathological, and clinical characteristics. J. Clin. Periodontol., 7:48, 1980.

23. Lindhe, J., Hiljenberg, B., Adielson, B., and Borjesson, I.: Use of metronidazole as a probe in the study of human periodontal disease. J. Clin. Periodontol., 10:100, 1983.

24. Listgarten, M. A., Lindhe, J., and Parodi, R.: The effect of sytstemic antimicrobial therapy on plaque and gingivitis in dogs. J. Periodont. Res., 14:65, 1979.

25. Lozdan, J., Sheiham, A., Pearlman, B. A., et al.: The use of nitrimidazine in the treatment of acute ulcerative gingivitis. A double-blind controlled trial. Br. Dent. J., 130:294, 1971.

26. Mazza, J. E., Newman, M. G., and Sims, T. N.: Clinical and antimicrobial effect of stannous fluoride on periodontitis. J. Clin. Periodontol., 8:203, 1981.

27. Mills, W. H., Thompson, G. W., and Beagrie, G. S.: Clinical evaluation of spiramycin and erythromycin in control of periodontal disease. J. Clin. Periodontol., 6:308, 1979.

28. Mousques, T., Listgarten, M. A., and Phillips, R. W.: Effect of scaling and root planing on the composition of the human subgingival microbial flora. J. Clin. Periodontol., 15:111, 1980.

29. Pattison, G., and Pattison, A.: Periodontal Instrumentation. Reston Publishing Co., Reston, VA, 1978.

30. Perry, D. A.: Fluorides and periodontal disease: a review of the literature. J. Western Soc. Periodontol., 30:92, 1982.

31. Saglie, F. R., Carranza, F. A., Jr., Newman, M. G., Cheng, L., and Lewin, K. J.: Identification of tissue-invading bacteria in human periodontal disease. J. Periodont. Res., 17:452, 1982.

32. Sinn, D. H.: Metronidazole in acute ulcerative gingivitis. Lancet, 1:1191, 1962.

33. Slots, J., Mashimo, P., Levine, M. J., and Genco, R. J.: Periodontal therapy in humans. I. Microbiological and clinical effects of a single course of periodontal scaling and root planing, and of adjunctive tetracycline therapy. J. Periodontol., 50:495, 1979.

34. Soh, L. L., Newman, H. N., and Strahan, J. D.: Effects of subgingival chlorhexidine irrigation on periodontal inflammation. J. Clin. Periodontol., 9:66, 1982.

35. Stewart, J. L., Briggs, R. L., Drisko, R. R., and Jamison, H. C.: Relative calculus and tooth structure loss with use of powerdriven scaling instruments. J. Am. Dent. Assoc., 83:840, 1971.

36. Tinanoff, N., Brady, J. M., and Gross, A.: The effect of NaF and SnF$_2$ mouthrinses on bacterial colonization of tooth enamel: TEM or SEM studies. Caries Res., 10:415, 1976.

37. Villa, P.: Degree of calculus inhibition by habitual tooth brushing. Helv. Odontol. Acta, 12:31, 1968.

38. Weiner, G. S., DeMarco, T. J., and Bissada, N. F.: Long-term effects of systemic antimicrobial therapy on plaque and gingivis in dogs. J. Periodontol., 50:619, 1979.

39. Wieder, S. G., Newman, H. N., and Strahan, J. D.: Stannous fluoride and subgingival chlorhexidine irrigation in the control of plaque and chronic periodontitis. J. Clin. Periodontol., 10:172, 1983.

40. Williams, R. C., et al.: Tetracyclone treatment of periodontal disease in the beagle dog. I. Clinical and radiographic course over 12 months—maximal effect on rate of alveolar bone loss. J. Dent. Res., 16:659, 1981.

41. Wolff, L. R., Bandt, C., Philstrom, B., and Brayer, H.: Phase contrast microscopic evaluation of subgingival plaque in combination with either conventional or antimicrobial home treatment of patients with periodontal inflammation. J. Periodont. Res., 17:537, 1982.

42. Wright, B. L.: The treatment of pyorrhea alveolaris and its secondary systemic infections by deep muscular injections of mercury. Dent. Cosmos, 57:1003, 1915.

43. Yoon, N. A., and Berry, C. W.: The antimicrobial effect of fluorides (acidulated phosphate, sodium and stannous) on *Actinomyces viscosus*. J. Dent. Res., 58:1824, 1979.

44. Yoon, N. A., and Berry, C. W.: An in vivo study of the effects of fluoride (SnF$_2$ 0.4%, APF 1.23% and neutral NaF 0.5%) on levels of organisms resembling *Actinomyces*, gingival inflammation and plaque accumulation. J. Dent. Res., 58:535, 1979.

Chapter 14

Plaque Control

Plaque control is the removal of microbial plaque. Plaque control also retards the formation of calculus. Removal of microbial plaque leads to the resolution of gingival inflammation in its early stages and cessation of tooth cleaning leads to its recurrence. Thus, plaque control is an effective way of treating and preventing gingivitis and is a critical part of all the procedures involved in the prevention of periodontal disease.

The most dependable way of controlling microbial plaque is by mechanical cleansing with a toothbrush and other hygiene aids. Considerable progress is being made with chemical inhibitors of plaque incorporated in mouthwashes or dentifrices, but mechanical oral hygiene procedures are still essential.

Plaque control is one of the keystones of the practice of dentistry, without which oral health can be neither attained nor preserved. *Every patient in every dental practice should be on a plaque control program.* For the patient with a healthy periodontium, plaque control means the preservation of health. For the patient

undergoing periodontal therapy, it means optimal healing following treatment. For the patient with treated periodontal disease, plaque control means maintenance of restored health.

TOOTHBRUSHES

The first bristle toothbrush appeared about the year 1500 in China; it was introduced to the Western world in 1640 and has since undergone little basic change. Generally, toothbrushes vary in size and design as well as in length, hardness, and arrangement of the bristles. The American Dental Association has described the range of dimensions of acceptable brushes: these have a brushing surface from 1 to 1.25 inches (25.4 to 31.8 mm) long and 5/16 to 3/8 inch (7.9 to 9.5 mm) wide, two to four rows of bristles, and 5 to 12 tufts per row.[2] A toothbrush should be able to reach and clean efficiently most areas of the mouth. The choice of brush is a matter of individual preference; there is no demonstrated superiority of any one type of brush. Ease of manipulation by the patient is an important factor in brush selection. The effectiveness of and potential injury from different types of brushes depend to a great degree on how the brushes are used.

Two kinds of bristle material are used in toothbrushes; *natural* (hog bristle) and *artificial filaments* made predominantly of nylon. The cleaning effect of the two types seems to be equally satisfactory. However, with regard to homogeneity of the material, uniformity of size, elasticity, resistance to fracture, and repulsion of water and debris, nylon filaments are clearly superior to natural bristles. Hog bristles, because of their tubular form, are significantly more susceptible to fraying, breaking, contamination with diluted microbial debris, softening, and loss of elasticity.

The bristles are grouped in tufts that are usually arranged in three or four rows. Four-row brushes (multitufted) contain more bristles and therefore tolerate more working pressure without flexing. The question of the most desirable bristle hardness is not settled. Diameters of commonly used bristles range from 0.007 inch (0.2 mm) for soft brushes to 0.012 inch (0.3 mm) for medium brushes and 0.014 inch (0.4 mm) for hard brushes.[19] Soft bristle brushes have gained wide acceptance because they tend to be less traumatic.

Opinions regarding the merits of hard and soft bristles are often inconclusive and contradictory.[20] Medium bristles seem to cleanse better than soft bristles.[9] Soft bristles are more flexible, cleanse beneath the gingival margin (sulcus cleansing),[4] and reach more of the proximal tooth surface, but they may not completely remove heavy plaque deposits.[16] Soft bristles, especially in a multitufted brush head, seem to cleanse better than hard bristles,[3] partly because of a "matting effect" produced by the combination of soft bristles and dentifrice[6] and also because the close proximity of the bristles in a multitufted brush enables the user to generate significantly higher brushing forces against the teeth than would be possible with two- or three-row brushes.

Overzealous brushing can lead to gingival recession; implantation of bristles into the gingiva, with ensuing abscess formation; overt bacteremia, especially in patients with pronounced gingivitis[15]; and wedge-shaped defects on the cervical area of root surfaces.[15, 32]

Patients should be advised that, in order to benefit from the cleaning efficiency of a toothbrush, it must be replaced as soon as the bristles begin to fray. Soft three-row brushes tend to wear out the fastest.[30] With conscientious, regular use of a brush, this occurs within 3 months.

Selecting the handle shape of a toothbrush is a matter of individual preference. A handle should be long enough to fit the palm of the hand. Straight handles are most common. Handles with contraangle shanks may provide the grasping hand with a better feeling of touch, since the working surface of the brush (i.e., the bristle ends) is on the direct imaginary extension of the long axis of the handle.

For most patients, a short-headed brush with straight-cut, round-ended, soft-to-medium nylon bristles arranged in three or four rows of tufts is recommended.

Powered Toothbrushes

In 1939, electrically powered toothbrushes were invented to make plaque control easier. There are many types of electric toothbrushes, some with reciprocal arcuate or back-and-forth motion, others with combinations of both, some with a circular motion, and some with an elliptical motion. Patients who can develop the ability to use a toothbrush properly usually do equally well with manual or electric brushes. Less diligent brushers do better with electric toothbrushes, which generate proper stroke motions automatically and require minimal operator effort.[18] Electric brushes are recommended for (1) individuals lacking manual dexterity, (2) small children, handicapped people, or hospitalized patients who need to have their teeth cleaned by someone else, and (3) patients with orthodontic appliances.

DENTIFRICES

Dentifrices are aids for cleaning and polishing tooth surfaces. They are used mostly in the form of pastes. Tooth powders and liquids are also available. The cleansing effect of any dentifrice is related to its content of

(1) abrasives such as calcium carbonate, calcium phosphate, calcium sulfate, sodium bicarbonate, sodium chloride, aluminum oxide, or silicate, and (2) detergents such as sodium lauryl sulfate and sodium lauryl sarcosinate. In addition, pastes contain humectants (glycerin, sorbitol), water, thickening agents (carboxymethylcellulose, alginate, amylose), flavoring, and coloring agents.[1]

There is considerable interest in improving dentifrices by using them as vehicles for chemotherapeutic agents to inhibit plaque, calculus, caries, or root sensitivity. Except for the pronounced caries preventive effect of fluorides incorporated in dentifrices, substances such as chlorhexidine, penicillin, dibasic ammonium phosphate, vaccines, vitamins, chlorophyll, formaldehyde, and strontium chloride have proved to be of little therapeutic value.

Existing literature suggests that hard tissue damage from oral hygiene procedures is mainly due to abrasive dentifrices, whereas gingival lesions can be produced by a toothbrush alone.[31] However, the fact that abrasions are more prevalent on maxillary than on mandibular teeth and are found more frequently on the left than on the right half of the dental arch[12, 22] indicates that abrasion may be caused by a *number of factors*. Dentifrices that provide the cleansing effectiveness required for plaque control, with a minimum of abrasion, should be selected for periodontal patients. Because the formulations of dentifrices are occasionally changed, the most current information can be obtained from the Council on Dental Therapeutics of the American Dental Association.[2]

TOOTHBRUSHING METHODS

There are many methods of toothbrushing. Numerous controlled studies have evaluated the effectiveness of the most common brushing techniques and have shown that no one method is clearly superior.[37]

Three methods of toothbrushing are presented here that, if properly performed, can accomplish the desired results. Each technique should be evaluated with regard to its feasibility in a given patient's dentition in order to arrive at a plaque control program that is tailored to the individual.

The Bass Method (Sulcus Cleansing)[5]

Place the head of a soft-to-medium brush parallel with the occlusal plane and with the "tip" of the brush distal to the last molar. Place the bristles at the gingival margin, establish an apical angle of 45° to the long axis of the teeth, *exert gentle vibratory pressure in the long axis of the bristles*, and force the bristle ends into the facial gingival sulci as well as into the interproximal embrasures (Fig. 14–1). This should produce perceptible blanching of the gingiva (Fig. 14–2). Activate the brush with a short back-and-forth motion *without dislodging the tips of the bristles*. Complete about 20 strokes in the same position. This cleans the teeth facially within the apical third of their clinical crowns, as well as within their adjacent gingival sulci and along the proximal surfaces as far as the bristles reach.

Lift the brush to move it (Fig. 14–3). Con-

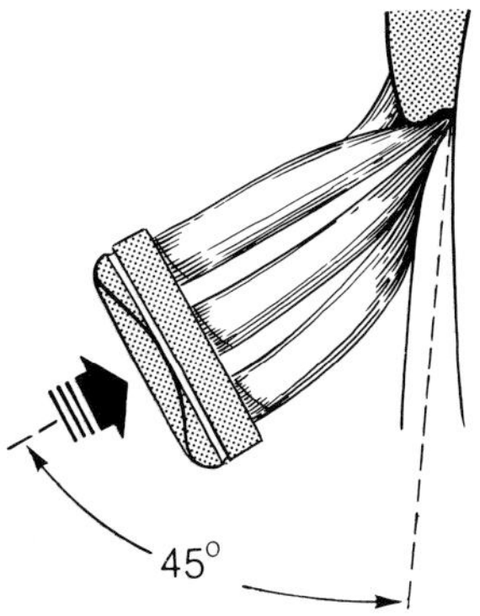

Figure 14–1. **Bass method.** Intrasulcus position of brush at 45° angle to long axis of tooth.

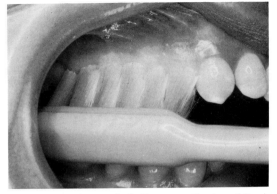

Figure 14–2. **Bass method.** Correct application of brush should produce perceptible blanching of the gingiva.

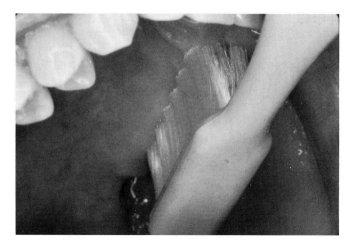

Figure 14–7. Bass method. Clinical aspect of palatal position on molars and premolars.

3. This technique can be *recommended for the routine patient* with or without periodontal involvement.

The Modified Stillman Method[39]

A medium-to-hard two- or three-row brush is placed with the bristle ends resting partly on the cervical position of the teeth and partly on the adjacent gingiva, pointing in an apical direction at an oblique angle to the long axis of the teeth. Pressure is applied laterally against the gingival margin so as to produce a perceptible blanching. The brush is activated with 20 short back-and-forth

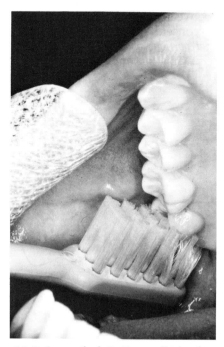

Figure 14–8. Bass method. Position on distal surface of the most distal molars.

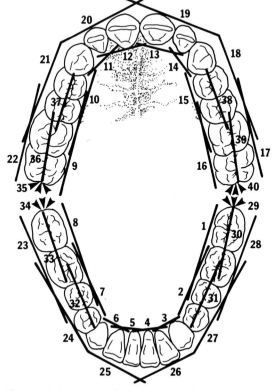

Figure 14–9. Bass method. Recommended sequence of brush positions.

strokes and is simultaneously moved in a coronal direction along the attached gingiva, the gingival margin, and the tooth surface. This process is repeated on all tooth surfaces, proceeding systematically around the mouth. To reach the lingual surfaces of the maxillary and mandibular incisors, the handle of the brush is held in a vertical position, engaging the "heel" of the brush.

The occlusal surfaces of molars and premolars are cleaned with the bristles perpendicular to the occlusal plane and penetrating deeply into the sulci and interproximal embrasures. With this technique, the sides rather than the ends of the bristles are used and penetration of the bristles into the gingival sulci is avoided. Therefore the Stillman method is *recommended for cleaning in areas with progressing gingival recession* and root exposure in order to prevent abrasive tissue destruction.

The Charters Method[8]

A medium-to-hard two- or three-row brush is placed on the tooth with the bristles pointed toward the crown at a 45° angle to the long axis of the teeth. To cleanse the occlusal surfaces, the bristle tips are placed in the pits and fissures and the brush is activated with *short* back-and-forth strokes.

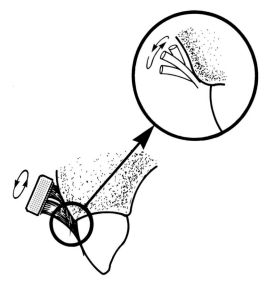

Figure 14–10. Charters method. The bristles are pressed sideward against teeth and gingiva. The brush is activated with short circular on back-and-forth strokes.

The procedure is repeated until all chewing surfaces are cleansed (Fig. 14–10).

The Charters method is *especially suitable for gingival massage*. When using a soft brush, this technique is also recommended for cleaning in areas of healing gingival wounds, following periodontal surgery.

Methods of Cleaning with Powered Brushes

The various mechanical motions built into electric brushes do not require special techniques of application provided the vibratory excursions of the bristle ends are small enough.

The three methods described for manual brushing are also suitable for powered tooth cleaning.

INTERDENTAL CLEANSING AIDS

The use of a toothbrush, regardless of the brushing method used, does not completely remove interdental plaque accumulation, either in persons with healthy periodontal conditions or in periodontally treated patients with open embrasures.[7, 17, 35] For optimal plaque control, toothbrushing must be supplemented with an effective method of interdental cleaning. Among the numerous aids available, dental floss and interdental cleansers such as wooden or plastic tips and interdental brushes are the most commonly used.

Dental Floss

Dental flossing is the most widely recommended method of cleansing proximal tooth surfaces. Floss is available as a multifilament nylon yarn that is either twisted or nontwisted, bonded or nonbonded, waxed or unwaxed, and thick or thin. Various individual factors, such as the tightness of tooth contacts, the roughness of tooth surfaces, and the patient's manual dexterity, determine the choice of dental floss, rather than the superiority of any one product. Clinical research has not shown any significant differences in the ability of the various types of floss to remove dental plaque. Thin, un-

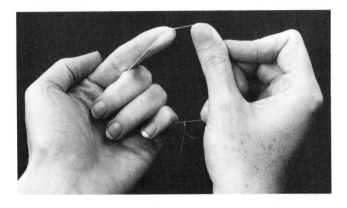

Figure 14–11. Dental flossing using the loop technique.

waxed floss passes more easily between teeth with tight contact areas. In addition, unwaxed floss produces a distinct squeaking sound when moved over a tooth surface that is clean. This can serve as an indicator of tooth cleanliness and may be valuable as an aid for instructing and motivating patients.

There are several ways of using dental floss. The following is recommended:

Use a piece of floss at least one foot long. Stretch it tightly between the thumb and forefinger (Fig. 14–11) and pass it gently through each contact area with a firm sideward sawing motion. It is sometimes helpful to tie the floss into a loop. Do not forcibly snap the floss past the contact area, because this will injure the interdental gingiva. Wrap the floss around the proximal surface of one tooth, at the base of the gingival sulcus (Fig.

14–12). Move the floss *firmly* along the tooth *up* to the contact area and *gently down* into the sulcus again, repeating this up-and-down stroke five or six times. Displace the floss across the interdental gingiva and repeat the procedure on the proximal surface of the adjacent tooth. Continue through the whole dentition, including the distal surface of the last tooth in each quadrant. When the working portion of the floss becomes soiled or begins to shred, move the index finger and thumb along to a fresh portion of floss.

The manipulation of dental floss can be simplified by using a floss holder. A floss holder should feature (1) one or two forks that are rigid enough to keep the floss taut even when it is moved past tight contact areas and (2) an effective and simple mounting mechanism that holds the floss firmly in

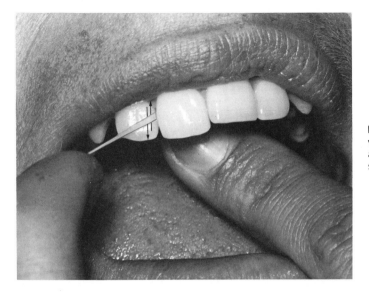

Figure 14–12. Dental flossing. The floss is wrapped around each proximal surface and activated with repeated up-and-down strokes.

place and yet allows quick rethreading of the floss whenever its working portion becomes soiled, stretched, or begins to shred.

The purpose of flossing is to remove plaque, not to dislodge fibrous threads of food wedged in between teeth or impacted in the gingiva. Chronic food impaction should be treated by correcting proximal tooth contacts and "plunger" cusps. Removing impacted food with dental floss simply provides temporary relief but permits the condition to become worse.

Interdental Cleansers

For cleaning in narrow gingival embrasures that are occupied by intact papillae and bordered by tight contact zones, dental floss is probably the most effective dental hygiene aid. Proper manipulation of the floss requires good dexterity, intensive instruction, and repeated monitoring. *However, concave root surfaces and furcations cannot be reached with dental floss. Therefore, special cleaning devices that adapt to irregular tooth surfaces better than does dental floss are recommended for cleaning large interproximal spaces.* A wide variety of interdental cleansers are available.

Interdental Brushes

Interdental brushes are cone-shaped brushes made of bristles mounted on handles, unitufted brushes, or miniature bottle brushes. Interdental brushes are particularly suitable for cleaning large, irregular, or concave tooth surfaces adjacent to wide interdental spaces. They are inserted interproximally and activated with short back-and-forth strokes in a linguofacial direction. For the most efficient cleansing, the diameter of the brush should be slightly larger than the gingival embrasures so that the bristles can exert pressure on the tooth surfaces.

Wooden Tips

Wooden tips are used either with a handle, such as the Perio-Aid, or without, such as the Stim-U-Dent.

The *Stim-U-Dent* is a soft wooden tip that is triangular in cross section. Held between the middle finger, index finger, and thumb, it is placed in the interdental spaces in such a way that the base surface of the triangle rests tangentially on the interproximal gingiva and the sides are in contact with the proximal tooth surfaces. The Stim-U-Dent is then moved in and out of the embrasure, removing soft deposits from the teeth and mechanically stimulating the papillary gingiva.

The *Perio-Aid* consists of a round, tapered end of a toothpick that is inserted in a handle for convenient application. Deposits are removed by using either the side or the end of the tip. This device is particularly efficient for cleaning along the gingival margin[35] and within gingival sulci or periodontal pockets. The small dimensions of the tip allow for exceptionally good visibility of the tooth surface being cleaned, which contributes substantially to the effectiveness of the Perio-Aid.

Selection of Interdental Cleansing Aids

In general, when selecting an interdental cleansing device, the largest device that fits into the embrasure spaces should be used (Fig. 14–13).

In embrasures totally occupied by the interdental papillae, dental floss should be used. It is the only device that can be passed through narrow spaces without forcing the papillae apically, which can induce undesired gingival recession.

In embrasures with slight to moderate recession, small interdental brushes such as the PROXABRUSH should be used. Wooden tips are also effective. Dental floss is less efficient in these cases because interproximal gingival recession usually leads to the exposure of concave root depressions that are missed by the floss.

In embrasures with extensive recession, larger devices such as unitufted brushes are recommended.

GINGIVAL MASSAGE

Massaging the gingiva with toothbrushes or interdental cleansers increases keratinization and improves circulation. However, ker-

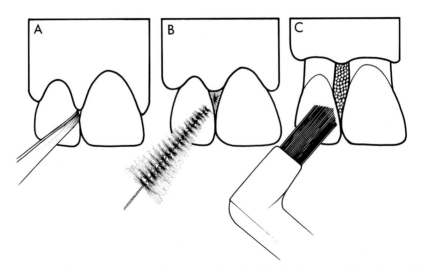

Figure 14–13. Interproximal embrasure types and corresponding interdental cleansers. A, Type I—no gingival recession: dental floss. B, Type II—moderate papillary recession: interdental brush. C, Type III—complete loss of papillae: unitufted brush.

atinization occurs in the oral gingiva and not in the sulcular gingiva, which is more vulnerable to microbial attack. The importance of this increased keratinization is not clear, because studies of chemotherapeutic mouthrinses have demonstrated that gingival health can be maintained in the absence of mechanical oral hygiene procedures.[27]

Gingival massage may be performed using the Charters method of brushing or with wooden or rubber stimulators. Massage with the latter consists of placing the stimulator against the papilla with the tip pointed interdentally, applying moderate pressure, and rotating the instrument in a circular motion.

ORAL IRRIGATION

Oral irrigators work by directing high-pressure steady or pulsating streams of water through a nozzle to the tooth surfaces. The pressure is generated by a built-in pump or by attaching the device to a water faucet. Oral irrigators clean nonadherent bacteria and debris from the oral cavity more effectively than toothbrushes and mouthrinses.[42] They are particularly helpful for removing nonstructured debris from inaccessible areas around orthodontic appliances and fixed prostheses. *However, water irrigation removes only negligible amounts of stainable plaque from tooth surfaces.*[13]

CHEMICAL INHIBITORS OF PLAQUE AND CALCULUS

Many agents have been tested for their ability to inhibit the quantitative or qualitative development of microbial deposits, calculus, or periodontal inflammation. Promising results have been reported with fluorides, chlorhexidine, alexidine, and other agents. The most commonly used mode of applying these agents has been topical, in the form of mouthrinses, dentifrices, gels, lozenges, and chewing gum.

The agent that has attracted the most attention is *chlorhexidine*, a diguanidohexane with pronounced antiseptic properties. The initial finding was that *two daily rinses with 10 ml of a 0.2 per cent aqueous solution of chlorhexidine gluconate* almost completely inhibited the development of dental plaque, calculus, and gingivitis[27] in the human model for experimental gingivitis. This has been confirmed by a number of short term clinical investigations.[41] In most of the studies, a mouthrinse has been employed as the preferred mode of application.[27, 41] Chlorhexidine incorporated into dentifrices, gels, and lozenges has proved so far to be considerably less, if at all, effective.

Aside from some local, reversible side effects, such as brown staining of teeth, tongue, and silicate and resin restorations,[11] transient impairment of taste perception, and discrete desquamation of the oral mucosa,[14] chlorhexidine appears to be one of the safest antiseptics known.[41] It has not so far shown any evidence of systemic toxicity in humans,[39] nor has it produced any appreciable resistance in oral microorganisms.[33]

Similarly promising results have been reported with alexidine, another bis-guanide that is closely related to chlorhexidine.[26]

DISCLOSING AGENTS

There are *solutions* and *wafers* capable of staining bacterial deposits on the surfaces of teeth, tongue, and gingivae (Fig. 14–14). They are excellent oral hygiene aids because they provide the patient with an educational and motivational tool to improve efficiency in plaque control.

Solutions

1. Basic fuchsin   6 grams
   Ethyl alcohol, 95%   100 ml
   Add two drops of solution to water in a dappen dish

2. Potassium iodide   1.6 grams
   Iodine crystals   1.6 grams
   Water   13.4 ml
   Glycerin   to make   30.0 ml

Solutions are applied to the teeth as concentrates on cotton swabs or diluted in mouthrinses. They usually produce heavy staining of bacterial plaque, gingivae, tongue, lips, fingers, and sink. Therefore, they are useful only in the dental office, where an impressive demonstration of bacterial deposits is desirable and excessive staining can be controlled or readily removed by prophylaxis. Except for a sodium fluorescein dye, which produces a yellow glowing of dental plaque only when exposed to a light source of a certain wavelength,[24] solutions are not frequently recommended for home use owing to this inconvenient intensive staining effect, which may act as a deterrent rather than as a motivator.

Wafers

FDC red #3 (erythrosine)   15 mg
Sodium chloride   0.747%

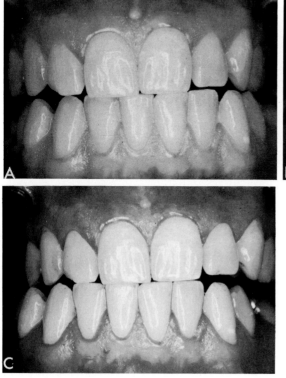
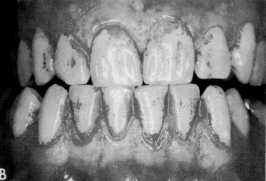

Figure 14–14. Effect of a disclosing agent. *A,* Unstained. *B,* Stained with a 6 per cent solution of basic fuchsin; plaque shows as dark particulate patches. *C,* Restained with basic fuchsin after thorough tooth cleaning.

Sodium sucaryl	0.747%
Calcium stearate	0.995%
Soluble saccharin	0.186%
White oil	0.124%
Flavoring (FDA approved)	2.239%
Sorbitol	to make 7.0 grams

Wafers are crushed between the teeth and swished around the mouth for about 30 seconds without swallowing. Because of the convenient mode of application, wafers are recommended specifically for home use.

It is obvious that the mere addition of disclosing agents to oral health instructions is not sufficient motivation for a patient to clean his teeth more effectively. Visual feedback can, however, be an important aspect of health education if used in conjunction with other methods.

FREQUENCY OF TOOTH CLEANING

In the controlled and supervised environment of clinical research, where trained individuals remove all visible plaque, gingival health can be maintained by one thorough cleaning with brush, floss, and toothpicks every 24 to 48 hours.[21, 23] In spite of such revealing data, clinical experience shows that most patients fall far short of such perfection. In the average cleaning effort, lasting just 2 minutes every day, only 40 per cent of the deposits are removed, leaving 60 per cent to promote rapid regrowth of the microbiota.[10] Numerous studies have reported improved periodontal health associated with increasing frequency of brushing up to twice per day.[36, 39] Three or more cleanings per day did not produce significantly better periodontal conditions. For practical purposes, *two brushings per day*, one of them performed very thoroughly, are recommended. *Emphasis must be placed on the efficiency rather than on the frequency of tooth cleaning*.

STEP-BY-STEP PROCEDURE FOR PLAQUE CONTROL

The daily mechanical removal of plaque by the patient appears to be the only practical means for improving oral hygiene on a long-term basis. A step-by-step procedure for teaching patients this self-therapy is suggested.

Step I: Motivation

Motivation for effective plaque control is one of the most critical and most difficult elements of long-term success of periodontal therapy. In most cases, it requires from patients the following efforts: (1) *receptiveness* to understanding the concepts of the pathogenesis, the treatment, and the prevention of periodontal disease; (2) *change of habits*, adopting a self-administered *daily* plaque control regimen; and (3) *behavioral changes*, adjusting the hierarchy of one's beliefs, practices, and values to accommodate the required new oral hygiene habits.

The patient must understand what periodontal disease is and its effects, his susceptibility to periodontal disease, and what he can do to achieve and maintain oral health. He must be willing and able to develop and use the manual skills that are necessary to establish a plaque control regimen. He must then want to keep his mouth clean for his own benefit. If these efforts are not made, long-term failure of any individual plaque control program is inevitable and leads to frustration for the clinician and the patient.

Step II: Education

Most patients think of cleaning the teeth as toothbrushing to remove food debris and to prevent tooth decay. Its importance in the prevention and treatment of periodontal disease is rarely recognized and must be explained. *Good oral hygiene is the most effective preventive and therapeutic procedure*. When individuals maintain good oral hygiene from 5 to 50 years of age, the effects of destructive periodontal disease can most likely be avoided during this period of life.[25]

Patients must be informed that periodic scaling and cleansing of the teeth in the dental office are necessary protective measures against periodontal disease, but only if these are combined with daily oral hygiene procedures at home. Therefore, time spent in the dental office teaching the patient how to cleanse his teeth is as valuable a service as cleaning his teeth for him. It must be explained that dental visits 2 or 3 times a year are not nearly as effective as is daily oral home care. Only a combination of regular office visits with conscientious home care significantly reduces gingivitis and loss of supporting periodontal tissues.[25, 28, 40]

The periodontal patient should be shown that periodontal disease has manifested itself *in his own mouth*. Stained dental plaque, the bleeding of inflamed gingiva, and a periodontal probe inserted into a pocket are impressive and convincing demonstration of the presence of pathogens and actual disease. It is of great educational value to have oral cleanliness and periodontal condition recorded periodically so that patients can utilize this feedback about their levels of performance. A plaque control record[29] is recommended as an index of the patient's level of performance.

Plaque Control Record

Disclosing solution is applied to all supragingival tooth surfaces. After the patient has rinsed, each tooth surface (except occlusal surfaces) is examined for the presence or absence of stained deposits at the dentogingival junction. If present, they are recorded by coloring the appropriate box in a diagram. After all teeth have been scored, an index is calculated by dividing the number of surfaces with plaque by the total number of teeth scored.

Step III: Instruction

With repeated instruction and supervision, patients can reduce the incidence of plaque and gingivitis far more effectively than with self-taught oral hygiene habits. However, instruction in how to clean the teeth must be more than a cursory chairside demonstration of the use of a toothbrush and oral hygiene aids. It is a painstaking procedure that requires patient participation, careful supervision with immediate correction of developing mistakes, and reinforcement during return visits until the patient demonstrates that he has developed the necessary proficiency.

PROPHYLAXIS

Conscientious oral home care substantially inhibits the formation of plaque, stain, and calculus but cannot completely prevent their occurrence, especially in patients with periodontal pockets and in heavy calculus formers. Therefore, periodic professional care consisting of complete mechanical removal of all deposits and repeated oral hygiene instruction is an integral part of a comprehensive plaque control program. It must be emphasized, however, that prophylaxis alone is insufficient for maintaining a healthy oral environment or preventing the progression of periodontal disease, even if administered frequently. Only a combination of scaling, root planing, and polishing at regular intervals of up to three months, reinforcement of oral hygiene instructions, and conscientious daily plaque control by patients has proved to be successful arresting treated periodontal disease and maintaining periodontal health.

References

1. Abrasivity of current dentifrices: Report of the Council of Dental Therapeutics. J. Am. Dent. Assoc., *81*:117, 1970.
2. Accepted Dental Therapeutics. 3rd ed. Chicago, American Dental Association, 1969–1970, p. 225.
3. Allet, B., Regolati, B., and Muhlemann, H. R.: Die Rolle der Griffabwinkelung auf die Reinigungskraft einer Zahnurste. Schweiz. Mschr. Zahnheilk., *82*:452, 1972.
4. Bass, C. C.: Optimum characteristics of dental floss for personal oral hygiene. Dent. Items Int., *70*:921, 1948.
5. Bass, C. C.: An effective method of personal oral hygiene. Part II. J. Louisiana State Med. Soc., *106*:100, 1954.
6. Bergenholtz, A.: Mechanical cleaning. *In* Frandsen, A. (ed.): Oral Hygiene. Copenhagen, Munskgaard, 1971, pp. 27–60.
7. Bergenholtz, A., Hugoson, A., Lundgren, D., and Ostgren, A.: The plaque-removing ability of various toothbrushes used with the roll technique. Svensk. Tandläk. T., *62*:15, 1969.
8. Charters, W. J.: Eliminating mouth infections with the toothbrush and other stimulating instruments. Dent. Digest, *38*:130, 1932.
9. Conroy, C. W.: Comparison of automatic and hand toothbrushes: cleaning effectiveness. J. Am. Dent. Assoc., *70*:921, 1965.
10. De la Rosa, M. R., Guerra, J. Z., Johnston, D. A., and Radike, A. W.: Plaque growth and removal with daily toothbrushing. J. Periodontol., *50*:661, 1979.
11. Eriksen, H. M., and Gjermo, P.: Incidence of stained tooth surfaces in students using chlorhexidine-containing dentifrices. Scand. J. Dent. Res., *81*:533, 1973.
12. Ervin, J. C., and Bucher, E. T.: Prevalence of tooth root exposure and abrasion among dental patients. Dent. Items Int., *66*:760, 1944.
13. Fine, D. H., and Baumhammers, A.: Effect of water pressure irrigation on stainable material on the teeth. J. Periodontol., *41*:468, 1970.
14. Flötra, L., Gjermo, P., Rolla, G., et al.: A four-month study on the effect of chlorhexidine mouth washes on 50 soldiers. Scand. J. Dent. Res., *80*:10, 1972.

15. Gillette, W. B., and Van House, R. L.: Ill effects of improper oral hygiene procedures. J. Am. Dent. Assoc., 101:476, 1980.

16. Gilson, C. M., Charbeneau, G. T., and Hill, H. C.: A comparison of physical properties of several soft toothbrushes. J. Michigan Dent. Assoc., 51:347, 1969.

17. Gjermo, P., and Flötra, L.: The effect of different methods of interdental cleaning. J. Periodont. Res., 5:230, 1970.

18. Glass, R. L.: A clinical study of hand and electric toothbrushing. J. Periodontol., 36:322, 1965.

19. Hine, M. K.: Toothbrush. Int. Dent. J., 6:15, 1956.

20. Hiniker, J. J., and Forscher, B. K.: The effect of toothbrush type on gingival health. J. Periodontol., 25:40, 1954.

21. Kelner, R. M., Wahl, B. R., Deasy, M. J., and Formicola, A. J.: Gingival inflammation as related to frequency of plaque removal. J. Periodontol., 45:303, 1974.

22. Kitchin, P.: The prevalence of tooth root exposure and the relation of the extent of such exposure to the degree of abrasion in different age classes. J. Dent. Res., 20:565, 1941.

23. Lang, N. P., Cumming, B. R., and Löe, H.: Toothbrushing frequency as it relates to plaque development and gingival health. J. Periodontol., 44:396, 1973.

24. Lang, N. P., Ostergaard, E. Q., and Löe, H.: A fluorescent plaque disclosing agent. J. Periodont. Res., 7:59, 1972.

25. Lindhe, J., and Nyman, S.: The effect of plaque control and surgical pocket elimination on the establishment and maintenance of periodontal health. A longitudinal study of periodontal therapy in cases of advanced disease. J. Clin. Periodontol., 2:67, 1975.

26. Lobene, R. R., and Soparkar, P. M.: The effect of an alexidine mouthwash on human plaque and gingivitis. J. Am. Dent. Assoc., 87:848, 1973.

27. Löe, H., and Schiött, C. R.: The effect of mouthrinses and topical application of chlorhexidine on the development of dental plaque and gingivitis in man. J. Periodont. Res., 5:79, 1970.

28. Nyman, S., Rosling, B., and Lindhe, J.: Effect of professional tooth cleaning on healing after periodontal surgery. J. Clin. Periodontol., 2:80, 1975.

29. O'Leary, T. J., Drake, R. B., and Naylor, J. E.: The plaque control record. J. Periodontol., 43:38, 1972.

30. Robertson, N. A. E., and Wade, A. B.: Effect of filament diameter and density in toothbrushes. J. Periodont. Res., 7:346, 1972.

31. Sangnes, G.: Traumatization of teeth and gingiva related to habitual tooth cleaning procedures. J. Clin. Periodontol., 3:94, 1976.

32. Sangnes, G., and Gjermo, P.: Prevalence of oral soft and hard tissue lesions related to mechanical tooth cleaning procedures. Community Dent. Oral Epidemiol., 4:77, 1976.

33. Schiött, C. R., Briner, W. W., and Löe, H.: Two years oral use of chlorhexidine in man. II. The effect on the salivary bacterial flora. J. Periodont. Res., 11:145, 1976.

34. Schiött, C. R., Löe, H., and Briner, W. W.: Two years oral use of chlorhexidine in man. IV. Effect of various medical parameters. J. Periodont. Res., 11:158, 1976.

35. Schmid, M. O., Balmelli, O., and Saxer, U. P.: The plaque-removing effect of a toothbrush, dental floss and a toothpick. J. Clin. Periodontol., 3:157, 1976.

36. Sheiham, A.: Dental cleanliness and chronic periodontal disease: studies in British populations. Br. Dent. J., 129:413, 1970.

37. Sheiham, A.: Prevention and control of periodontal disease. International Conference on Research in the Biology of Periodontal Disease. Chicago, June 12-15, 1977, p. 324.

38. Stillman, P. R.: A philosophy of the treatment of periodontal disease. Dent. Digest, 38:314, 1932.

39. Suomi, J. D.: Periodontal disease and oral hygiene in an institutionalized population: report of an epidemiology study. J. Periodontol., 40:5, 1969.

40. Suomi, J. D., Greene, J. C., Vermillion, J. R., et al.: The effect of controlled oral hygiene procedures on the progression of periodontal disease in adults: results after two years. J. Periodontol., 40:416, 1969.

41. Symposium on chlorhexidine in the prophylaxis of dental diseases (Löe, H., ed.) J. Periodont. Res., Suppl. No. 12, 1973.

42. Toto, P. D., Evans, C. L., and Sawinski, V. J.: Effects of water jet rinse and toothbrushing on oral hygiene. J. Periodontol., 40:296, 1969.

Chapter 15

Principles of Periodontal Surgery

RATIONALE

The effectiveness of periodontal therapy depends on both the therapeutic elimination of factors that favor accumulation of bacterial plaque and on the daily removal of plaque by patients through the use of home care procedures. If one or both of these goals is not met, treatment will fail. A number of factors may make it difficult or even impossible to totally eliminate bacterial plaque by the patient and the therapist. These include the following:

1. Deep pockets. It is very difficult to deplaque the apical areas of deeper pockets.

2. Complex pockets. These pockets run tortuous courses and cannot be completely debrided unless the tissues are torn and separated.

3. Furcation involvements. The extension of pockets into furcation areas increases accessibility problems because of the difficulty of introducing and positioning instruments adequately.

The purpose of the surgical phase of therapy is to correct morphologic problems and ensure accessibility for complete removal of plaque and calculus.

Dental hygienists must have an understanding of surgical techniques in order to comprehend the overall objectives of periodontal therapy. Often it is not adequate treatment to perform Phase I therapy and progress to a maintenance regimen. This knowledge will enable the hygienist to educate patients about the benefits of total periodontal treatment and to participate in all aspects of therapy.

METHODS OF POCKET ELIMINATION

Pocket elimination (Fig. 15–1) is a technical procedure that can be accomplished in three general ways:

Reattachment techniques offer the ideal result, since they eliminate pocket depth by reuniting the gingiva to the tooth at a position coronal to the bottom of the pre-existing

209

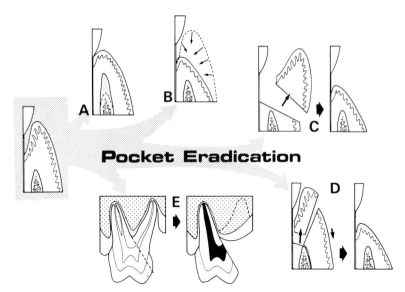

Pocket Eradication

Figure 15–1. Different methods of pocket eradication. From upper left, clockwise, reattachment and bone regeneration, shrinkage after scaling and curettage, gingival excision (gingivectomy), pocket wall apically displaced by a flap operation, and root resection. (*From* Takei, H. H., and Carranza, F. A.: General principles of periodontal surgery. *In* Steiner, R. B., and Thompson, R. D. (eds.): Oral Surgery and Anesthesia. Philadelphia, W. B. Saunders Co., 1977, pp. 132–150.)

pocket. Reattachment is usually associated with filling-in of bone and regeneration of the periodontal ligament and cementum.

Removal of the lateral wall of the pocket is the most common method. The lateral wall of the pocket can be removed using any of the following techniques:

1. Retraction or shrinkage, in which scaling and root planing procedures resolve the inflammatory process by causing gingival shrinkage and pocket depth reduction.

2. Surgical removal performed by the gingivectomy technique.

3. Apical displacement with flap surgery.

Removal of the tooth side of the pocket can also result in pocket elimination. This is accomplished by tooth extraction or by partial tooth extraction (hemisection, or root resection).

Criteria for Method Selection

Scientific criteria to establish the indications for each technique are difficult to determine. Longitudinal studies following a significant number of cases over a significant number of years, standardizing multiple factors and different parameters, would be needed and are almost impossible to con-

duct. Clinical experience, however, has suggested criteria for selecting the method to be used to eliminate the pocket in individual cases.

Gingival Pockets

Two factors must be considered: (1) the character of the pocket wall, and (2) the pocket accessibility.

The pocket wall can be either edematous or fibrotic. Edematous tissue will shrink after the elimination of local factors, thereby reducing or totally eliminating pocket depth. Pockets having fibrotic walls will not be appreciably reduced in depth after scaling and root planing. Only after long periods of adequate plaque control their depth may be somewhat reduced. Therefore fibrotic gingival pockets are more likely to require surgical intervention.

Pocket elimination must be based on total elimination of the responsible local factors. Patient and operator accessibility for plaque control then becomes an important consideration. The following table will clarify the rationale for the selection of a particular pocket eradication method for gingival pockets:

Accessibility	Pocket Wall Edematous	Fibrotic
Good	Curettage	Gingivectomy
Fair	Gingivectomy	Gingivectomy

Suprabony Pockets

In order to reduce suprabony pockets, two problems must be considered: (1) the presence or absence of an adequate band of attached gingiva and (2) the presence of bone deformities requiring some type of surgical correction. The following table is a summary of the rationale for the selection of a particular treatment technique in suprabony pockets:

Adequate Attached Gingiva		Inadequate Attached Gingiva	
No Bone Deformities	*Bone Deformities*	*No Bone Deformities*	*Bone Deformities*
Closed or open root planing or gingivectomy	Muco-periosteal apically positioned flap with osseous contouring	Mucosal apically positioned flap or gingival extension with free soft tissue auto-graft	Muco-periosteal apically positioned flap with osseous contouring

Infrabony Pockets

Treatment of infrabony pockets may be directed to obtaining bone regeneration and reattachment or to contouring the remaining bone to an acceptable morphology. The decision depends mainly on the exact shape of the bony defect, considering the number of walls, width, and general configuration. The only way to determine the shape of the bone is by visual inspection. Therefore the technique indicated for the treatment of infrabony pockets will be the mucoperiosteal flap, with osseous surgery aimed at bone regeneration or bone removal. This technique may also be combined with mucogingival procedures when an inadequate amount of attached gingiva is present.

GENERAL CONSIDERATIONS

Surgical periodontal procedures are usually performed in the dental office. On some occasions periodontal surgery is performed in the hospital setting. The preparation of patients and the general considerations that are common to all periodontal surgical techniques are presented in this section. Specific techniques are described in the next chapter.

Preparation of the Patient

Reevaluation After Phase I Therapy

Every patient is subject to the initial or preparatory phase of therapy, which basically consists of thorough scaling and root planing and the removal of all irritants responsible for the periodontal inflammation. This will (1) eliminate some lesions entirely; (2) render the tissues more firm and consistent, thus permitting a more accurate and delicate surgery; and (3) acquaint the patient with the office, the operator, and the assistants, thereby reducing the patient's apprehension and fear.

The reevaluation phase consists of reprobing and reexamining all the pertinent findings that previously indicated the need for the surgical procedure. Their persistence will confirm the indication. Decisions are made at this time with reference to the number of surgical procedures to be performed, the dates for all the procedures, the expected outcome, and the postoperative care that will be needed. All this is discussed with the patient and final decisions made.

Premedication

Some patients will need special premedication because of systemic diseases or extreme anxiety. Antibiotics should be administered prophylactically to all patients with heart disease, diabetes, and certain other conditions. This subject is discussed in detail in Chapter 11. For patients who do not have any of these special conditions, the value of routinely administering antibiotics for periodontal surgery has not been clearly demonstrated.

Informed Consent

The patient should be informed at the time of the initial visit about the diagnosis, the prognosis, the different possible treatments with their expected results, and all the pros and cons of each approach. At the time of surgery, the patient should again be informed, verbally and in writing, about the procedure to be performed; the patient should indicate his agreement to the procedure by signing the consent form.

Planning for Emergencies

All office personnel should be trained to handle emergency situations that may arise. Emergency drugs and equipment must be readily available at all times.

Syncope is the most common emergency. It is a transient loss of consciousness due to a reduction in cerebral blood flow, usually caused by fear and anxiety. Syncope is often preceded by a feeling of weakness, and then the patient develops pallor, sweating, coldness of the extremities, dizziness, and slowing of the pulse. The patient should be placed in a supine position with the legs elevated; tight clothing should be loosened and a wide open airway ensured. The administration of oxygen is useful. Unconsciousness persists only for a few seconds.

A history of previous syncopal attacks during dental appointments should be explored before treatment is begun, and, if these are reported, extra efforts should be made to relieve the patient's fear and anxiety. The reader is referred to other texts such as the work by G. R. Allen[1] for a complete analysis of this important topic.

SURGICAL CONSIDERATIONS

Sedation and Anesthesia

Periodontal surgery should be painless. The patient should be assured of this at the outset and should be thoroughly anesthetized by means of block and infiltration injections of local anesthetic agents. Injections directly into the interdental papillae may be helpful.

Apprehensive patients often require special management. The history, physical condition, and personality of the patient should be taken into consideration in order to determine the medications required, if any. Diazepam (Valium), 10 mg orally before surgery, can be helpful. Intravenous sedation with diazepam or inhalation analgesia with nitrous oxide–oxygen is also helpful in some cases. The use of some drugs requires that the patient come to the dental office accompanied by a responsible adult who can drive the patient home after surgery. Therefore the patient and office personnel must plan ahead when these agents are to be employed.

Scaling and Root Planing

Although scaling and root planing will have been performed previously as part of Phase I therapy, all exposed root surfaces should be carefully explored and planed as needed as part of the surgical procedure. In particular, areas of difficult access, such as furcations or deep pockets, often have rough areas of residual calculus. The assistant, who is separating the tissues and using the aspirator, can also, from a different angle, look for calculus on visible surfaces.

Hemostasis

An aspirator is indispensable for performing periodontal surgery. It provides the operator with a clear view of each root surface, which is necessary for thorough removal of deposits and planing. Further, it permits the accurate appraisal of the extent and pattern of soft tissue and bone involvement and prevents the seepage of blood into the floor of the mouth and oropharynx.

Periodontal surgery produces profuse bleeding during the initial incisional steps. However, after the existing granulation tissue has been removed, the bleeding is considerably reduced. Packing with gauze squares and the use of aspiration are necessary to keep the field dry.

Periodontal Dressings (Periodontal Packs)

After the surgical periodontal procedures are completed, the area is covered with a surgical pack. In general, dressings have no curative properties; they assist healing by protecting the tissue rather than by providing "healing factors." The pack serves the following functions:

1. Controls postoperative bleeding.

2. Minimizes the likelihood of postoperative infection and hemorrhage.

3. Provides some splinting of mobile teeth.

4. Facilitates healing by preventing surface trauma during mastication and irritation from plaque and food debris.

5. Protects against pain induced by contact of the wound with food or with the tongue during mastication.

Types of Dressings

Numerous types of dressings have been proposed for periodontal use. The most common types of dressing are zinc oxide–eugenol and noneugenol packs.

Zinc Oxide–Eugenol Packs. These are based on *the reaction of zinc oxide and eugenol.* They include the Wondr-Pak developed by Ward[16] in 1923 and several others that modified Ward's original formula. The addition of accelerators, such as zinc acetate, gives the dressing a better working time. Other substances that have been added include asbestos, used as a binder and a filler, and tannic acid. It has been shown, however,

that asbestos can induce lung diseases and that tannic acid may lead to liver damage; therefore, both substances should be avoided. Zinc oxide–eugenol type dressings are supplied as a liquid and a powder that are mixed prior to use. Some of them may be prepared ahead of time, wrapped in wax paper, and frozen for prolonged storage. The presence of eugenol in this type of pack may induce an allergic reaction that produces reddening of the area and burning pain in some patients.

Noneugenol Packs. The reaction between a *metallic oxide and fatty acids* is the basis for Coe-Pak (Fig. 15–2), which is the most widely used type of noneugenol dressing in the United States. This is supplied in two tubes that are mixed immediately before use until a uniform color is obtained. Fingers should be lubricated with petrolatum (Vaseline). Coe-Pak can be handled and molded 3 to 5 minutes after mixing and remains workable for 15 to 20 minutes. Working time can be shortened by adding a small amount of zinc oxide powder to the pink paste (from the accelerator tube) before spatulating. This dressing does not contain asbestos or eu-

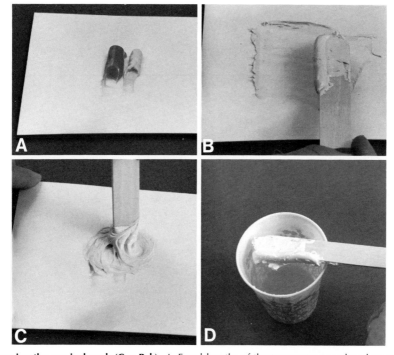

Figure 15–2. Preparing the surgical pack (Coe-Pak). A, Equal lengths of the two pastes are placed on paper pad. B, Mix with a wooden tongue depressor for 2 or 3 minutes until C, the paste loses its tackiness. D, Paste is placed in a paper cup of water at room temperature. With lubricated fingers it is then rolled into cylinders and placed on the surgical wound.

genol, thereby avoiding the problems associated with these substances.

Retention of Packs

Periodontal dressings are usually kept in place mechanically by interlocking in interdental spaces and by joining the lingual and facial portions of the pack.

Around isolated teeth or when there are several missing teeth in an arch, retention of the pack may be difficult. Numerous reinforcements, splints and stents for this purpose have been described.[5, 6]

Application of Periodontal Dressing

Zinc oxide packs are mixed with eugenol or noneugenol liquids on a wax paper pad with a wooden tongue depressor. The powder is gradually incorporated with the liquid until a thick paste is formed.

Coe-Pak is prepared by mixing equal lengths of paste from the accelerator and base tubes until the resulting paste is a uniform color. In 2 to 3 minutes the paste loses its tackiness and can be handled with lubricated fingers.

The pack is then rolled into two strips approximately the length of the treated area. The end of one strip is bent to fit around the distal surface of the last tooth. The remainder of the strip is brought forward along the facial surface to the midline and gently pressed into place along the incised gingival margin and interproximally. The second strip is applied from the lingual surface. It is joined to the pack at the distal surface of the last

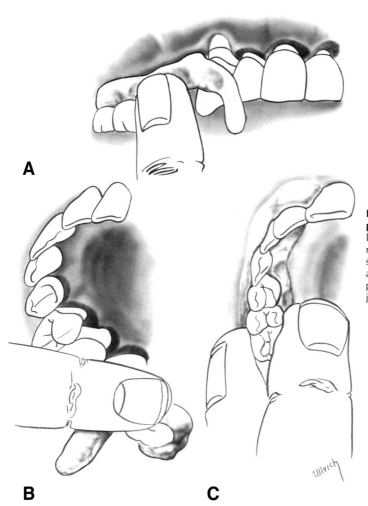

A

B

C

Figure 15–3. Inserting the periodontal pack. *A,* Strip of pack is hooked around last molar and pressed into place anteriorly. *B,* Lingual pack joined to the facial strip at the distal surface of the last molar and fitted into place anteriorly. *C,* Gentle pressure on facial and lingual surfaces joins pack interproximally.

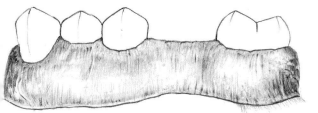

Figure 15–4. Continuous pack covers edentulous space.

tooth and then brought forward along the cut gingival margin to the midline. The strips are joined interproximally by applying gentle pressure on the facial and lingual surfaces of the pack (Fig. 15–3). For isolated teeth separated by edentulous spaces, the pack should be made continuous from tooth to tooth, covering the edentulous areas (Fig. 15–4).

The pack should cover the gingiva, but overextensions onto uninvolved mucosa should be avoided. *Excess pack irritates the mucobuccal fold and floor of the mouth and interferes with the tongue.* Overextension also jeopardizes the remainder of the pack because it tends to break off, taking pack from the operated area with it. *Pack that interferes with the occlusion should be trimmed away before the patient is dismissed* (Fig. 15–5). Failure to do this causes discomfort and jeopardizes retention of the pack.

As a general rule, the pack is kept on for 1 week after surgery. This guideline is based upon the timetable of healing and on clinical experience. It is not a rigid requirement; the period may be extended, or the area may be repacked for an additional week.

Fragments of the surface of the pack may break off postoperatively, but this presents no problem. If a portion of the pack is lost from the operated area and the patient is uncomfortable, it is usually best to repack the area. To repack, remaining pack is removed, the tissue gently washed with warm water, and a topical anesthetic applied before replacing the pack. Patients may develop pain from an overextended margin that irritates the vestibule, floor of the mouth, or tongue. Any excess pack should be trimmed away, making sure that the new margin is not rough.

Postoperative Instructions

After the pack is placed, printed instructions should be given to the patient. Important points should be stressed verbally. An example of written postoperative instructions follows:

POSTOPERATIVE INSTRUCTIONS

The operation which has been performed on your gums will help you keep your teeth. The following information has been prepared to answer questions you may have about how to take care of your mouth. Please read the instructions carefully—our patients have found them very helpful.

When the anesthesia wears off, you may have slight discomfort—not pain. Two acetaminophen (Tylenol) tablets will usually keep you comfortable. You may repeat every 4 hours if necessary.

We have placed a periodontal pack over your gums to protect them from irritation. The pack prevents pain, aids healing, and enables you to carry on most of your usual activities in comfort. The pack will harden in a few hours, after which it can withstand most of the forces of chewing

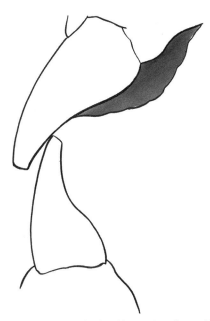

Figure 15–5. The pack should not interfere with the occlusion.

without breaking off. It may take a little while to become accustomed to it.

For your benefit the pack should remain in place as long as possible. *Do not remove it*. If particles of the pack chip off during the week, do not be concerned as long as you do not have pain. If a piece of the pack breaks off and you are in pain, or if a rough edge irritates your tongue or cheek, please call the office. The problem can be easily remedied by replacing the pack. The pack will be removed at your next appointment.

For the first 3 hours after the operation avoid hot foods in order to permit the pack to harden. After this, eat anything you can manage without chipping the pack. Eggs, Jell-O, cereals, soups, milk, fish, hamburger, or any semisolid or finely minced foods are suggested. Avoid citrus fruits or fruit juices, highly spiced foods, and alcoholic beverages. They will cause pain. Food supplements and/or vitamins are generally not necessary. We will prescribe them if needed.

Do not smoke—the heat and smoke will irritate your gums and delay healing. If at all possible, use this opportunity to give up smoking. Smokers have more gum disease than nonsmokers.

Rinsing is not part of the treatment, but it will help to make your mouth feel refreshed. *Do not rinse today*. Beginning tomorrow, you may rinse as often as you wish with one of the popular, pleasant-flavored mouthwashes. Do not use it in concentrated form; dilute it—1/3 mouthwash to 2/3 warm water.

Clean the parts of your mouth which have been treated in previous weeks, using the methods in which you were instructed. The gums most likely will bleed more than they did before the operation. This is perfectly normal in the early stage of healing and will gradually subside. Do not stop cleaning because of it.

Follow your regular daily activities, but avoid excessive exertion of any type. Golf, tennis, skiing, bowling, swimming, or sunbathing should be postponed until 2 days after the operation.

You may experience a slight feeling of weakness or chills during the first 24 hours. This should not be cause for alarm but should be reported at the next visit.

Swelling is not unusual, particularly in areas which required extensive surgical procedures. The swelling generally subsides in 3 or 4 days. If the swelling is painful or appears to become worse, please call the office.

There may be occasional blood stains in the saliva for the first 4 or 5 hours after the operation. This is not unusual and will correct itself. If there is considerable bleeding beyond this, take a piece of gauze, form it into the shape of a U, hold it in the thumb and index finger, apply it to both sides of the pack, and hold it there under pressure for 20 minutes. Do not remove it during this period to examine it. If the bleeding does not stop at the

end of 20 minutes, please contact the office. *Do not try to stop the bleeding by rinsing*.

If any other problems arise, please call the office, telephone no. _____.

Management During the First Postoperative Week

Properly performed, periodontal surgery presents no serious postoperative problems. Unfavorable sequelae are the exception rather than the rule. However, several circumstances may arise that will cause the patient to call or return to the office.

1. *Persistent bleeding after surgery*. The pack should be removed, the bleeding points located, and the bleeding stopped with pressure, electrosurgery, or electrocautery. After the bleeding is stopped, the pack is replaced.

2. *Sensitivity to percussion*. Sensitivity to percussion may be caused by the extension of inflammation into the periodontal ligament. The patient should be questioned regarding the progress of the symptoms. Progressively diminishing severity is a favorable sign. The pack should be removed and the gingiva checked for localized areas of infection or irritation, which should be cleaned or incised to provide drainage. Particles of calculus that may have been overlooked should be removed. Relieving the occlusion is usually helpful. Sensitivity to percussion may also be caused by excess pack which interferes with the occlusion. Removal of the excess usually corrects the condition.

3. *Swelling*. Sometimes within the first 2 postoperative days patients report a soft, painless swelling of the cheek in the area of operation. There may be lymph node enlargement, and the temperature may be slightly elevated. The area of operation itself is usually symptom-free. This type of involvement results from a localized inflammatory reaction to the operative procedure. It generally subsides by the fourth postoperative day, without necessitating removal of the pack. Penicillin, 250 mg every 4 hours for 48 hours, is helpful as a prophylactic measure for subsequent surgeries.

4. *Feeling of weakness*. Occasionally patients report having experienced a "washed out," weakened feeling for about 24 hours after the operation. This represents a systemic reaction to a transient bacteremia induced by

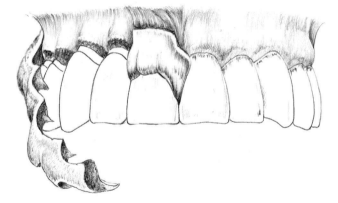

Figure 15–6. Removal of the periodontal pack.

the operative procedure. It is prevented by premedication with penicillin, 250 mg every 4 hours, beginning 24 hours before the next operation and continuing for a 24-hour postoperative period.

Postoperative Visits

When the patient returns after 1 week, the pack is taken off (Fig. 15–6) by inserting an instrument along the margin and exerting gentle lateral pressure. Pieces of pack retained interproximally and particles which adhere to the tooth surfaces are removed gently with scalers. Particles may be enmeshed in the cut surface and should be carefully picked off with fine cotton pliers. The entire area should be syringed with warm water to remove superficial debris.

If a *gingivectomy* has been performed, the cut surface will be covered with a friable meshwork of new epithelium which should not be disturbed. After a *flap operation*, the areas corresponding to the incisions will be epithelialized but may bleed readily when touched; they should not be disturbed. Pockets should not be probed. The facial and lingual mucosa may be covered with a grayish-yellow or white granular layer of food debris that has seeped under the pack. It is easily removed with a moist cotton pellet. The root surfaces will probably be sensitive to a probe or to thermal changes, and the teeth may be stained.

When to Repack

After the pack is removed, it is usually not necessary to replace it. However, it is advisable to repack for an additional week for patients with (1) low pain thresholds who are particularly uncomfortable when the pack is removed, (2) unusually extensive periodontal involvement, or (3) slow healing. Clinical experience and judgment will help to decide whether to repack the area or leave the initial pack on longer than 1 week.

Tooth Mobility

Tooth mobility is increased immediately after surgery, but by the fourth week it diminishes below the pretreatment level.

Final Check on Smoothness of Root Surfaces

One week after the pack is removed from the final quadrant, all root surfaces should be checked to see that they are smooth and firm. A rubber cup polish may be used for the final smoothing of the roots at this time.

Postoperative Oral Hygiene Care

Care of the mouth by the patient between the treatment of the first and the final areas, as well as after surgery is completed, is extremely important. It begins after the pack is removed from the first operation. The patient has been through a presurgical period of instructed plaque control and should be reinstructed at this time.

Vigorous brushing during the first week after the pack is removed is not feasible. However, the patient is informed that plaque and food accumulation will retard healing and is advised *to try to keep the area as clean as possible* by the gentle use of interdental cleansers and dental floss and light water irrigation. Brushing is resumed gradually as healing of the tissues permits, and the vigor of the overall hygiene regimen is increased as healing progresses. Patients should be told that there will most likely be more gingival bleeding than before the operation, that it is perfectly normal and will subside as healing progresses, and that it should not deter them from following their oral hygiene regimen.

Chlorhexidine mouthrinses or topical application of chlorhexidine with Q-tips for the first few postoperative weeks is helpful in postoperative care.

Management of Postoperative Pain

Periodontal surgery performed following the basic principles outlined here should produce only minor pain and discomfort.[14] However, in some cases severe pain may be present; its control then becomes an important part of patient management.[11]

In general, procedures that involve extensive and/or prolonged bone surgery are more likely to induce postoperative pain than more conservative procedures such as the so-called modified Widman flap or gingivectomy.

A common source of postoperative pain is *overextension of the periodontal pack* onto the soft tissue beyond the mucogingival junction or onto the frena. Overextended packs cause localized areas of edema, usually noticed 1 to 2 days after surgery. Removal of excess pack is followed by resolution in about 24 hours.

When severe postoperative pain is present, the patient should be seen at the office immediately. The area should be anesthetized by infiltration or topically, the pack removed, and the wound examined. Postoperative pain related to *infection* will induce localized lymphadenopathy and a slight elevation in temperature. It should be treated with systemic antibiotics and analgesics. Extensive and excessively prolonged exposure and dryness of bone will also induce severe pain. This may necessitate narcotic analgesics, such as oxycodone compounds (Percodan) or meperidine hydrochloride (Demerol).

Treatment of Sensitive Roots

Root sensitivity is a relatively common problem in periodontal practice. It may occur spontaneously when the root becomes exposed through gingival recession or pocket formation, or it may appear after scaling and root planing, and surgical procedures. It is manifested as pain induced by cold or hot temperatures, more commonly the former; by citrus fruits or sweets; or by contact with toothbrushes or dental instruments.

It occurs more frequently in the cervical area of the root, where the cementum is extremely thin or nonexistent, exposing the dentin. Scaling and root planing procedures remove this thin cementum, inducing the sensitivity.

The transmission of stimuli from the surface of the dentin to the nerve endings located in the dental pulp or in the pulpal region of the dentin could occur through the odontoblastic process or owing to a hydrodynamic mechanism by means of displacement of fluid in dentinal tubules. The latter process seems more likely and would explain the importance of burnishing desensitizing agents in order to obturate the dentinal tubules.

A very important factor for reducing or eliminating sensitivity is adequate plaque control. However, sensitivity may prevent plaque control, and therefore a vicious circle may be created.

Desensitizing Agents

A number of agents have been proposed to control root sensitivity. Pattison and Pattison[12] list the following possible mechanisms of action for desensitizing agents: (1) precipitation or denaturing of organic material at the exposed end of the odontoblastic process, (2) deposition of an inorganic salt at the exposed end of the dentinal tubules, (3) stimulation of secondary dentin formation within the pulp, and (4) suppression of pulpal inflammation.

The patient should be informed about the possibility of root sensitivity before treatment is undertaken. The following information on how to cope with the problem should also be given:

1. Sensitivity appears because of the exposure of dentin, which is inevitable if calculus and plaque and their products, buried in the tissue, are to be removed.

2. Sensitivity usually disappears slowly over a few weeks.

3. Plaque control is very important for the reduction of sensitivity.

4. Desensitizing agents do not produce immediate relief. They have to be used for several days or even weeks to produce results.

Clinical evaluation of the many desensitizing agents proposed has proved very difficult, in part because it is difficult to measure and compare different persons' pain, because sensitivity disappears by itself after a time, and because desensitizing agents take a few weeks to act.

Desensitizing agents can be applied by the patient at home or by the dentist or hygienist in the dental office.

Agents Used by the Patient. The most common agents used by the patient for desensitization are dentifrices. The following agents in dentifrices have been reported to be useful: strontium chloride (Sensodyne),[2, 13] sodium monofluorophosphate (Colgate),[8] formaldehyde (Thermodent),[3] polyglycol (Protect), and potassium nitrate (Denquel).

An aqueous solution of 2 per cent sodium fluoride can also be used instead of a dentifrice; the patient should be cautioned not to swallow it. Fluoride rinsing solution and gels can also be used after the usual plaque control procedures.[15] Currently 0.05% fluoride rinses are available as non-prescription items and may be helpful for densensitization.

Agents Used in the Dental Office. Fluoride solutions and pastes are the agents of choice. In addition to their desensitivity properties they have the advantage of anticaries activity, which is particularly important for patients with a tendency to develop root caries.

High concentration fluoride paste consists of equal parts of sodium fluoride, kaolin, and glycerin. This paste is applied as follows:

1. Isolate the tooth or teeth requiring desensitization and dry them with cotton pellets.

2. Burnish the paste with an instrument; leave it for 2 minutes.

3. Remove the paste with warm water and rinse thoroughly.

The patient may feel an initial sensation of cold or pain that may require anesthesia prior to the application of the paste.

Iontophoresis can be used to deliver sodium fluoride into the tooth structure.[4] The results with this method are controversial.

Other desensitizing agents for office use are zinc chloride, 8 per cent solution; liquid phenol; formaldehyde; ammoniacal silver nitrate; a mixture of sodium carbonate monohydrate, 2.5 grams, and potassium carbonate, 12.5 mg; and sodium silicofluoride.[7, 9] Except for the last two, these agents should not be used on freshly cut dentin.

Corticosteroid hormones have also been used for desensitizing exposed root surfaces.[10] They probably act by reducing the inflammatory reaction of the pulp.

References

1. Allen, G. D.: Dental Anesthesia and Analgesia (Local and General). 2nd ed. Baltimore, Williams & Wilkins, 1979.
2. Blitzer, B.: A consideration of the possible causes of dental hypersensitivity: treatment by a strontiumion dentifrice. Periodontics, 5:318, 1967.
3. Forrest, J. O.: A clinical assessment of three desensitizing toothpastes containing formalin. Br. Dent. J., 114:103, 1963.
4. Gangarosa, L.: Iontophoretic application of fluoride by tray techniques for desensitizing multiple teeth. J. Am. Dent. Assoc., 95:50, 1981.
5. Hirschfeld, A. S., and Wasserman, B. H.: Retention of periodontal packs. J. Periodontol., 29:199, 1958.
6. Holmes, C. H.: Periodontal pack on single tooth retained by acrylic splint. J. Am. Dent. Assoc., 64:831, 1962.
7. Hunter, G. C., Jr., Barringer, M., and Spooner, G.: Analysis of desensitization of dentin by sodium silicofluoride and Gottlieb's solution by use of radioactive silver nitrate. J. Periodontol., 32:333, 1961.
8. Kanouse, M. C., and Ash, M. M., Jr.: The effectiveness of a sodium monofluorophosphate dentifrice on dental hypersensitivity. J. Periodontol., 40:38, 1969.
9. Massler, M.: Desensitization of cervical cementum and dentin by sodium silicofluoride. J. Dent. Res., 34:761, 1955.
10. Mosteller, J. H.: Use of prednisolone in the elimination of postoperative thermal sensitivity. J. Prosthet. Dent., 12:1176, 1962.
11. Murphy, N. C., and DeMarco, T. J.: Controlling pain in periodontal patients. Dent. Survey, 55:46, 1979.
12. Pattison, G. L., and Pattison, A. M.: Periodontal Instrumentation. Reston, Va., Reston Publishing Company, 1979.
13. Ross, M. R.: Hypersensitive teeth: effect of strontium chloride in a compatible dentifrice. J. Periodontol., 32:49, 1961.
14. Strahan, J. D., and Glenwright, H. D.: Pain experience in periodontal surgery. J. Periodont. Res., 1:163, 1967.
15. Tarbet, W. J., Silverman, G., Stolman, J. W., and Fratarcangelo, P. A.: A clinical evaluation of a new treatment for dentinal hypersensitivity. J. Periodontol., 51:535, 1980.
16. Ward, A. W.: Inharmonious cusp relation as a factor in periodontoclasia. J. Am. Dent. Assoc., 10:471, 1923.

Chapter 16

Surgical Techniques

GINGIVAL CURETTAGE

The word *curettage* is used in periodontics to mean the scraping of the gingival wall of a periodontal pocket to separate diseased soft tissue. *Scaling* refers to the removal of deposits from tooth surfaces, and *root planing* means smoothing the root to remove infected and necrotic tooth substance. Scaling and root planing may inadvertently include various degrees of curettage. However, they are different procedures, with different rationales and indications, and should be considered as separate parts of periodontal treatment.

Curettage hastens healing by reducing the task of the body's enzymes and phagocytes, which ordinarily remove tissue debris during healing. Also, by removing the epithelial lining of the periodontal pocket, curettage removes a barrier to reattachment of the periodontal fibers to the root surface. It has been reported that bacteria invade the pocket lining and the junctional epithelium in advanced periodontal disease.[29] Curettage removes these areas of bacterial penetration.

Some degree of irritation and trauma to the gingiva is unavoidable in curettage, even if it is performed with extreme care. In such cases, the injurious effects are of microscopic proportion and generally do not significantly affect healing. Overzealous curettage causes postoperative pain and retards healing.

A differentiation has been made between gingival and subgingival curettage. *Gingival curettage* consists of the removal of the inflamed soft tissue lateral to the pocket wall, whereas *subgingival curettage* refers to the procedure that is performed apical to the epithelial attachment, severing the connective tissue attachment down to the osseous crest (Fig. 16–1).

It is important to note that some degree of curettage is done unintentionally when scaling and root planing are performed. This is called *inadvertent curettage*. This section con-

221

days,[18, 22, 43] and restoration of the junctional epithelium occurs in animals as early as 5 days after treatment. Immature collagen fibers appear within 21 days. Healthy gingival fibers severed from the tooth by scaling, root planing, and curettage[17] and tears in the sulcular epithelium[17, 26] and junctional epithelium are repaired in the healing process.

Several investigators have reported that in monkeys[3] and in humans[42] treated by scaling and curettage, healing results in the formation of a long, thin junctional epithelium with no new connective tissue attachment. Sometimes this long epithelium is interrupted by "windows" of connective tissue attachment.[3]

Opinions differ regarding whether scaling and curettage consistently remove the pocket lining and the junctional epithelium. Some report that scaling and root planing tear the epithelial lining of the pocket without removing it or the junctional epithelium. But both epithelial structures,[16, 17] and sometimes underlying inflamed connective tissue,[18] are removed by curettage. Others report that the removal of pocket lining and junctional epithelium by curettage is not complete.[31, 39, 43]

Clinical Appearance of the Gingiva After Curettage

Immediately after scaling and curettage, the gingiva appears hemorrhagic and bright red.

After 1 week, the gingiva appears reduced in height because of an apical shift in the position of the gingival margin. The gingiva is also slightly redder than normal, but much less so than in previous days.

After 2 weeks, and with proper oral hygiene by the patient, the normal color, consistency, surface texture, and contour of the gingiva are attained, and the gingival margin is well adapted to the tooth.

GINGIVECTOMY

The term *gingivectomy* means excision of the gingiva. By removing the diseased pocket wall which obscures the tooth surface, gingivectomy provides the visibility and accessibility that are essential for the complete removal of calculus and thorough smoothing of the roots. By removing diseased tissue and

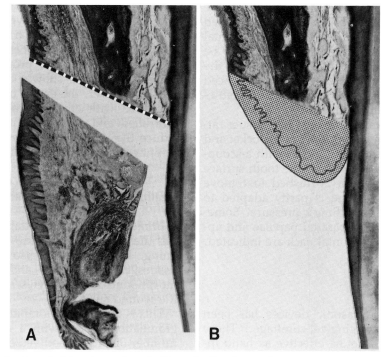

Figure 16–4. Gingivectomy incision close to bone facilitates healing that produces physiologic gingival contour. *A,* Labial incision close beyond the pocket and close to the bone. *B,* Diagrammatic representation of healed gingiva with physiologic contour and normal sulcus.

local irritants, it also creates a favorable environment for gingival healing and the restoration of a physiologic gingival contour.

Indications and Contraindications

The gingivectomy technique is indicated in the following cases[8]:

1. Elimination of suprabony pockets, regardless of their depth, if the pocket wall is fibrous and firm. This is because fibrous gingival tissue does not shrink after scaling and curettage, and therefore some form of surgical treatment is necessary to eliminate the pocket.

2. Elimination of gingival enlargements.

3. Elimination of suprabony periodontal abscesses.

These findings contraindicate the use of the gingivectomy technique:

1. The need for bone surgery or even for examination of the bone shape and morphology.

2. The location of the bottom of the pocket apical to the mucogingival junction.

When used for the purposes for which it is intended, the gingivectomy technique is a most effective form of treatment.

Technique

The pockets on each surface are explored with a periodontal probe and marked with a pocket marker. The gingiva is then resected with periodontal knives, a scalpel, or scissors (Figs. 16–4 and 16–5).

The gingivectomy incision is started apical to the points marking the course of the pockets[41] and directed coronally to a point between the base of the pocket and the crest of the bone. The incision should be beveled at approximately 45 degrees to the tooth surface. This is most important where the pocket wall is enlarged and fibrous, such as on the palatal surface in the molar area. The gingival margin is detached at the line of

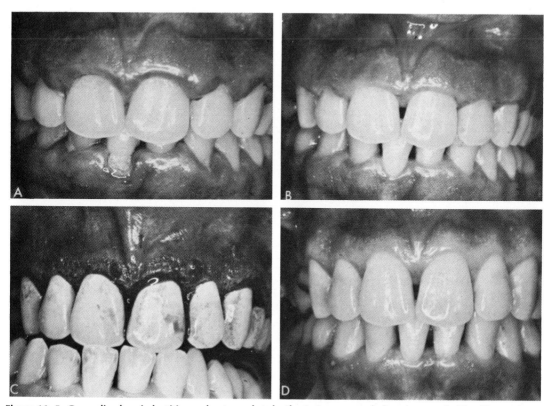

Figure 16–5. Generalized periodontitis, moderate pocket depth. *A,* Appearance before therapy. *B,* After Phase I therapy. *C,* After excision of gingival pocket wall. *D,* After 1 month of healing (courtesy of Dr. C. A. Dotto, Sao Paulo, Brazil). (*From* Takei, H. H., and Carranza, F. A.: General principles of periodontal surgery. *In* Steiner, R. B., and Thompson, R. D. (eds.): Oral Surgery and Anesthesia. Philadelphia, W. B. Saunders Co., 1977, pp. 132–150.)

incision with surgical hoes and scalers, and granulation tissue is removed. Thorough scaling and root planing is performed to remove any remaining calculus and necrotic cementum. The area is then covered with a periodontal pack.

Healing

The initial response after gingivectomy is the formation of a protective surface clot; the underlying tissue becomes acutely inflamed, with some necrosis. The clot is replaced by granulation tissue. After 12 to 24 hours, epithelial cells at the margins of the wound migrate over the granulation tissue to separate it from the contaminated surface layer of the clot. Surface epithelialization is generally complete after 5 to 14 days. During the first 4 weeks after gingivectomy, keratinization is less than it was prior to surgery.

Electrosurgery

Gingivectomy incisions can also be performed by use of electrosurgery. The advantage of this instrument is that electrosurgery permits adequate contouring of the tissue and controls hemorrhage.

There are several disadvantages to the use of electrosurgery. It cannot be used in patients who have noncompatible or poorly shielded cardiac pacemakers. Also, the treatment causes an unpleasant odor. If the electrosurgery point touches the bone, irreparable damage can be done,[1] further, the heat generated by injudicious use can cause tissue damage and loss of periodontal support when the electrode is used close to bone. When the electrode touches the root, areas of cementum burn are produced.[44]

It is recommended that the use of electrosurgery be limited to superficial procedures such as removal of gingival enlargements, gingivoplasty, relocating frenum and muscle attachments, and incising periodontal abscesses and pericoronal flaps. *It should not be used for procedures that involve proximity to the bone,* such as treatment of infrabony pockets, flap operations, or mucogingival surgery.

Gingivoplasty

Gingival and periodontal diseases often produce deformities in the gingiva which interfere with normal food excursion, collect irritating plaque and food debris, and prolong and aggravate the disease process. Gingival clefts and craters, shelf-like interdental papillae caused by acute necrotizing ulcerative gingivitis, and gingival enlargement are examples of such deformities. *Artificially reshaping the gingiva to create physiologic gingival contours is termed gingivoplasty.*[9]

The gingivoplasty technique is similar to

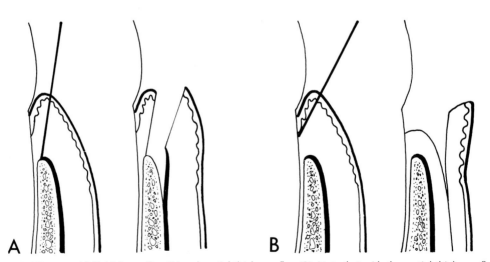

Figure 16–6. Diagram of full thickness flap *(A)* and partial thickness flap *(B).* Note that with the partial thickness flap the bone remains covered by periosteum.

the gingivectomy technique; however, its purpose is different. Gingivectomy is performed in order to eliminate periodontal pockets and includes reshaping as part of the technique. Gingivoplasty is done in the absence of pockets with the sole purpose of recontouring the gingiva.

Gingivoplasty may be done with periodontal knives, scalpels, rotary diamond stones, or electrosurgery. It creates a tapered gingival margin with an escalloped marginal outline, thins the attached gingiva, and forms vertical interdental grooves and shapes the interdental papillae to provide sluiceways for the passage of food.

PERIODONTAL FLAP SURGERY

Rationale

The periodontal flap consists of surgically separating a section of gingiva and/or mucosa from the underlying tissues in order to provide visibility of and access to the bone and root surface (Fig. 16-6). Once the flap is elevated, one or more of the following purposes can be accomplished:

a. Thorough scaling and planing of the exposed root surfaces, followed by replacement of the flap in its original positon. This technique is known as "flap curettage," the "unrepositioned flap technique," or the "modified Widman flap."

b. Displacement of the flap to cover a denuded root surface, called the "laterally sliding flap," or to regenerate attached gingiva in a position apical to that of the pre-existent pocket, the "apically positioned flap."

c. Osseous surgery consisting of recontouring the existing bone, or procedures to enhance the possibility of bone regeneration.

Incisions

Periodontal flaps utilize horizontal and vertical incisions. *Horizontal incisions* are directed along the margin of the gingiva in a mesial or a distal direction. Two types of horizontal incisions have been recommended: the internal bevel incision,[6] which starts at a distance from the gingival margin and is aimed at the bone crest; and the crevicular incision, which starts at the bottom of the pocket and is directed to the bone margin. The *internal bevel incision* is the incision basic to all periodontal flap procedures; it is the incision from which the flap will be reflected to expose the underlying bone and root (Fig. 16-7A). The internal bevel incision accomplishes three very important objectives: it (1) removes the pocket lining; (2) conserves the relatively uninvolved outer surface of the gingiva, which, if apically positioned, will become attached gingiva; and (3) creates a sharp, thin flap margin for adaptation to the bone-tooth junction.

A surgical scalpel is used for this incision. That portion of the gingiva left around the tooth contains the epithelium of the pocket lining and the adjacent granulomatous tissue. It will be discarded after the crevicular and interdental incisions are performed.

The *crevicular incision* (Fig. 16-7B) is made from the base of the pocket to the crest of the bone. This incision, together with the initial incision, will form a V-shaped wedge ending at the crest of bone. The incision is carried around the entire tooth.

Figure 16-7. The three incisions necessary for flap surgery. *A,* Internal bevel (1); *B,* crevicular (2); *C,* interdental (3).

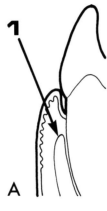
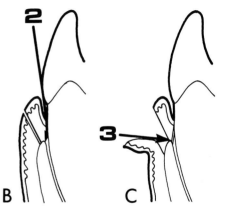

A periosteal elevator can now be inserted into the initial internal bevel incision and the flap separated from the bone. With this access, the surgeon is now able to make the *interdental incision* (Fig. 16–7C) to separate the collar of gingiva which is left around the tooth. The Orban knife is usually used for this incision. The incision is made not only around the facial and lingual radicular area but also interdentally, connecting the facial and lingual segments, to completely free the gingiva around the tooth.

These three incisions will now allow the removal of the gingiva around the tooth, including the pocket epithelium and the adjacent granulomatous tissue. A curette or a large scaler is used for this purpose. After removal of the large pieces of tissue, the remaining connective tissue in the osseous lesion should be carefully curetted out so that the entire root and the bone surface adjacent to the teeth can be seen.

Vertical or *oblique releasing incisions* can be utilized on either one or both ends of the horizontal incision, depending on the design and purpose of the flap. Vertical incisions at both ends are necessary if the flap is to be repositioned. Vertical incisions must extend beyond the mucogingival line, reaching the alveolar mucosa, to allow for the release and repositioning of the flap.

Elevation of the Flap

Periodontal flaps are classified as either full thickness (mucoperiosteal) or partial thickness (mucosal) flaps (Fig. 16–6). In *full thickness flaps*, all of the soft tissue, including the periosteum, is reflected to expose the underlying bone. This complete exposure of and access to the underlying bone is indicated if osseous surgery is contemplated. The full thickness flap is reflected by means of a blunt dissection. A periosteal elevator is used to separate the mucoperiosteum from the bone by moving it mesially, distally, and apically until the desired reflection is accomplished.

The *partial thickness flap* includes reflection of the epithelium and a layer of the underlying connective tissue. The bone remains covered by a layer of connective tissue, including the periosteum. Sharp dissection is necessary to reflect the partial thickness flap.

A surgical scalpel is utilized to separate the flap carefully. The partial thickness flap is indicated when the flap is to be positioned apically or when the operator does not desire to expose bone.

Flaps can also be classified as (1) repositioned or positioned flaps and (2) unrepositioned flaps, depending on the placement of the flap at the conclusion of the surgical procedure. An *unrepositioned flap* is placed in the position it had before surgery, whereas a *repositioned flap* can be placed apical, coronal, or lateral to its original position.

Distal Molar Surgery

The treatment of periodontal pockets on the *distal surface of terminal molars* is frequently complicated by the presence of bulbous fibrous tissue over the maxillary tuberosity or prominent retromolar pads in the mandible. Deep vertical defects are also commonly present in conjunction with the redundant fibrous tissue. Some of these osseous lesions may result from incomplete repair after the extraction of impacted third molars.

The gingivectomy incision is the most direct approach in treating distal pockets which have no osseous lesions and have adequate attached gingiva. However, the flap approach is less traumatic postsurgically, since it results in a primary closure wound rather than the open secondary wound left by a gingivectomy incision. In addition, it produces attached gingiva and provides access for examination and, if needed, correction of the osseous defect.[2, 27] The initial incision for the distal wedge procedure is shown in Figure 16–8.

Suturing Techniques

There are many types of sutures, suture needles, and materials;[4, 15] the following methods, using a 3/8 circle reverse cutting needle and 3-0 black braided silk, fill most needs in periodontal surgery.

Interdental Ligation

Two types of interdental ligation can be used: (1) the direct or loop suture (Fig. 16–9), also called the simple interrupted suture, and (2) the figure eight suture (Fig. 16–10).

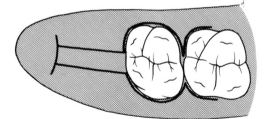

Figure 16–8. Distal molar surgery. A typical incision design for a surgical procedure distal to the maxillary second molar.

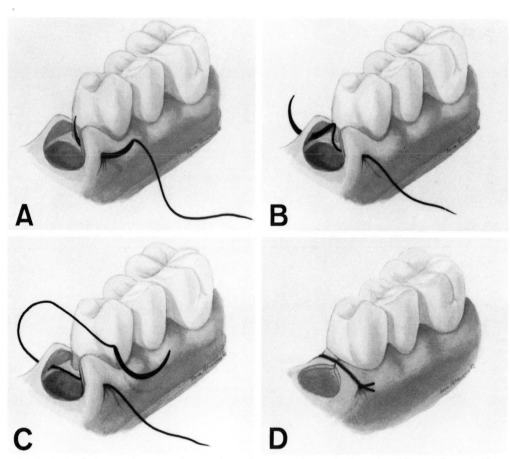

Figure 16–9. A simple loop or interrupted suture is used to approximate the buccal and lingual flaps. *A,* The needle penetrates the outer surface of the first flap. *B,* The undersurface of the opposite flap is engaged, and *C,* the suture is brought back to the initial side, where *D,* the knot is tied.

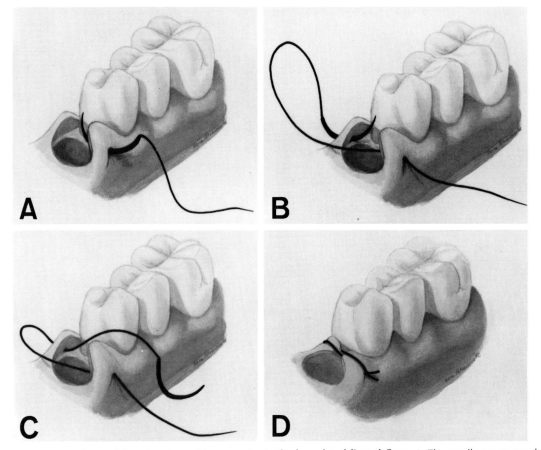

Figure 16–10. A figure eight suture is used to approximate the buccal and lingual flaps. *A,* The needle penetrates the outer surface of the first flap and *B,* the outer surface of the opposite flap. *C,* The suture is brought back to the first flap, and *D,* the knot is tied.

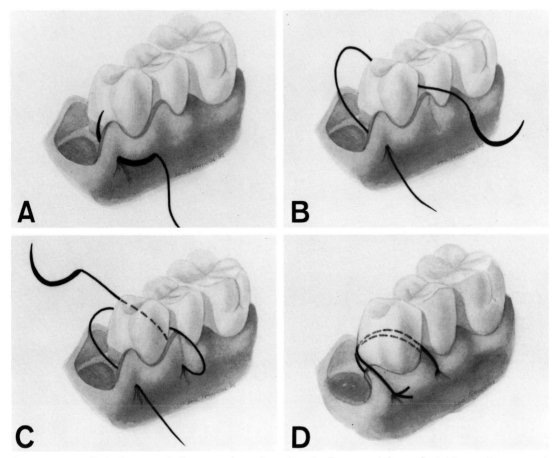

Figure 16–11. A single, interrupted sling suture is used to adapt the flap around the tooth. *A,* The needle engages the outer surface of the flap and *B,* encircles the tooth. *C,* The outer surface of the same flap of the adjacent interdental area is engaged, and *D,* the suture is returned to the initial site and the knot tied.

Sling Ligation

The sling ligation can be used for a flap on one surface of a tooth, involving two or more interdental spaces (Fig. 16–11).

Horizontal Mattress Suture

This suture is often used for the interproximal areas of diastemata or for wide interdental spaces in order to properly adapt the interproximal papilla against the bone. Two sutures are often necessary.

Continuous Independent Sling Suture

This is used when there is both a facial and a lingual flap involving many teeth (Fig. 16–12). The suture is initiated on the facial papilla closest to the midline, since this is the easiest place to position the final knot. A continuous sling suture is laced for each papilla on the facial surface. When the last tooth is reached, the suture is anchored around it to prevent any pulling of the facial sutures when the lingual flap is sutured around the teeth in a similar fashion. The suture is again anchored around the last tooth prior to the final knot. This type of ligature does not produce a pull on the lingual flap when the latter is sutured. The two flaps are completely independent of each other owing to the anchoring around both the initial and the final tooth. The flaps are tied to the teeth and not to each other because of the sling sutures.

Anchor Suture

The closing of a flap mesial or distal to a tooth, as in the mesial or distal wedge procedures, is best accomplished by the anchor

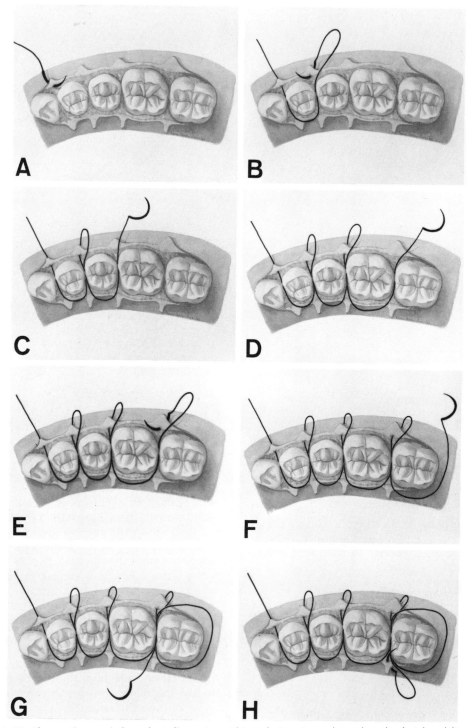

Figure 16–12. The continuous, independent sling suture. This technique is used to adapt the facial and lingual flaps without tying the facial flap to the lingual flap. The teeth are utilized to suspend each flap independently.

Illustration continued on opposite page

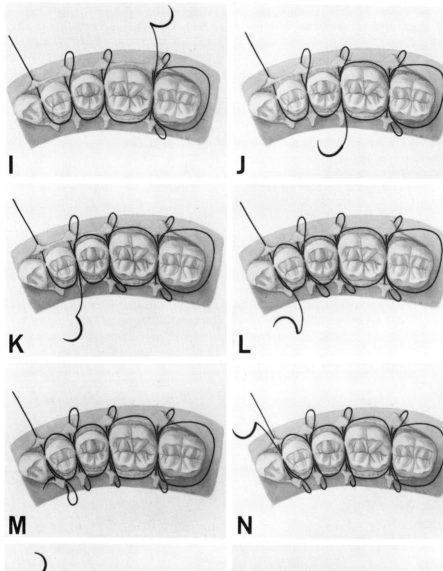

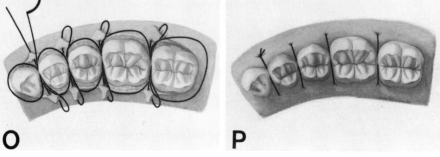

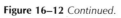

Figure 16–12 *Continued.*

suture (Fig. 16–13). This suture closes the facial and lingual flaps and adapts them tightly against the tooth. The needle is placed at the line angle area of the facial or lingual flap adjacent to the tooth, anchored around the tooth, passed beneath the opposite flap, and tied.

OSSEOUS SURGERY

Osseous surgery may be defined as the procedure by which changes in the alveolar bone can be accomplished to rid it of deformities created by the periodontal disease process or other related factors, such as exostosis and tooth supraeruption. It is performed after the flap is elevated.

Osseous surgery can be either additive or subtractive in nature. *Additive osseous surgery* includes the procedures directed at restoring the alveolar bone to original levels, whereas *subtractive methods* are designed to restore the form of preexisting alveolar bone to the level existing at the time of surgery or slightly more apical to it.

The morphology of osseous defects will greatly determine the treatment technique to be used. One-wall angular defects usually have to be recontoured surgically. Three-wall defects, particularly if they are narrow and deep, can be successfully treated by techniques that aim at reattachment and bone regeneration. Two-wall angular defects can be treated by either method, depending on their depth, width, and general configuration.

Osseous Resective Surgery

Osseous resective surgery is the most predictable pocket reduction technique. However, it is performed at the expense of bony tissue and attachment level.[38, 45] The goal of osseous resective therapy is reshaping the marginal bone to resemble the alveolar process undamaged by periodontal disease. The technique is accomplished in combination with apically repositioned flaps, and the procedure eliminates periodontal pocket depth and improves tissue contour to provide a more easily maintainable environment. *The major rationale for osseous resective surgery is centered on the tenet that discrepancies in levels and shapes of the bone and gingiva predispose to*

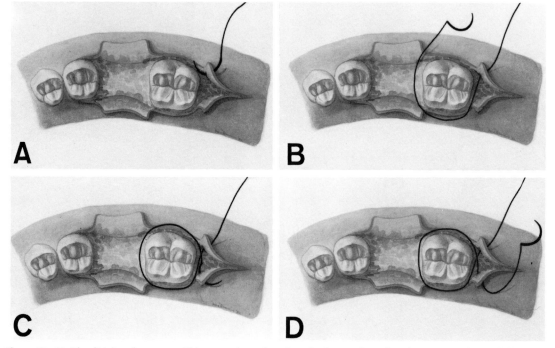

Figure 16–13. The distal anchor suture. This suture is used to close the flaps and to adapt them against the tooth following mesial or distal wedge surgery.

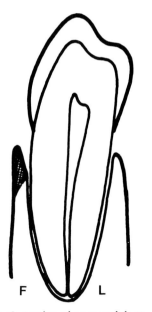

F   L

Figure 16–14. Correction of osseous defects. A one-wall defect located on the facial surface (F) is reduced by osteoplasty, resulting in no additional loss of bone support for the tooth. A one-wall defect located on an interproximal surface requires ostectomy for reduction, thereby reducing support for the adjoining tooth. (L = lingual surface.)

the recurrence of pocket depth postsurgically.[23] Although this concept is not universally accepted,[46] and despite the fact that the procedure induces loss of radicular bone in the healing phases, *there are cases in which recontouring of bone is the only logical treatment choice.*

Procedures used to correct osseous defects have been classified in two groups: osteoplasty and ostectomy[7] (Fig. 16–14). *Osteoplasty* refers to reshaping the bone without removing tooth-supporting bone. *Ostectomy* (or osteoectomy) includes the removal of tooth-supporting bone. Either or both of these procedures may be necessary to produce the desired result.

Methods of Osseous Resective Surgery

Osseous resective surgery is an extremely precise, demanding technique. It is fundamentally an attempt to gradualize the bone sufficiently to allow soft tissue structure to follow the contour of the bone. The soft tissue will predictably attach to the bone within certain specific dimensions.

The topography that is encountered after periodontal flap reflection varies greatly. When all soft tissue is removed around the teeth, there may be large exostoses, ledges, troughs, craters, vertical defects, or combinations of any of these. Each osseous situation presents uniquely challenging problems, especially if reshaping to the optimum level is contemplated.

A number of hand and rotary instruments have been used for osseous resective surgery. Whichever is used, care and precision are required to prevent excessive bone removal or root damage.

There is considerable difference of opinion regarding the wisdom of artificially remodeling bone in the treatment of periodontal disease. The biologic expense of selective recession and attachment loss must be constantly weighed against the benefits of pocket reduction when a patient is considered for osseous resective surgery.

Osseous Regenerative Surgery

The other major area of osseous surgery is osseous regeneration. This technique is less predictable than osseous resection, but the rewards include not only the elimination of the periodontal pocket but also the restoration of the periodontal apparatus by filling in the osseous defect and restoring smooth physiologic bone contours (Fig. 16–15). The likelihood of obtaining this "bone fill" depends in large measure on the architecture of and the number of bony walls in the defect. The more a defect is surrounded by bone, the more likely is regeneration.

Reconstructive periodontics can be subdivided into two major areas: non-graft associated new attachment and graft-associated new attachment.

Non–Graft Associated New Attachment

Conservative treatment consisting of scaling and root planing and possibly flap surgery can result in regeneration of bone in periodontal defects. The likelihood of obtaining this bone fill depends on the architecture of the defect and results are not consistent. The technique requires thorough scaling and root planing of the affected areas because any residual calculus or irritants will prevent new attachment. The usefulness of locally or systemically administered antibiotics,

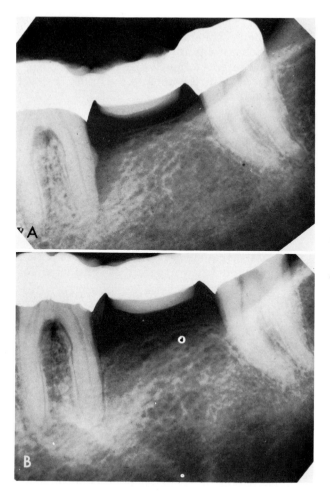

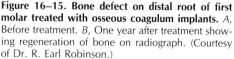

Figure 16–15. Bone defect on distal root of first molar treated with osseous coagulum implants. *A,* Before treatment. *B,* One year after treatment showing regeneration of bone on radiograph. (Courtesy of Dr. R. Earl Robinson.)

though logical, has yet to be confirmed through research.

Graft-Associated New Attachment

Periodontal reconstruction using non-graft material is best accomplished in the three-wall pocket and the periodontal and endodontal abscess.[19] However, the defects left by most periodontal diseases are not of three-wall configuration. Therefore, grafting modalities for restoring these more numerous defects have been investigated.

Periodontal defects as sites for bone transplantation differ from osseous cavities surrounded by bony walls. Saliva and bacteria may easily penetrate along the root surface, and epithelial cells may proliferate into the defect, resulting in contamination and possible exfoliation of the grafts. Therefore, the principles established to govern transplantation of bone into closed osseous cavities may

not be fully applicable to transplantation of bone into periodontal defects.

The considerations that govern the selection of a material have been defined by Schallhorn:[35]

1. Biologic acceptability.
2. Predictability.
3. Clinical feasibility.
4. Minimal operative hazards.
5. Minimal postoperative sequelae.
6. Patient acceptance.

Naturally, it is difficult to find a material with all these characteristics, and to date there is no "ideal" material or technique. Once the material is placed in the bony defect, it may act in a number of ways. It may have no effect; it may act only as a scaffolding material for the host to lay down new bone; it may actively induce bone formation; or through its own viability, it may deposit new bone in the defect.

Many graft materials have been developed

and tried in various forms. Bone or bone-forming tissue obtained from the same patients have the advantage of immunologic acceptance. Sources of autogenous bone include that from healing extraction wounds,[28] edentulous ridges,[11] bone trephined from within the jaw without damaging tooth roots, newly formed bone in wounds especially created for the purpose,[10] and bone removed during osteoplasty and ostectomy. Extraoral sources, such as iliac autografts, have also been tried.[34]

All the bone grafting techniques require presurgical scaling, occlusal adjustment as needed, and exposure of defects with full thickness flaps. Incisions must be planned to allow tissue to cover the bony area completely after suturing. The use of antibiotics for a few days after the procedure is generally recommended.

In addition to bone graft materials, many different non–bone graft materials have been tried for restoration of the periodontium. Among them are dura,[5] cartilage,[33] cementum,[32] dentin,[36] plaster of Paris,[37] and sclera.[13] However, none of these materials offers predictable regeneration of lost bone.

Bioceramics, such as tricalcium phosphate and hydroxylapatite, have acquired wide popularity in recent years. Porous ceramics in powder or solid form have been suggested as substitutes for bone grafts in the treatment of periodontal defects. This material seems to be well tolerated by the organism, and bone apposition occurs directly on the ceramic lattice.[14] Analysis of the clinical effectiveness of these materials through research has been limited[21, 24, 40] but is promising.[12]

MUCOGINGIVAL SURGERY

Mucogingival surgery is performed as an adjunct to regular pocket elimination or as an independent procedure for the purpose of widening the zone of attached gingiva when an insufficient amount is present. The width of the attached gingiva varies in different individuals and on different teeth in the same individual. "Attached gingiva" is not synonymous with "keratinized gingiva," since the latter also includes the free gingiva. The width of the attached gingiva is determined by subtracting the depth of the sulcus or pocket from the distance from the crest of the margin to the mucogingival junction.

Rationale

The rationale for mucogingival surgery is predicated upon the assumption that a minimum width of attached gingiva is required for optimal gingival health to be maintained. However, several studies[4a, 43a] have challenged the view that a wide attached gingiva is more protective against the accumulation of plaque than a thin or a nonexistent zone.

No minimum width of attached gingiva has been established as a standard necessary for gingival health. Persons who practice excellent oral hygiene may maintain healthy areas with almost no attached gingiva.

Reduced or absent attached gingiva may be due to several factors:

1. *The base of the periodontal pocket is apical or close to the mucogingival line.* In these cases, some attached gingiva must be created to separate the healed gingival sulcus from the alveolar mucosa and to prevent pockets from recurring. The functional adequacy of the attached gingiva can be predicted by the following *tension test*: Retract the cheeks and lips laterally with the fingers. If such tension pulls the marginal gingiva from the teeth, the attached gingiva is too narrow and should be widened when the pockets are treated.

2. *Frena and muscle attachments encroach upon periodontal pockets and pull them away from the tooth surface.* Tension from such attachments (a) distends the gingival sulcus and fosters the accumulation of irritants that lead to gingivitis and pocket formation and (b) aggravates the progression of periodontal pockets and causes their recurrence after treatment. The problem is more common on facial surfaces, but it occasionally occurs on lingual surfaces.

3. *Recession causes denudation of root surfaces,* often creating a functional as well as an esthetic problem. The tension test should also be used in cases of progressive gingival recession to check the effect of soft tissue tension on the gingival margin. Clinical examination and probing will reveal areas of root denudation.

Techniques

Several different types of procedures are currently performed in order to widen the zone of attached gingiva.

Gingival Extension Operation

The gingival extension procedure consists of the surgical apical displacement of the mucogingival line. In order to prevent the mucogingival line from creeping back coronally during postoperative healing, two methods have proved useful: the placement of a *free mucosal autograft (commonly called the free gingival graft)* (Fig. 16–16) and the so-called *fenestration procedure.* This procedure consists of

a partial thickness flap with removal of the periosteum and exposure of bone in a rectangular area at the base of the operative field. Its purpose is to create a scar, which is firmly bound to the bone, that will prevent coronal displacement of the mucogingival line. Fenestration procedures are seldom performed. The graft procedure is more predictable and heals with fewer problems. It is usually preferred even though two surgical sites are required.

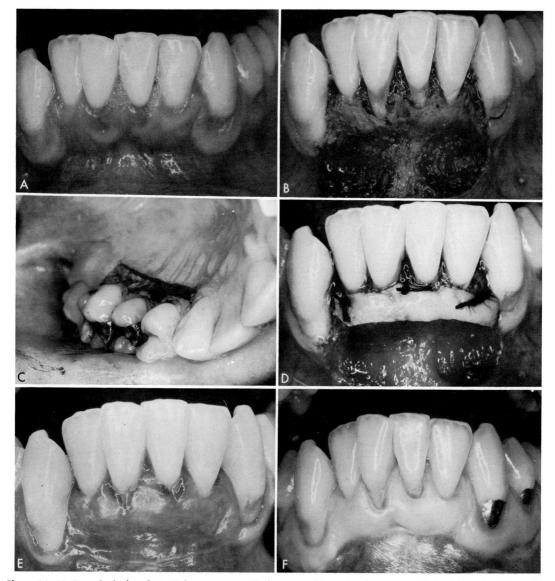

Figure 16–16. Free gingival graft. *A,* Before treatment. Pockets extend into alveolar mucosa. *B,* Recipient site prepared for graft. *C,* Graft obtained from the palate. *D,* Graft sutured in position. *E,* After 2 weeks. *F,* After 1 year. Note the widened zone of attached gingiva.

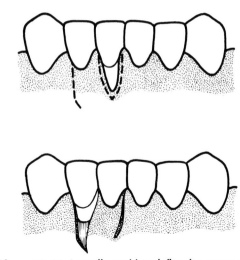

Figure 16–17. **Laterally positioned flap for coverage of denuded root.** *Top,* Incisions removing gingival margin around exposed root and outlining flap. *Bottom,* After recipient site is prepared by removing surface epithelium, flap is separated, transferred, and sutured.

Free gingival grafts are commonly performed to increase the width of attached gingiva. They require the surgical preparation of the recipient site, obtaining a partial thickness (1.5 to 2 mm) graft from a donor site (usually the palate), transfer of the graft to the recipient site, and suturing it in place. Both the donor and recipient sites must be protected with periodontal dressing.

Apical Displacement of the Existing Pocket Wall

With this technique, the pocket wall becomes attached to the cementum and/or bone and takes on the appearance and function of attached gingiva. This operation utilizes the apically positioned flap, either partial thickness or full thickness, for the combined purposes of eliminating pockets and widening the zone of attached gingiva. When apically positioned flaps are used to correct mucogingival deformities, they avoid some of the limitations of gingival extension operations and require less extensive surgical interference.[6]

Operations to Cover Denuded Roots

Laterally displaced flaps from attached gingiva of adjoining teeth or from adjacent edentulous ridges are used to cover denuded root surfaces. The laterally positioned flap for root coverage is shown in Figure 16–17.

Removal of Frena

A frenum may need to be removed if its attachment is too close to the gingival mar-

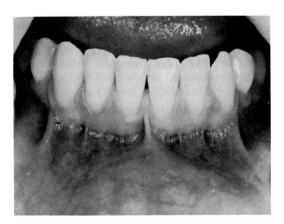

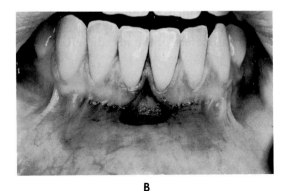

B

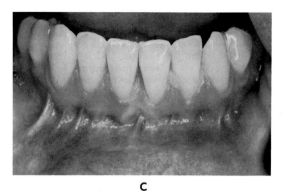

C

Figure 16–18. **Frenectomy technique.** *A,* Frenum attached close to the gingival margin. *B,* Frenum removed. *C,* Healing after six months.

Chapter 17

Maintenance Therapy

RATIONALE FOR MAINTENANCE THERAPY

Preservation of the periodontal health of treated patients requires as positive a program as does the elimination of periodontal disease. After Phase I therapy is completed, patients are placed on a schedule of periodic recall visits for evaluation and maintenance care to prevent recurrence of disease (Figs. 17–1 and 17–2).

Transfer from active treatment status to the maintenance program is a definitive step that requires educating patients about the purpose of the maintenance program. Patients who are not maintained in a supervised recall program subsequent to active treatment will show obvious signs of recurrent periodontitis.[2] In fact, one study described tooth loss three times as great in treated patients who do not return for regular recall visits as in those who do.[10] It is meaningless simply to inform patients that they are to return for periodic recall visits without emphasizing their significance and describing what behavior is expected between visits.

The maintenance phase of periodontal treatment *starts immediately after the completion of Phase I therapy* (Fig. 17–2). While the patient is in the maintenance phase, the necessary surgical and restorative procedures are performed. This will ensure that all areas of the mouth will retain the degree of health attained after Phase I therapy.

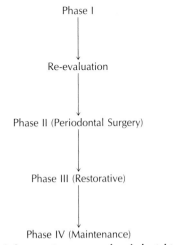

Phase I

Re-evaluation

Phase II (Periodontal Surgery)

Phase III (Restorative)

Phase IV (Maintenance)

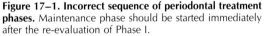

Figure 17–1. Incorrect sequence of periodontal treatment phases. Maintenance phase should be started immediately after the re-evaluation of Phase I.

243

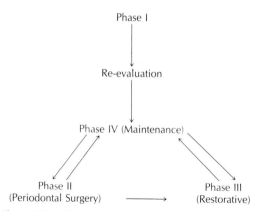

Figure 17–2. Correct sequence of periodontal treatment phases.

MAINTENANCE PROGRAM

Periodic recall visits form the foundation of a meaningful long-term prevention program. The interval between visits is initially set at 3 months but may be varied according to the patient's needs.

Periodontal care at each recall visit comprises three parts (Table 17–1). The first concern is examination and evaluation of the patient's current oral health. The second part includes the necessary maintenance treatment and oral hygiene reinforcement. The third part involves scheduling the patient for the next recall appointment, further periodontal treatment, or restorative dental procedures. The time required for patients with multiple teeth in both arches is approximately 1 hour.[27] This allows adequate time for greeting the patient, setup, and cleanup.

Examination and Evaluation

The recall examination is similar to the initial evaluation of the patient. However, since the patient is not new to the office, the examiner will primarily be looking for changes that have occurred since the last evaluation. The oral mucosa should be carefully inspected for pathologic conditions. Updating of changes in the medical history, evaluation of restorations, caries, prostheses, occlusion, tooth mobility, gingival status, and periodontal pockets are important parts of the recall appointment. Analysis of the current oral hygiene status of the patient is also essential.

A complete series of intraoral radiographs is taken when needed, depending on the initial severity of the case and the findings at the recall visit. These can be compared with previous· radiographs in order to check the bone height, repair of osseous defects, signs of trauma from occlusion, periapical pathology, and caries.

Plaque Control

Plaque control in the patient's mouth should be evaluated using disclosing agents. Patients should perform their hygiene regimen immediately before the recall appointment so that its effectiveness can be assessed. Plaque control must be reviewed and corrected until the patient demonstrates the necessary proficiency, even if it requires additional instruction sessions. Patients instructed in plaque control have less plaque and gingivitis than uninstructed patients.[2, 29, 30]

Treatment

The required scaling and root planing are performed, followed by polishing of the teeth. Irrigation with antimicrobial agents, such as stannous fluoride (1.64%),[19] may be performed in maintenance patients with remaining pockets.[13, 19, 27]

TABLE 17–1. MAINTENANCE RECALL PROCEDURES

Part I: Examination (approximate time, 17 minutes)[27]
  Medical history changes
  Oral pathology examination
  Oral hygiene status
  Gingival changes
  Pocket depth changes
  Mobility changes
  Occlusal changes
  Dental caries
  Restorative and prosthetic status

Part II: Treatment (approximate time, 35 minutes)[27]
  Oral hygiene reinforcement
  Scaling and root planing
  Polishing
  Chemical irrigation

Part III: Schedule Next Procedure (approximate time, 1 minute)[27]
  Schedule next recall visit
  Schedule further periodontal treatment
  Schedule or refer for restorative or prosthetic treatment

TABLE 17–2. SYMPTOMS AND CAUSES OF RECURRENCE OF DISEASE

Symptom	Possible Causes
Increased inflammation	Poor oral hygiene Subgingival calculus Inadequate restorations Deteriorating or poorly designed prostheses Systemic disease modifying host response to plaque
Recession	Toothbrush abrasion Inadequate keratinized gingiva Frenum pull Orthodontic therapy
Increased mobility with no change in pocket depth and no radiographic change	Occlusal trauma due to lateral occlusal interference Bruxism High restoration Poorly designed or worn-out prostheses Poor crown-to-root ratio
Increased pocket depth with no radiographic change	Poor oral hygiene Infrequent recall Subgingival calculus Poorly fitting partial denture Mesial inclination into edentulous space Failure of new attachment surgery Cracked teeth Grooves in teeth New periodontal disease
Increased pocket depth with increased radiographic bone loss	Poor oral hygiene Subgingival calculus Infrequent recall visits Inadequate or deteriorating restorations Poorly designed prostheses Inadequate surgery Systemic disease modifying host response to plaque Cracked teeth Grooves in teeth New periodontal disease

RECURRENCE OF PERIODONTAL DISEASE

Occasionally, lesions may recur. This can usually be traced to inadequate plaque control on the part of the patient. It should be understood, however, that it is the clinician's responsibility to teach, motivate, and control the patient's oral hygiene technique and that the patient's failure is also the clinician's failure. Periodontal surgery should not be undertaken unless the patient has shown proficiency and willingness to cooperate by performing adequate plaque control.[28]

Other causes of recurrence are the following (Table 17–2):

1. Inadequate or insufficient treatment that has failed to remove *all* the potential factors favoring plaque accumulation. Incomplete calculus removal in areas of difficult access is a common source of problems.

2. Inadequate restorations placed after the periodontal treatment was completed.

3. Failure of the patient to return for periodic checkups. This may be due to the patient's conscious or unconscious decision not to continue treatment or to the clinician's not having emphasized the need for periodic maintenance.

4. Presence of some systemic diseases that may affect host resistance to previously acceptable levels of plaque.

A failing case can be recognized by the following signs:

1. Recurring inflammation revealed by gingival changes and bleeding of the sulcus upon probing.

2. Increasing depth of sulci, leading to the recurrence of pocket formation.

3. Gradual increases in bone loss, as determined by the radiograph.

4. Gradual increases in tooth mobility, as ascertained by clinical examination.

The decision to retreat a periodontal patient should not be made at the preventive maintenance appointment but should be postponed for 1 to 2 weeks.[5] Often the patient's mouth will look a great deal better at that time, due to the resolution of edema and improved tone of the gingiva following treatment.

CLASSIFICATION OF POSTTREATMENT PATIENTS

The first year following periodontal therapy is important in terms of indoctrinating the patient in a recall pattern and reinforcing oral hygiene. In addition, it may take several months to accurately evaluate the results of some periodontal surgical procedures. Consequently, some areas may have to be re-

TABLE 17–3. RECALL INTERVALS FOR VARIOUS CLASSES OF RECALL PATIENTS

Classification	Characteristics	Recall Interval
First year	First-year patient—routine therapy and uneventful healing	3 months
	or	
	First-year patient—difficult case with complicated prosthesis, furcation involvement, poor crown-to-root ratios, questionable patient cooperation	1 to 2 months
Class A	Excellent results maintained well for 1 year or more Patient displays good oral hygiene, minimal calculus, no occlusal problems, no complicated prostheses, no remaining pockets, and no teeth with less than 50 per cent of alveolar bone remaining	6 months to 1 year
Class B	Generally good results maintained reasonably well for 1 year or more, but patient displays some of the following factors: 1. Inconsistent or poor oral hygiene 2. Heavy calculus formation 3. Systemic disease that predisposes to periodontal breakdown 4. Some remaining pockets 5. Occlusal problems 6. Complicated prostheses 7. Ongoing orthodontic therapy 8. Recurrent dental caries 9. Some teeth with less than 50 per cent of alveolar bone support	3 to 4 months (decide on recall interval on the basis of the number and severity of negative factors)
Class C	Generally poor results following periodontal therapy and/or several negative factors from the following list: 1. Inconsistent or poor oral hygiene 2. Heavy calculus formation 3. Systemic disease that predisposes to periodontal breakdown 4. Remaining pockets 5. Occlusal problems 6. Complicated prostheses 7. Recurrent dental caries 8. Periodontal surgery indicated but not performed for medical, psychologic, or financial reasons 9. Many teeth with less than 50 per cent of alveolar bone support 10. Condition too far advanced to be improved by periodontal surgery	1 to 3 months (decide on recall interval on the basis of the number and severity of negative factors; consider re-treating some areas or extracting the severely involved teeth)

treated because the results are not optimal. Furthermore, the first-year patient will often present etiologic factors that may have been overlooked and that may be more amenable to treatment at this stage. For these reasons, the recall interval for first-year patients should not be longer than 3 months.

The patients who are on a periodontal recall schedule are a varied group. Several categories of maintenance patients and suggested recall intervals are described in Table 17–3. One must realize that patients can improve or relapse to a different classification with the reduction or exacerbation of periodontal disease. When one dental arch is more involved than the other, the patient is classified by the arch that is more severely involved.

In summary, maintenance care is a critical phase of therapy. The long-term preservation of the dentition is closely associated with the frequency and quality of recall maintenance.

Referring to the Periodontal Specialist

The majority of periodontal care of the population belongs in the general dental office. This is because of the overwhelming number of patients with periodontal disease and the intimate relationship between periodontal disease and restorative dentistry.

The number of caries per capita has dwindled in the last 20 years by about 50 per cent, and there is some evidence that the decline will continue.[27] Caries reduction has occurred because of the use of fluorides. As more people retain their teeth throughout their lifetimes, and as the proportion of older people in the population increases, more teeth will be at risk for periodontal disease. Therefore, an ever greater number of periodontal patients is expected in future years.

This expected increase in the number of periodontal patients will require a greater understanding of periodontal problems and an increased level of expertise in treatment on the part of general dentists and dental hygienists. However, there will always be a need for specialists to treat particularly difficult cases, patients with systemic health problems, and situations in which a complex prosthetic treatment requires the greatest assurance of reliable results.

Where to draw the line between the cases to be treated in the general dental office and those to be referred to a specialist will vary for different practitioners and for different patients. The diagnosis will indicate the type of periodontal treatment required. If the periodontal destruction necessitates surgery on the distal surfaces of second molars, extensive osseous surgery, or involved bone grafting, the patient will usually be best treated by a specialist. However, patients who require localized areas of gingivectomy or flap curettage can usually be treated sucessfully in the general dental office.

In many instances it will be obvious that referral of patients to a specialist is necessary; other patients will clearly have problems that can be treated in the generalist's office. However, for some patients, it is very difficult to decide if treatment by a specialist is required. Any patient who does not plainly belong in the categories of treatment by a generalist should be a candidate for referral to a specialist.[22]

The decision as to whether a patient's periodontal problem should be treated in a general practice should be guided by the degree of risk that the patient will lose a tooth or teeth for periodontally related reasons. The most important factors in the decision are the extent and location of the periodontal deterioration present. Teeth with pockets of 5 mm or more, measured from the cemento-enamel junction, may have a prognosis of rapid decline. The location of the periodontal deterioration is also an important factor in determining the risk of tooth loss. Teeth with furcation lesions may be at risk even when there is more than 50 per cent bone support remaining. Therefore, cases in which strategic teeth fall into these categories are usually best treated by specialists.

Even if the patient is treated by a periodontist, an important question remains: Should the maintenance phase of therapy be performed by the general practitioner or by the specialist? This should be determined by the amount of periodontal deterioration present. Class A recall patients (see Table 17–3) should be maintained by the general dentist, whereas Class C patients should be maintained by the specialist. Class B patients fall into the gray area in between and can alternate recall visits between the general and specialty offices. The severity of the patient's disease should dictate whether the general practitioner or the specialist should perform the maintenance therapy.

RESULTS OF PERIODONTAL TREATMENT

The prevalence of periodontal disease and the high tooth mortality due to this disease raise an important question: Is periodontal treatment effective in preventing and stopping the progressive destruction of periodontal disease? Evidence is now overwhelming that periodontal therapy is effective in preventing the disease, slowing the destruction of the periodontium, and reducing tooth loss.

Prevention and Treatment of Gingivitis

For many years, the belief that good oral hygiene is necessary for the successful prevention and treatment of gingivitis has been widespread among periodontists. In addition, worldwide epidemiologic studies have confirmed a close relationship between the incidence of gingivitis and lack of oral hygiene.[6, 7]

Conclusive evidence of the relation of oral hygiene and gingivitis in healthy dental students has been demonstrated.[15, 31] After 9 to 21 days without oral hygiene, experimental subjects with previously excellent oral hygiene and healthy gingiva developed heavy accumulations of plaque and generalized mild gingivitis. When oral hygiene was reinstituted, the plaque in most areas disappeared in 1 or 2 days, and the gingival inflammation in these areas disappeared 1 day after the plaque had been removed. This evidence demonstrates that gingivitis is reversible and can be resolved by effective daily plaque removal.

A number of long-term studies have shown that gingival health can be maintained by a combination of effective oral hygiene and dental scaling.[1, 3, 9, 11, 17, 29, 30] A 3-year study of 1248 subjects in California confirmed that the progression of gingival inflammation can be retarded if high levels of oral hygiene are maintained.[29, 30] Experimental and control groups were computer matched on the basis of periodontal and oral hygiene status, past caries experience, age, and sex. One group was given a series of frequent oral prophylaxis treatments, combined with oral hygiene instruction. Subjects in the control groups received no attention from the study team except for annual examinations. After 3 years, the increase in plaque and debris in the control group was four times as great as that in the experimental group. Similarly, gingivitis scores were much higher in the control subjects than in the matching experimental group. *Therefore, it has been established that chronic marginal gingivitis can be controlled by good oral hygiene and oral prophylaxis.*

Prevention and Treatment of Loss of Attachment

Although periodontal therapy has been employed for more than 100 years, it is only within the last 15 years or so that a number of studies have been conducted to determine the effect of treatment on reducing the progressive loss of periodontal support for the natural dentition.

Prevention of Loss of Attachment

A longitudinal investigation to study the natural development and progression of periodontal disease has been conducted.[16] This study compared a large group of individuals who had enjoyed a lifetime of preventive care in Norway to a group in Sri Lanka who had experienced no dental care. The study showed that the Norwegian group, as the members approached 40 years of age, had a mean individual loss of attachment of slightly above 1.5 mm, with a mean annual rate of attachment loss of 0.08 mm for interproximal surfaces and 0.10 mm for buccal surfaces. As the Sri Lankans approached 40 years of age, the mean individual loss of attachment was 4.50 mm, with a mean annual rate of progression of 0.30 mm for interproximal surfaces and 0.20 mm for buccal surfaces. This study suggested that without intervention initial periodontal lesions will continue to progress.

In a 3-year study of 1248 subjects,[29, 30] the control group who did not receive oral hygiene instructions and frequent prophylaxes showed loss of attachment at a rate more than 3.5 times that of the experimental group receiving preventive care. This clearly demonstrated that *loss of attachment can be reduced by good oral hygiene and frequent dental prophylaxis*.

Treatment of Loss of Attachment

The studies cited previously involved treatment of populations without extensive periodontal disease. A longitudinal study of patients with moderate to advanced periodontal disease, conducted at the University of Michigan, showed that the progression of periodontal disease can be stopped for a period of 3 years postoperatively regardless of the modality of treatment.[23–25] Even for long-term observations, the average loss of attachment was only 0.3 mm over 7 years.[24] These results indicate a more favorable prognosis for treatment of advanced periodontal lesions than was previously assumed.

Another study conducted on 75 patients with advanced periodontal disease showed that plaque control and surgical pocket elimination stopped further alveolar bone loss during the 5-year observation period.[12] The meticulous plaque control practiced by the patients in this study was considered a major factor in the excellent results produced.

None of these studies used a control group, because leaving periodontal disease untreated cannot be justified. However, in a private practice study,[4] an effort was made to find and evaluate patients with diagnosed moderate to advanced periodontitis who did not follow through with recommended periodontal therapy. Thirty patients ranging in age from 25 to 71 years were found and evaluated after periods ranging from 18 to 115 months. All of these untreated patients had progressive increases in pocket depth and radiographic evidence of progressive bone resorption. It can be concluded that periodontal treatment has been very effective in reducing loss of attachment.

TOOTH MORTALITY

The ultimate test of the effectiveness of periodontal treatment is whether tooth loss can be prevented. There are now enough studies from both private practice and research institutions to document that loss of teeth is retarded or prevented by therapy.

The combined effect of subgingival scaling every 3 to 6 months and controlled oral hygiene has been evaluated over a 5-year period.[17] Tooth loss was significantly reduced for all patients. This study showed that frequent subgingival scalings reduced tooth loss even when oral hygiene was "not good."

In a University of Michigan study, 104 patients with a total of 2604 teeth were evaluated for tooth mortality.[23–25] After 1 to 7 years of treatment, 53 teeth were lost for various reasons. Thirty-two teeth were lost during the first and second years after initiation of treatment. The remaining 21 teeth were lost in a random pattern over the next 6 years. The loss of teeth due to advanced periodontal disease following treatment was only about 2 per cent.

Another study tested the effectiveness of periodontal therapy in cases of advanced disease.[12] Seventy-five subjects were studied who had lost 50 per cent or more of their periodontal support. Treatment consisted of oral hygiene, scaling, extraction of untreatable teeth, periodontal surgery, and prosthetic treatment where indicated. After completion of periodontal treatment, none of the patients showed any further loss of periodontal support and no teeth were extracted in the 5-year posttreatment period. It should be pointed out that the patients in this study were selected because of their capacity to meet high requirements of plaque control following repeated instruction in oral hygiene techniques. This fact did not detract from the validity of the study, but it demonstrated the etiologic importance of bacterial plaque. The results showed that periodontal surgery coupled with a detailed plaque control program prevented further progression of periodontal breakdown even in patients with severely reduced periodontal support.

Several studies in private practice have attempted to measure tooth loss following periodontal therapy. In one series, 180 patients who had been treated for chronic destructive periodontal disease were evaluated 2 to 20 years after treatment, an average of 8.6 years.[26] The average age of the patients before treatment was 43.7 years. From the beginning of treatment to the time of the survey, 65 per cent of the patients lost no teeth. A total of 141 teeth were lost by the remaining 35 per cent of patients for several reasons, including periodontal disease, caries, and nonperiodontal causes. The study showed periodontal care helped to retain most teeth, because an average of slightly less than one tooth (0.9) was lost per patient.

Another private practice study evaluated patients who had been treated 5 or more years previously and had continued to receive regular preventive periodontal care.[20, 21] The average length of time since treatment for the 442 patients studied was 10.1 years. Two thirds of the patients were over 40 at the time of treatment. These patients were seen for preventive periodontal care an average of every 4.6 months. The total tooth loss due to periodontal disease was 178 of over 11,000 teeth. More important, 78 per cent of the patients did not lose a single tooth following periodontal therapy, and 11 per cent lost only one tooth. Considering that over 600 teeth had furcation involvements at the time of the original treatment and that well over 1000 teeth had less than half of the alveolar bone support remaining, the tooth loss was very low. During the same period, only 45 teeth were lost through caries or pulpal involvement (Fig. 17–3).

Even more surprising were the statistics for teeth with less than optimal prognoses. Only 85 (14 per cent) of a total of 601 teeth with furcation involvement were lost, and 117 teeth (11 per cent) were lost of 1039 teeth with half or less of their bone support remaining. Of the teeth listed as having a guarded prognoses, only 126 (12 per cent) of 1043 were lost over this average 10-year period. From the standpoint of the average tooth mortality per patient, it was demonstrated that 0.72 teeth were lost per patient per 10 years.

Also in a private practice study, 600 patients were followed over a period between 15 and 53 years after periodontal therapy.[8] The majority (76.5 per cent) had advanced periodontal disease at the start of treatment. There was a total of 15,666 teeth, an average of 26 teeth per patient. During the follow-up period, an average of 22 years, 1312 teeth were lost. Of this number, 1110 were lost for periodontal reasons. The average tooth mortality per patient was 2.2 teeth; converted to a 10-year rate, the average was one tooth lost per 10 years for each patient.

An effort has also been made to find and evaluate patients with diagnosed moderate to advanced periodontitis who did not follow

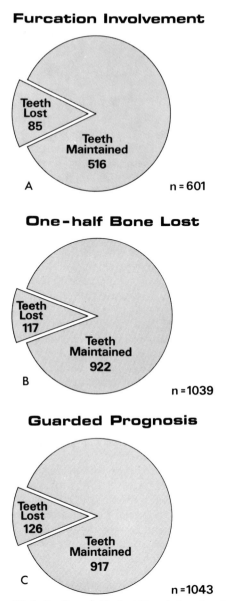

Figure 17–3. Tooth mortality in 442 periodontal patients treated over a period of 10 years. (Data from Dr. R. G. Oliver.)

through with recommended periodontal therapy in a private practice.[4] Patients with untreated periodontal disease were losing teeth at a rate greater than 0.61 teeth per year (6.1 teeth per 10 years).

Comparison of these tooth mortality studies with other epidemiologic surveys is hazardous, since few involve treatment and few are longitudinal. However, it has been shown that average tooth loss due to all causes in the general population was 5.2

teeth per 10 years after the age of 35.[18] In patients over 40, the rate increased to 6 teeth per 10 years. The United States Public Health Service surveys indicated that about 4.3 teeth are lost per 10 years after the age of 35 in the general population.[7, 14] It is clear that tooth loss in the general population far exceeds that in the treated periodontal patients.

CONCLUSION

In summary, the prevalence of periodontal disease and the high tooth mortality due to this disease emphasize the need for effective treatment. Treatment can prevent the disease and stop the progression of bone destruction once periodontitis is present. In addition, there is overwhelming evidence that periodontal therapy greatly reduces tooth mortality. Every dental practitioner should be familiar with the philosophy and techniques of periodontal therapy because failure to diagnose and treat periodontal disease, or to make periodontal treatment available to patients, will result in unnecessary dental problems and tooth loss.

References

1. Axelsson, P., and Lindhe, J.: Effect of controlled oral hygiene procedures on caries and periodontal disease in adults. Results after 6 years. J. Clin. Periodontol., 8:239, 1981.
2. Axelsson, P., and Lindhe, J.: The significance of maintenance care in the treatment of periodontal disease. J. Clin. Periodontol., 8:281, 1981.
3. Bay, I., and Møller, I. J.: The effect of a sodium monofluorophosphate dentifrice on the gingiva. J. Periodont. Res., 3:103, 1968.
4. Becker, W., Berg, L., and Becker, E. B.: Untreated periodontal disease: a longitudinal study. J. Periodontol., 50:234, 1979.
5. Chace, R.: Retreatment in periodontal practice. J. Periodontol., 48:410, 1977.
6. Greene, J. C.: Periodontal disease in India: report of an epidemiological study. J. Dent. Res., 39:302, 1960.
7. Greville, T. N. E.: United States Life Tables by Dentulous or Edentulous Condition, 1971, and 1957–58. Dept. of Health Education and Welfare, Publication No. (HRA) 75-1338, August, 1974.
8. Hirschfeld, L., and Wasserman, B.: A long-term survey of tooth loss in 600 treated periodontal patients. J. Periodontol., 49:225, 1978.
9. Hoover, D. R., and Lefkowitz, W.: Reduction of gingivitis by toothbrushing. J. Periodontol., 36:193, 1955.
10. Lietha-Elmer, E.: Langsfristge Ergebnisse regelmässig betreuter und unbetreuter Parodontosepatienten. Schweiz. Mschr. Zahnheilk., 87:613, 1977.
11. Lightner, L. M., O'Leary, J. T., Drake, R. B., Crump, P. O., and Allen, M. F.: Preventive periodontic treatment procedures: result over 46 months. J. Periodontol., 42:555, 1971.
12. Lindhe, J., and Nyman, S.: The effect of plaque control and surgical pocket elimination on the establishment and maintenance of periodontal health. A longitudinal study of periodontal therapy in cases of advanced disease. J. Clin. Periodontol., 2:67, 1975.
13. Lindhe, J., Heijl, L., Goodson, J. M., and Socransky, S. S.: Local tetracycline delivery using hollow fiber devices in periodontal therapy. J. Clin. Periodontol., 6:141, 1979.
14. Linder, F. E., et al.: Decayed Missing and Filled Teeth in Adults. United States—1960–1962. Public Health Service Publication No. 1000, Series 11, No. 23, February, 1967.
15. Löe, H., Theilade, E., and Jensen, S. B.: Experimental gingivitis in man. J. Periodontol., 36:177, 1965.
16. Löe, H., Anerud, A., Boysen, H., and Smith, M.: The natural history of periodontal disease in man. J. Periodontol., 49:607, 1978.
17. Lovdal, A., Arno, A., Schei, O., and Waerhaug, J.: Combined effect of subgingival scaling and controlled oral hygiene on the incidence of gingivitis. Acta Odontol. Scand., 19:537, 1961.
18. Marshall-Day, C. D., Stephens, R. G., and Quigley, L. F.: Periodontal disease: prevalence and incidence. J. Periodontol., 26:185, 1955.
19. Mazza, J. E., Newman, M. G., and Sims, T. N.: Clinical and antimicrobial effect of stannous fluoride on periodontitis. J. Clin. Periodontol., 8:213, 1981.
20. McFall, W. T., Jr.: Tooth loss with and without periodontal therapy. Periodont. Abstracts, 17:8, 1969.
21. Oliver. R. C.: Personal communication, 1977.
22. Parr, R. W., Pipe, P., and Watts, T.: Periodontal Maintenance Therapy. Berkeley, Praxis Publishing Company, 1974.
23. Ramfjord, S. P., Knowles, J. W., Nissle, R. R., Burgett, F. G., and Shick, R. A.: Results following three modalities of periodontal therapy. J. Periodontol., 46:522, 1975.
24. Ramfjord, S. P., Knowles, J. W., Nissle, R. R., Shick, R. A., and Burgett, F. G.: Longitudinal study of periodontal therapy. J. Periodontol., 44:66, 1973.
25. Ramfjord, S. P., and Nissle, R. R.: The modified Widman flap. J. Periodontol., 45:601, 1974.
26. Ross, I. F., Thompson, R. H. Jr., and Galdi, M.: The results of treatment: a long term study of one hundred and eighty patients. Parodontologie, 25:125, 1971.
27. Schallhorn, R. G., and Snider, L. E.: Periodontal maintenance therapy. J. Am. Dent. Assoc., 103:227, 1981.
28. Sternlicht, H. C.: Evaluating long-term periodontal therapy. Texas Dent. J., 92:4, 1974.
29. Suomi, J. D., West, J. D., Chang, J. J., and McClendon, B. J.: The effect of controlled oral hygiene procedures on the progression of periodontal disease in adults: radiographic findings. J. Periodontol., 42:562, 1971.
30. Suomi, J. D., Greene, J. C., Vermillion, J. R., Doyle, J., Chang, J. J., and Leatherwood, E. C.: The effect of controlled oral hygiene on the progression of periodontal disease in adults: results after the third and final year. J. Periodontol., 42:152, 1971.
31. Theilade, E., Wright, W. H., Jensen, S. B., and Löe, H.: Experimental gingivitis in man. II. J. Periodont. Res., 1:1, 1966.

Epidemiologic surveys conducted throughout the world point to the wide distribution of gingival and periodontal disease.[81, 83] These diseases have been recognized in almost every culture; paleontologic studies indicate that periodontal disease existed as early as 2000 B.C.[77, 109] It is important for the clinician to understand the extent and distribution of these diseases in order to grasp the magnitude of treatment responsibility for the dental profession.

Dental epidemiology is the study of the *pattern (distribution)* and *dynamics* of dental diseases in a human population. *Pattern* implies that certain people are vulnerable to a disease and that the association between that disease and individuals can be described by variables such as age, sex, racial/ethnic group, occupation, social characteristics, place of residence, susceptibility, and exposure to specific agents, to name a few. The term *dynamics* refers to a temporal pattern or distribution and is concerned with trends, cyclic patterns, and the time elapsed between the exposure and the onset of disease.[89] *Incidence* is defined as the rate of occurrence of new disease in a population during a given period of time. *Prevalence* is the proportion of persons affected by a disease at a specific point in time, as described in cross-sectional surveys.

Russell defined the *purpose of dental epidemiology as "not so much the study of disease as a process as it is a study of the condition of the people in whom the disease occurs."*[84] Epidemiology identifies populations at risk and improves understanding of disease processes that can lead to methods of control and prevention. It also provides methods for evaluating clinical trials of preventive and curative measures.

Epidemiologic indices are indispensable tools that quantitate clinical conditions on graduated scales, facilitating comparisons between populations examined by the same criteria and methods. Unlike the absolute or definitive diagnosis that can be made for an individual patient, an epidemiologic index, represented as a numerical value, will estimate the *relative* prevalence or occurrence of the clinical condition. The *criteria* of good epidemiologic indices are that they must be easy to use, permit the examination of many people in a short period of time, define clinical conditions objectively, be highly reproducible in assessing a clinical condition when used by one or more examiners, be amenable to statistical analysis, and be strongly correlated to the clinical stages of the diseases under investigation. The epidemiology of periodontal disease has been vexed by subjective diagnostic parameters. Dental caries is far easier to evaluate objectively. Calibration or standardization of the examiners, the key to reliable findings, has been much easier to achieve with caries indices.

In general, there are two types of dental indices. One measures the *number* or *proportion* of people in a population with or without a specific condition at a point or interval of time. The second measures the *number of people affected* and the *severity of the condition* at a point or interval in time.[84] The second type of index has the advantage of assessing the diseases on a graduated scale and is more commonly used to evaluate periodontal disease.

Many indices are available for recording and quantitating the signs of periodontal disease; however, only indices of historical importance or those frequently used will be described in this chapter. (Two excellent symposium publications[15, 17] are available for in-depth study of dental indices.)

The four types of indices described here evaluate the following:

Gingival inflammation
Periodontal destruction
Plaque accumulation
Calculus accumulation

INDICES USED TO ASSESS GINGIVAL INFLAMMATION

Papillary-Marginal-Attachment Index
(Schour and Massler[93])

Originally the severity of gingivitis was believed to be correlated with the amount of gingiva affected by disease. The Papillary-Marginal-Attachment (PMA) Index[93] was used to count the number of affected gingival units with gingivitis by dividing the facial gingiva into three gingival scoring units: the mesial dental papilla (P), the gingival margin (M), and the attached gingiva (A).[92, 93] For each gingival unit, the presence of inflammation was scored 1, and the absence 0; the P, M, and A numerical values were totaled separately, added together, and expressed numerically as the PMA Index *score per person*. Usually only the maxillary and mandibular incisors, canines, and premolars were examined. The index was later modified to include a severity component; the papillary units were scored on a scale of 0 to 5, and the marginal and attached gingival units were scored on a scale of 0 to 3.[49] This index was valuable for its broad application to epidemiologic surveys and clinical trials and because of its capacity for use on individual patients. The severity criteria have also been the basis for other indices.

Indices based on modifications of the PMA Index include those developed by Muhlemann and Mazor,[59] Lobene,[40] and Suomi and Barbano.[100]

Periodontal Index (Russell[79])

The Periodontal Index (PI) was intended to estimate deeper periodontal disease than the PMA Index by measuring the presence and severity of gingival inflammation, pocket formation, and masticatory function. All of the gingival tissue around each tooth, which is the scoring unit in this index, is scored by the criteria presented in Table 18–1. Because the PI measures both reversible and irreversible aspects of periodontal disease, it is an epidemiologic index with a true biologic gradient.[84] A PI *score per individual* is determined by adding all of the tooth scores and dividing the total by the number of teeth examined.

Much of the data on the distribution of

TABLE 18–1. THE PERIODONTAL INDEX (PI) (Russell[79])

Score	Criteria and Scoring for Field Studies	Additional X-ray Criteria Followed in the Clinical Test
0	NEGATIVE. There is neither overt inflammation in the investing tissues nor loss of function due to destruction of supporting tissues.	Radiographic appearance is essentially normal
1	MILD GINGIVITIS. There is an overt area of inflammation in the free gingivae, but this area does not circumscribe the tooth.	
2	GINGIVITIS. Inflammation completely circumscribes the tooth, but there is no apparent break in the epithelial attachment.	
4	(Used when radiographs are available.)	There is early, notchlike resorption of the alveolar crest.
6	GINGIVITIS WITH POCKET FORMATION. The epithelial attachment has been broken and there is a pocket (not merely a deepened gingival crevice due to swelling in free gingivae). There is no interference with normal masticatory function; the tooth is firm and has not drifted.	There is horizontal bone loss involving the entire alveolar crest, up to half of the length of the tooth root.
8	ADVANCED DESTRUCTION WITH LOSS OF MASTICATORY FUNCTION. The tooth may be loose, may have drifted, may sound dull on percussion with a metallic instrument, and may be depressible in its socket.	There is advanced bone loss, involving more than one half of the length of the tooth root, or a definite infrabony pocket with widening of the periodontal ligament. There may be root resorption, or rarefaction at the apex.

RULE: When in doubt, assign the lesser scores.

$$\text{Periodontal Index Score per Person} = \frac{\text{Sum of individual scores}}{\text{Number of teeth present}}$$

Clinical Condition	Group PI Scores*	Stage of Disease
Clinically normal supportive tissues	0 to 0.2	
Simple gingivitis	0.3 to 0.9	
Beginning destructive periodontal disease	0.7 to 1.9	Reversible
Established destructive periodontal disease	1.6 to 5.0	
Terminal disease	3.8 to 8.0	Irreversible

*From reference 76.

periodontal disease in the United States and throughout the world has been measured using the PI. This important index is also used in the National Health Survey (NHS),[34] the largest ongoing health survey in the United States.

Gingivitis Component of the Periodontal Disease Index (Ramfjord)[74]

The Periodontal Disease Index (PDI) is similar to the PI in that both are used to measure the presence and severity of periodontal disease. The PDI combines the assessments of gingivitis and gingival sulcus depth on six selected teeth (numbers 3, 9, 12, 19, 25, and 28). Calculus and plaque are also measured in order to provide a comprehensive assessment of periodontal status. Gingivitis components are described here; periodontal disease components are described in a later section.

The tissue circumscribing each of the six selected teeth is assessed using the criteria described in Table 18–2. The six index teeth have been verified as reliable indicators of the conditions of various regions of the mouth. The Gingivitis Index score per person, the gingival status component of the

TABLE 18–2. CRITERIA FOR SEVERAL COMPONENTS OF THE
PERIODONTAL DISEASE INDEX (Ramfjord[74])

Gingival Status (Gingivitis Index)

0 = Absence of signs of inflammation.
1 = Mild to moderate inflammatory gingival changes, not extending around the tooth.
2 = Mild to moderately severe gingivitis extending all around the tooth.
3 = Severe gingivitis characterized by marked redness, swelling, tendency to bleed, and ulceration.[75]

Crevicular Measurements

A. If the gingival margin is on the enamel, measure from the gum margin to the cemento-enamel junction and record the measurement. If the epithelial attachment is on the crown and the cemento-enamel junction cannot be felt by the probe, record the depth of the gingival sulcus on the crown. Then record the distance from the gingival margin to the bottom of the pocket if the probe can be moved apically to the cemento-enamel junction without resistance or pain. The distance from the cemento-enamel junction to the bottom of the pocket can then be found by subtracting the first from the second measurement.
B. If the gingival margin is on the cementum, record the distance from the cemento-enamel junction to the gingival margin as a minus value. Then record the distance from the cemento-enamel junction to the bottom of the gingival sulcus as a plus value. Both loss of attachment and actual sulcus depth can easily be assessed from the scores.[75]

Periodontal Disease Index (PDI) Criteria for Surveys

If the gingival sulcus in none of the measured areas extended apically to the cemento-enamel junction, the recorded score for gingivitis is the PDI score for that tooth. If the gingival sulcus in any of the two measured areas extended apically to the cemento-enamel junction but not more than 3 mm (including 3 mm in any area), the tooth is assigned a PDI score of 4. The score for gingivitis is then disregarded in the PDI score for that tooth. If the gingival sulcus in either of the two recorded areas of the tooth extends apically to from 3 to 6 mm (including 6 mm) in relation to the cemento-enamel junction, the tooth is assigned a PDI score of 5 (again, the gingivitis score is disregarded). Whenever the gingival sulcus extends more than 6 mm apically to the cemento-enamel junction in any of the measured areas of the tooth, the score of 6 is assigned as the PDI score for that tooth (again disregarding the gingivitis score).[75]

Shick-Ash Modification[98] of Plaque Criteria

0 = Absence of dental plaque.
1 = Dental plaque in the interproximal or at the gingival margin covering less than one third of the gingival half of the facial or lingual surface of the tooth.
2 = Dental plaque covering more than one third but less than two thirds of the gingival half of the facial or lingual surface of the tooth.
3 = Dental plaque covering two thirds or more of the gingival half of the facial or gingival surface of the tooth.

Calculus Criteria

0 = Absence of calculus.
1 = Supragingival calculus extending only slightly below the free gingival margin (not more than 1 mm).
2 = Moderate amount of supra- and subgingival calculus or subgingival calculus alone.
3 = An abundance of supra- and subgingival calculus.[75]

TABLE 18–3. CRITERIA FOR THE GINGIVAL INDEX (LÖE AND SILNESS[41]) AND THE PLAQUE INDEX (SILNESS AND LÖE[99])

Gingival Index (GI)

0 = Normal gingiva.
1 = Mild inflammation, slight change in color, slight edema; *no bleeding on palpation.*
2 = Moderate inflammation, redness, edema, and glazing; *bleeding on palpation.*
3 = Severe inflammation, marked redness and edema; ulcerations; *tendency to spontaneous bleeding.*

Plaque Index (PlI)

0 = No plaque in the gingival area.
1 = A film of plaque adhering to the free gingival margin and adjacent area of the tooth. The plaque may be recognized only by running a probe across the tooth surface.
2 = Moderate accumulation of soft deposits within the gingival pocket and on the gingival margin and/or adjacent tooth surface, which can be seen by the naked eye.
3 = Abundance of soft matter within the gingival pocket and/or on the gingival margin and adjacent tooth surface.

PDI, is obtained by adding scores of the gingival units and dividing by the number of teeth present.[75]

Gingival Index (Löe and Silness)[41]

The Gingival Index (GI) was developed to assess the severity of gingivitis in four areas around each tooth. The gingival tissue is divided into four scoring units: distal-facial papilla, facial margin, mesial-facial papilla, and the entire lingual gingival margin. A blunt instrument, usually a periodontal probe, is used to assess the bleeding potential of the four gingival units according to the criteria presented in Table 18–3.

The total of the scores around each tooth is the GI score for the *area.* The GI score for the *tooth* is the total scores around each tooth divided by four. Totaling all of the scores per tooth and dividing by the number of teeth examined provides the GI *score per person.* The numerical scores of the GI may be associated with varying degrees of clinical gingivitis as follows:

Gingival Scores	Condition
0.1-1.0	Mild gingivitis
1.1-2.0	Moderate gingivitis
2.1-3.0	Severe gingivitis

The index can be used to determine the prevalence and severity of gingivitis in epidemiologic surveys, as well as in the individual dentition. For this reason the GI has been used in many controlled clinical trials of preventive or therapeutic agents.[23]

Indices of Gingival Bleeding

Two indices that combine the clinical parameters of inflammation and bleeding have been described. The Sulcus Bleeding Index (SBI) of Mühlemann and Mazor[59] uses bleeding upon gentle probing as the criterion of gingival inflammation. In 1971, Mühlemann and Son[60] modified the original criteria, resulting in a scale of 0 to 5 for assessing inflammation and sulcular bleeding. The Mühlemann indices are predicated on the assumption that sulcular bleeding is the first sign of inflammation. Alternatively, the GI of Löe and Silness[41] uses the presence of slight color change and the absence of bleeding when a blunt instrument is used to palpate the soft tissue wall at the gingival margin to indicate initial gingival inflammation. Although the correlation between inflammation and bleeding is not perfect, the histologic evidence for associating inflammation with the GI criteria is stronger than that for the SBI. From the epidemiologic viewpoint, it is better to measure single parameters than to combine several into one measure. Conveniently, the criteria for the GI can easily be separated into an index of gingival inflammation and an index of gingival bleeding without destroying the integrity of the scoring system.

Several other indices of gingival bleeding are worthy of mention. The Bleeding Points Index (Lenox and Kopczyk[39]) was developed to assess oral hygiene performance. It measures the presence or absence of gingival bleeding interproximally and on the facial and lingual surfaces of each tooth. The technique requires drawing a periodontal probe horizontally through the gingival crevices of teeth, and after 30 seconds examining the gingiva for bleeding. The Gingival Bleeding Index of Carter and Barnes[14] assesses the presence or absence of gingival bleeding at the interproximal spaces, using unwaxed dental floss. The floss is thought to assess larger areas of gingiva more quickly than a periodontal probe, and it can be used by the clinician or the patient and therefore is a potentially valuable tool for self-assessment. The Gingival Bleeding Index (GBI) of Ainamo and Bay[1] was developed as a practical technique for the practitioner to assess patient progress in plaque control. The presence or absence of gingival bleeding is determined by gentle probing of the gingival crevice with a periodontal probe. The appearance of bleeding within 10 seconds is a positive score and the patient's score is expressed as the percentage of positive scores of the total number of gingival margins examined.

In conclusion, gingival bleeding indices provide more objective indications of inflammation than gingival color changes and provide evidence of recent plaque exposure.[39] The indices that utilize palpation or dental floss are suitable for diagnosis and assessing individual progress in plaque control; however, indices that utilize probing of the gingival sulcus better assess periodontal treatment effects.

INDICES USED TO MEASURE PERIODONTAL DESTRUCTION

The destruction of bone is the most important criterion for assessing the severity of periodontal disease.[72] The approaches to measuring bone loss discussed here are gingival crevice measurements, radiographic evaluations, gingival recession measurements, and assessment of tooth mobility.

Gingival Sulcus Measurement Component of the Periodontal Disease Index (Ramfjord[75])

Ramfjord's technique of measuring gingival sulcus depth with a calibrated periodontal probe is the most quantitative method currently available for assessing periodontal support. It requires measuring the distance from the cementoenamel junction to the free gingival margin and the distance from the free gingival margin to the bottom of the gingival sulcus or pocket. The difference between the two measurements yields the gingival *sulcus depth*, which translates into level of attachment. These measurements are useful in epidemiologic surveys, longitudinal

studies of periodontal disease, and clinical trials of preventive and therapeutic agents.[76]

The probe used for the sulcus depth measurements is graduated in 3-mm increments, with all measurements rounded to the nearest millimeter. Any measurement close to 0.5 mm is rounded to the lower whole number, which has resulted in "underscoring" but has increased the reproducibility of the measurements. Placement of the periodontal probe in a standardized position relative to the tooth and the gingival crevice is crucial for the accuracy of this system. Measurements are made on the facial surface, equidistant between the mesial and distal surfaces; the mesial-facial surface at the interproximal contact area; the lingual surface, equidistant between the mesial and distal surfaces; and the distal-lingual surface at the interproximal contact area.[75] Omission of the distal-lingual measurement does not significantly decrease the accuracy of the Periodontal Disease Index (PDI) score.[76] The criteria for making sulcular determinations appear in Table 18–2. The PDI score for the *individual* is obtained by totaling the scores of the teeth and dividing the total by the number of teeth examined (a maximum of six).[75]

Radiographic Approaches to Measuring Bone Loss

The use of radiographs would seem to overcome some of the criticisms of the subjective clinical measurements in dental epidemiology. Radiographs present permanent records of interdental bone levels, they may have less variability than poorly standardized dental examination procedures; and they offer the advantage of allowing crown and root measurements to be made. However, they are not useful in the buccal or lingual assessment of bone level, they do not provide adequate information on soft tissue attachment, and differences in angulation make comparisons difficult.[19]

Only a few indices have been specifically designed to evaluate the radiographic evidence of periodontal disease, because time constraints in epidemiologic studies make taking radiographs inconvenient. However, techniques for making reasonably accurate measurements from radiographs have been developed for longitudinal studies.

Techniques Used to Obtain More Accurate Measurements of Radiographs

Miller and Seidler[54, 55] used a scale of 0 to 5 to assess tooth-to-marginal bone level ratios from radiographs. A percentage value was used as the index of periodontal disease. Schei et al.[91] introduced a graded scale to estimate bone loss using the cemento-enamel junction as a point of reference. Bjorn et al.[8, 9] developed a method involving the projection of radiographs at a fixed distance onto a screen with a graded scale of 20 divisions. The number of divisions between the most coronal level of bone and the apical base of the bone was counted.

Another, more practical method to assess radiographs is the use of a wire grid with 1-mm squares, which is attached to the film packet before exposure.[21, 101] Either direct observation or projection of the radiograph permits measurements relative to the cemento-enamel junction, rounded to the nearest 0.5 mm.

Techniques Used to Measure Horizontal Tooth Mobility

Miller[53] described a subjective method for assessment of horizontal tooth mobility by evaluating a tooth, which is held between two instruments, on a scale of 0 to 3. The numerical values correspond to movement in 1-mm increments. This approach is useful in clinical diagnosis and treatment planning, but is of little value in longitudinal or clinical studies. (The reader is referred to an excellent review of this subject by Timothy O'Leary.[62])

Several complex electronic devices have been developed[37, 38, 65, 67, 69, 70] but the time required to use them is prohibitive for epidemiologic surveys or large clinical trials. Muhlemann[56, 57] developed two instruments for measuring tooth mobility, the macroperiodontometer and microperiodontometer. Many studies have been completed using the first device, but its value is limited to specific areas of the mouth.[58] The latter device is more difficult to master, and its results are less reproducible.[62]

The Periodontometer (United States Air Force School of Aerospace Medicine) developed by O'Leary and Rudd[63] has been used more extensively than any other device to measure tooth mobility. It measures the facial or palatal deflection of teeth in increments of 0.0001 inch when 500 grams of force are applied. Its use requires two investigators, extensive training, and a minimum of 8 to 10 minutes per quadrant. Therefore, it is only employed in clinical trials.[62]

INDICES USED TO MEASURE PLAQUE ACCUMULATION

In general, most of the indices used to measure plaque accumulation utilize a numerical scale to measure the extent of the tooth surface covered by plaque and debris. Although there are subtle differences in the definitions of plaque, debris, and materia alba used in various indices, the terms *plaque* and *debris* will be used interchangeably here.

Plaque Component of the Periodontal Disease Index (Ramfjord[75])

The plaque component of the Periodontal Disease Index (PDI) is used to evaluate six teeth, numbered 3, 9, 12, 19, 25, and 28, after staining with a disclosing solution. The presence and extent of plaque is measured on a scale of 0 to 3 on all interproximal facial and lingual surfaces of the index teeth. The criteria are suitable for longitudinal studies of periodontal disease,[75] and although the plaque component is not a part of the PDI score, it is helpful in the total assessment of periodontal status.

Shick and Ash[98] modified the original criteria of Ramfjord by excluding consideration of the interproximal areas of the teeth and "restricting the scoring of plaque to the gingival half"[76] of the facial and lingual surfaces of the index teeth. The criteria for the Shick-Ash modification of the Ramfjord plaque criteria appear in Table 18–2.

The plaque *score per person* is obtained by totaling all of the individual tooth scores and dividing this sum by the number of teeth examined. These modified plaque criteria are suitable for clinical trials of preventive or therapeutic agents.

Simplified Oral Hygiene Index
(Green and Vermillion[29])

Early in the development of the indices used to measure gingivitis and periodontal disease, it became apparent that the data lacked meaning or significance unless the level of oral hygiene or cleanliness was evaluated as a separate component. The lack of a simple, objective set of criteria that minimized examiner variability prompted Green and Vermillion to develop the Oral Hygiene Index (OHI).[28] They evaluated full mouth examinations and selected six index tooth surfaces that were representative of all anterior and posterior segments. This modification was called the Simplified Oral Hygiene Index (OHI-S).[29] The OHI-S measures the surface area of the tooth covered by debris and calculus. The imprecise term *debris* was used because it was not practical to observe the soft deposits microscopically and make the subtle distinctions between plaque, debris, and materia alba. In addition, determining the weight and thickness of the soft deposits is not possible in epidemiologic studies and led to the assumption that the dirtier the mouth, the greater the tooth surface area covered by debris. This also implies that the longer oral hygiene practices are neglected, the greater the tooth surface area that will be covered by debris.

The OHI-S consists of two components: a Simplified Debris Index (DIS) and a Simplified Calculus Index (CIS). Each component is assessed on a scale of 0 to 3. Only a mouth mirror and dental explorer, with no disclosing agent, are used for the examination. The six tooth surfaces examined in the OHI-S are the facial surfaces of the teeth numbered 3, 8, 14, and 24 and the lingual surfaces of the teeth numbered 19 and 30. Each tooth surface is divided horizontally into gingival, middle, and incisal thirds.

For the DIS a dental explorer is placed on the incisal third of the tooth and moved toward the gingival third according to the criteria illustrated in Figure 18–1. The DIS *score per person* is obtained by totaling the debris score per tooth surface and dividing by the number of surfaces examined.

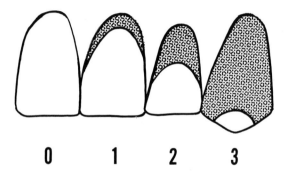

Figure 18–1. Criteria for scoring oral debris (DIS) component of the Simplified Oral Hygiene Index (OHI-S). (From Greene, J. C., and Vermillion, J. R.: J. Am. Dent. Assoc., 68:7, 1964.)

0—No debris or stain present.
1—Soft debris covering not more than one third of the tooth surface, or the presence of extrinsic stains without other debris regardless of surface area covered.
2—Soft debris covering more than one third but not more than two thirds of the exposed tooth surface.
3—Soft debris covering more than two thirds of the exposed tooth surface.

The CIS assessment is performed by gently placing a dental explorer into the distal gingival crevice and drawing it subgingivally from the distal contact area to the mesial contact area. The criteria for scoring the calculus component of the OHI-S are shown in Figure 18–2. The CIS *score per person* is obtained by totaling the calculus scores per tooth surface and dividing the total by the number of surfaces examined. The OHI-S *score per person* is the total of the DIS and CIS scores per person.

The clinical levels of oral cleanliness for debris associated with group DIS scores are as follows[27]:

Good = 0.0–0.6
Fair = 0.7–1.8
Poor = 1.9–3.0

The clinical levels of oral hygiene associated with group OHI-S scores are as follows[27]:

Good = 0.0–1.2
Fair = 1.3–3.0
Poor = 3.1–6.0

The OHI-S is easy to use because the criteria are objective, examinations may be performed quickly, and high levels of repro-

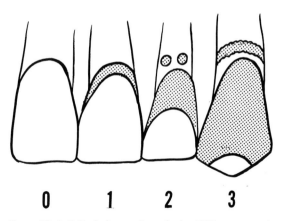

Figure 18–2. Criteria for scoring calculus (CIS) component of the Simplified Oral Hygiene Index (OHI-S). (From Greene, J. C., and Vermillion, J. R.: J. Am. Dent. Assoc., 68:7, 1964.)

0—No calculus present.

1—Supragingival calculus covering not more than one third of the exposed tooth surface.

2—Supragingival calculus covering more than one third but not more than two thirds of the exposed tooth surface or the presence of individual flecks of subgingival calculus around the cervical portion of the tooth or both.

3—Supragingival calculus covering more than two thirds of the exposed tooth surface or a coninuous heavy band of subgingival calculus around the cervical portion of the tooth or both.

ducibility are possible with minimum examiner training sessions.[27] For these reasons it has been used extensively throughout the world and has contributed greatly to our understanding of periodontal disease. There is a very high correlation ($r = 0.82$)[95] between the OHI-S and Russell's Periodontal Index, making it possible, if one of the two scores is known, to calculate the other using regression analysis.[26] The OHI-S has been used in epidemiologic surveys[47] and for longitudinal evaluations of dental health education programs. It is also useful to evaluate individual oral cleanliness and, to a more limited extent, for clinical trials.

Turesky-Gilmore-Glickman Modification[105] of the Quigley-Hein[73] Plaque Index

In 1962, Quigley and Hein[73] presented results from a plaque index that focused attention on the gingival third of the tooth surface.

TABLE 18–4. TURESKY-GILMORE-GLICKMAN MODIFICATION[105] OF THE QUIGLEY-HEIN PLAQUE INDEX[73]

0 = No plaque.
1 = Separate flecks of plaque at the cervical margin of the tooth.
2 = A thin, continuous band of plaque (up to 1 mm) at the cervical margin.
3 = A band of plaque wider than 1 mm but covering less than one third of the crown.
4 = Plaque covering at least one third but less than two thirds of the crown.
5 = Plaque covering two thirds or more of the crown.[46]

They examined the facial surfaces of the anterior teeth, employing a basic fuchsin mouthwash and a numerical scoring system of 0 to 5.

Turesky and associates[105] strengthened the objectivity of the Quigley-Hein criteria by redefining the scores of the gingival third area. The Turesky-Gilmore-Glickman modification of the Quigley-Hein criteria appears in Table 18–4. They assessed plaque on the facial and lingual surfaces of all of the teeth after using a disclosing agent. A plaque *score per person* was obtained by totaling all of the plaque scores and dividing by the number of surfaces examined. This system of scoring plaque is relatively easy to use because of the objective definitions of each numerical score. The strength of this plaque index is its application to longitudinal studies and clinical trials of preventive and therapeutic agents.

Glass Criteria for Scoring Debris[24]

Glass[24] developed a system for measuring the presence and extent of debris accumulation in order to evaluate toothbrushing efficacy. All of the teeth were scored, with the facial and lingual surfaces scored as a unit. Glass also developed criteria for measuring gingival changes, tooth stain, and calculus accumulation. The debris criteria are the following:

0 = No visible debris
1 = Debris visible at gingival margin—but discontinuous—less than 1 mm in height

2 = Debris continuous at gingival margin—greater than 1 mm in height
3 = Debris involving entire gingival third of tooth
4 = Debris generally scattered over tooth surface

The debris index *score per person* is obtained by totaling all of the debris scores per tooth and dividing by the number of teeth examined. The strength of this index is in clinical trials of preventive or therapeutic agents[46] because it places emphasis on the gingival third of the tooth.

Patient Hygiene Performance Index
(Podshadley and Haley[71])

The Patient Hygiene Performance (PHP) Index[71] was the first index developed for the sole purpose of assessing an individual's performance in removing debris after toothbrushing instruction. It assesses the presence or absence of debris as 1 or 0, respectively, on the six OHI-S teeth. The PHP Index is relatively more sensitive than the OHI-S because it divides each tooth surface into five areas: three longitudinal thirds—distal, middle, and mesial—with the middle third subdivided horizontally into incisal, middle, and gingival thirds. Scoring is preceded by the use of a disclosing agent. The PHP *score per person* is obtained by totaling the five subdivision scores of each tooth surface and dividing the total by the number of tooth surfaces examined. This index is easy to use because of its dichotomous criteria and can be performed quickly. Although it can be used in group studies of health education, its chief value lies in its application as an education aid.

Two other indices with a similar purpose are the Plaque Control Record of O'Leary et al.[64] and the plaque portion of the Bleeding Points Index of Lenox and Kopczyk.[39]

Plaque Index (Silness and Löe[99])

The Plaque Index (PlI) is unique among the indices because it ignores the coronal extent and assesses only the *thickness* of plaque at the gingival area of the tooth. Since it was developed as a component to parallel the Gingival Index (GI) of Löe and Silness,[41] it involves the same scoring units of the teeth: distal-facial, facial, mesial-facial, and lingual surfaces. A mouth mirror, dental explorer, and air drying of the teeth are used to assess plaque. Unlike most indices, it does not exclude or substitute for teeth with gingival restorations or crowns and all teeth or only selected ones may be measured. The criteria for the PlI of Silness and Löe appear in Table 18–3.

The PlI score for the *area* is obtained by totaling the four plaque scores per tooth. If the sum of the PlI scores per tooth is divided by four, the PlI score for the *tooth* is obtained. The PlI *score per person* is obtained by adding the PlI scores per tooth and dividing the sum by the number of teeth examined. The PlI may be obtained for a segment of the mouth or a group of teeth in a similar manner.

The strength of the PlI is in its application to longitudinal studies and clinical trials. In spite of the studies that have been conducted to ensure the reliability of the PlI data, the assessment of plaque thickness is so subjective that it requires highly trained and experienced examiners to ensure valid data.[46]

INDICES USED TO MEASURE CALCULUS

In general, the indices used to assess calculus may be divided into those appropriate for epidemiologic surveys; those appropriate for longitudinal studies, involving examinations every 3 to 6 months; and those useful in short-term clinical studies of 6 weeks or less.

Calculus Component of the Simplified Oral Hygiene Index (Greene and Vermillion[29])

The Simplified Calculus Index (CIS) component of the Simplified Oral Hygiene Index (OHI-S) was presented in detail in the section "Indices Used to Measure Plaque Accumulation" because it is less separable from its scoring system than any of the other indices that combine several component measures. The CIS component is applicable to epidemiologic surveys and longitudinal studies of periodontal disease.[27] Figure 18–2 presents the specific criteria of the OHI-S used to assess calculus.

Calculus Component of the Periodontal Disease Index (Ramfjord[74])

The calculus component of the Periodontal Disease Index (PDI) assesses the presence and extent of calculus on six index teeth, numbers 3, 9, 12, 19, 25, and 28, with a numerical scale of 0 to 3. A mouth mirror and a dental explorer and/or a periodontal probe are used in the examination. The criteria for assigning a score to each tooth surface are listed in Table 18–2.

The calculus scores per tooth are totaled and the total is then divided by the number of teeth examined to yield the calculus *score per person*. Like the Simplified Calculus Index (CIS) of the OHI-S, the calculus component of the PDI has a high degree of examiner reproducibility, can be performed quickly, and is best applied in epidemiologic surveys and longitudinal studies.[75]

Probe Method of Calculus Assessment (Volpe et al.[107])

The Probe Method of Calculus Assessment was developed to assess the quantity of supragingival calculus formed in longitudinal studies. A periodontal probe graduated in millimeter divisions is used to measure the deposits of calculus on the lingual surfaces of the six mandibular anterior teeth. The smallest unit used to record the presence of calculus is 0.5 mm. For proper examination, a mouth mirror is needed and air is used to dry the teeth. Measurements are made in three planes: gingival, distal, and mesial. The gingival measurement is made with the probe held parallel to the long axis of the tooth and equidistant from the mesial and distal surfaces. The probe should be simultaneously in contact with the calculus and the incisal edge of the tooth. The distal measurement is made by holding the probe diagonally so that the tip is in contact with the distal aspect of the tooth and the portion toward the shank of the probe is bisecting the mesial-incisal line angle of the tooth. The opposite is true for the mesial measurement. The measurement may be calculated and expressed as the measurement score, the tooth score, or the subject score. The *measurement score* is simply the total of all of the scores divided by the number of measurements made. The *tooth score* is the total of all of the scores divided by the number of teeth scored. The *subject score* is the total of all of the scores (subjects with fewer than six teeth are excluded).[106]

The Probe Method of Calculus Assessment has been shown to possess a high degree of inter- and intra-examiner reproducibility. However, extensive training under an experienced investigator is required to master this technique.

Calculus Surface Index (Ennever et al.[20])

The Calculus Surface Index (CSI) is one of two indices that are used in short-term clinical trials of calculus inhibitory agents. The objective of this type of study is the rapid determination of the effects of specific agents on reducing or preventing supra- or subgingival calculus formation. The CSI was designed to assess the presence or absence of supra- and/or subgingival calculus on the four mandibular incisors but has also been applied to the six mandibular anterior teeth. The presence or absence of calculus scored 0 or 1 is determined by visual or tactile examination. The surface of each incisor is divided into four scoring units. The labial surface is one unit, and the lingual surface is divided longitudinally into three units: the distal-lingual third, the lingual third, and the mesial-lingual third. The total number of surfaces with calculus is considered the CSI score *per person*. This index has been shown to have good intra-examiner reproducibility, and the examination can be performed in a relatively short period of time. Scoring four mandibular incisors per person, the maximum calculus score would be 16.[106]

A companion index to the CSI is the Calculus Surface Severity Index (CSSI).[20] This index quantifies on a scale of 0 to 3 the calculus present on the surfaces examined for the CSI. The criteria for the CSSI are as follows[18]:

0 = No calculus present
1 = Calculus observable, but less than 0.5 mm in width and/or thickness
2 = Calculus not exceeding 1.0 mm in width and/or thickness
3 = Calculus exceeding 1.0 mm in width and/or thickness

Marginal Line Calculus Index
(Mühlemann and Villa[61])

Another index used in short-term clinical trials of anti-calculus agents is the Marginal Line Calculus Index (MLCI). This index measures the accumulation of supragingival calculus on the gingival third of the tooth, specifically along the margin of the gingiva.

Using a mouth mirror to examine and air to dry the teeth, the cervical areas on the lingual surfaces of the four mandibular incisors are examined. The cervical third of each lingual surface is divided into a distal half and a mesial half. Each half is examined for the extent of calculus covering the surface, and a score on a scale of percentages is assigned as follows: 0, 12.5, 25, 50, 75, and 100 per cent. The MLCI *score per tooth* is determined by averaging the two units for each tooth. The MLCI *score per person* is determined by totaling the scores per tooth and dividing the total by the number of teeth examined. The MLCI has shown good reproducibility.[106]

RELIABILITY OF DENTAL INDICES

Reliability of epidemiologic indices is the ability of an index to repeatedly measure a condition in the same subject and give the same score. It is essential to the interpretation of epidemiologic data. Reliability is a matter of degree, since all measurements are subject to method and observer error or variability. Repeat examinations by one examiner will allow assessment of *intra-examiner variability*, and repeated examinations comparing two

or more examiners will measure *inter-examiner variability*. Unreliable measures make prevalence estimates from surveys questionable and mask true differences between groups in longitudinal studies. *Reliability* is considered the more general term; *reproducibility* or *repeatability* is usually restricted to repeat examination data.[78] The reader is referred to an excellent discussion of this subject by Clemmer and Barbano.[16]

An understanding of the reliability of periodontal indices dictates that all studies should incorporate some system to measure reliability, describe it in publications, and report the results.

DESCRIPTIVE EPIDEMIOLOGY OF GINGIVAL AND PERIODONTAL DISEASES

Prevalence of Gingivitis

In general, the prevalence and severity of gingivitis increases with age, beginning at approximately 5 years of age, reaching the highest point in puberty, and then very gradually decreasing but remaining relatively high throughout life (Fig. 18–3).[32] The rapid increase in the incidence of gingivitis prior to 10 years of age is associated with the eruption of the permanent dentition.[52] Surveys of the prevalance and severity of gingivitis in children and young adults are summarized in Table 18–5.

Prevalence of Periodontal Disease

On a worldwide basis, the United States ranks relatively low in the magnitude and prevalence of periodontal disease. Table 18–6 shows mean PI scores by various population groups throughout the world.[83]

Although there is no method of determining the absolute extent of periodontal disease in the United States population, sufficient data exist to allow relatively accurate estimates of prevalence. In adults 18 to 79 years of age in the 1960 to 1962 cycle of the National Health Survey (NHS), three of four (73.9 per cent) had some form of periodontal disease, and one of four (25.4 per cent) had destructive periodontal disease.[34] Data from the

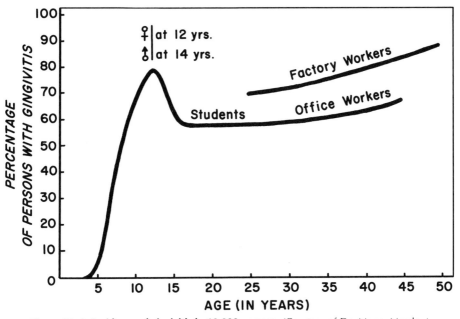

Figure 18–3. Incidence of gingivitis in 10,000 persons. (Courtesy of Dr. Maury Massler.)

HANES I survey (1971 to 1974) suggest that two of four adults (49.7 per cent) have some form of periodontal disease, and one of four (25.4 per cent) has destructive periodontal disease.[32] The decrease in periodontal disease noted here is probably attributable to a decrease in gingivitis, whereas the prevalence of destructive disease has remained almost constant. *As more people retain their teeth throughout their lifetimes, and as the proportion of older people increases, more teeth will be at risk for periodontal disease. It is commonly believed that the prevalence of destructive periodontal disease will increase in the future.*

Prevalence of Juvenile Periodontitis

It is difficult to arrive at a statement of prevalence for juvenile periodontitis because of the lack of uniform criteria for recognizing and classifying juvenile periodontitis and the small sample size of the documented study groups. One study conducted in Finland using strict diagnostic criteria found the prevalence to be 0.1 per cent.[90] This study did not include a black population, in which the prevalence is thought to be higher.

FACTORS AFFECTING THE PREVALENCE AND SEVERITY OF GINGIVITIS AND PERIODONTAL DISEASE

Personal and Environmental Factors

Age

The prevalence of periodontal disease increases with increasing age.[83] Figure 18–4 shows the distribution of periodontal disease, with and without pockets.[33, 34, 87] The prevalence of periodontal disease is approximately 45 per cent at 10 years of age, 67 per cent at 20 years, 70 per cent at 35 years, and 80 per cent at 50 years. Although these estimates may be high, the lower values reported by the HANES I survey may be too low: approximately 15 per cent at 10 years of age, 38 per cent at 20 years, 46 per cent at 35 years, and 54 per cent at 50 years.[32] *However, both surveys show gradual increases in the prevalence of periodontal disease, suggesting that few people escape the ravages of this disease.* The distribution of periodontal disease with pockets is approximately 1 per cent at 10 years of age, 10 per cent at 20 years, 20 per cent at 35

TABLE 18–5. PREVALENCE OF GINGIVITIS IN CHILDREN AND YOUNG ADULTS

Investigators	Year	Group Studied	No. Children in Group	Age Group	Percentage of Persons Affected with Gingivitis
McCall[18]	1933	New York	4600	1–14 yrs	98.0
Messner et al.[20]	1938	Children in 26 states of United States	1,438,318	6–14 yrs	3.5–8.6
Marshall-Day and Tandan[16]	1940	Middle-class children in Lahore, India	756	approx. 13 yrs	68.0
Marshall-Day[11]	1940	Fluoride endemic area in northern India	203	5–18 yrs	59.6
King[8]	1940	Isle of Lewis	2280	6–15 yrs	90.0
Campbell and Cook[2]	1942	Dundee Hospital in Scotland	1924		2.2
Marshall-Day[12]	1944	Boys in Kangra district of India (poor nutrition)	200	approx. 13 yrs	81.0
Marshall-Day and Shourie[13]	1944	Low to middle-class school children in India	613	5–15 yrs	80.0
King et al.[10]	1944	English boys	403	11–14 yrs	
				Group A	77.4
				Group B	87.6
	1944	Gibraltar evacuees in England	135	10–14 yrs	85.2
King[9]	1945	Primary school children in Dundee, Scotland	103	12–14 yrs	90.0
	1945	Harpenden Institution, England	170	11–14 yrs	Groups vary 56.4–97.5
Marshall-Day and Shourie[14]	1947	Low- to middle-class male school children in Lahore, India	1054	9–17 yrs	99.4
Marshall-Day and Shourie[14]	1947	Girls of high socioeconomic level in Lahore, India	179	9–17 yrs	73.3
Schour and Massler[25]	1947	Four communities in Italy suffering from malnutrition	682	6–10 yrs	40.3
			721	11–20 yrs	55.3
Marshall-Day and Shourie[15]	1948	Puerto Rico	1648	6–18 yrs	60.0–79.0
Massler et al.[17]	1950	Suburban Chicago school children	804	5–14 yrs	64.3
Marshall-Day and Shourie[15]	1950	Virgin Islands (91% black population)	823	6–18 yrs	57.0
			860	5–13 yrs	26.9
Stahl and Goldman[28]	1953	School children in Massachusetts	1300	13–17 yrs	29.0
Russell[24]	1957	Urban United States White	6682	5–9 yrs	10.8
			15,922	10–14 yrs	25.5
			4031	15–19 yrs	37.3
		Black	37	5–9 yrs	8.1
			494	10–19 yrs	28.7

1. Bowden, D. E. J., Davies, R. M., Holloway, P. J., et al.: A treatment need survey of a 15-year-old population. Br. Dent. J., *134*:375, 1973.
2. Campbell, H. G., and Cook, R. P.: Incidence of Gingivitis at Dundee Dental Hospital. Year Book of Dentistry. Chicago, Year Book Publishers, 1942.
3. Downer, M. C.: Dental caries and periodontal disease in girls of different ethnic groups: a comparison in a London secondary school. Br. Dent. J., *128*:379, 1970.
4. Dutta, A.: A study on prevalence of periodontal disease and dental caries amongst the school-going children in Calcutta. J. All India Dent. Assoc., *37*:367, 1965.
5. Greene, J. C.: Periodontal disease in India: report of an epidemiological study. J. Dent. Res., *39*:302, 1960.
6. Jamison, H. C.: Prevalence of periodontal disease of the deciduous teeth. J. Am. Dent. Assoc., *66*:207, 1963.
7. Jorkjend, L., and Birkeland, J. M.: Plaque and gingivitis among Norwegian children participating in a dental health program. Community Dent. Oral Epidemiol., *1*:41, 1973.
8. King, J. D.: Dental Disease in the Isle of Lewis. Medical Research Council, Special Report Series, No. 241. London, His Majesty's Stationery Office, 1940.
9. King, J. D.: Gingival disease in Dundee. Dent. Record, *65*:9, 32, 55, 1945.
10. King, J. D., Franklyn, A. B., and Allen, I.: Gingival disease in Gibraltar evacuee children. Lancet, *1*:495, 1944.
11. Marshall-Day, C. D.: Chronic endemic fluorosis in Northern India. Br. Dent. J., *68*:409, 1940.
12. Marshall-Day, C. D.: Nutritional deficiencies and dental caries in northern India. Br. Dent. J., *76*:115, 143, 1944.
13. Marshall-Day, C. D., and Shourie, K. L.: The incidence of periodontal disease in the Punjab. Indian J. Med. Res., *32*:47, 1944.
14. Marshall-Day, C. D., and Shourie, K. L.: Hypertrophic gingivitis in Indian children and adolescents. Indian J. Med. Res., *35*(4):261, 1947.
15. Marshall-Day, C. D., and Shourie, K. L.: Gingival disease in the Virgin Islands. J. Am. Dent. Assoc., *40*:175, 1950.
16. Marshall-Day, C. D., and Tandan, G. C.: The incidence of dental caries in the Punjab. Br. Dent. J., *69*:389, 1940.

TABLE 18–5. PREVALENCE OF GINGIVITIS IN CHILDREN AND YOUNG ADULTS *Continued*

Investigators	Year	Group Studied	No. Children in Group	Age Group	Percentage of Persons Affected with Gingivitis
Green[5]	1960	School boys in low socioeconomic area of India	1613	11–17 yrs	96.9
		School boys in low socioeconomic area of Atlanta, Georgia	577	11–17 yrs	92.0
Zimmerman and Baker[30]	1960	White children from Maryland	529	6–12 yrs	35.0
		Black children from Texas	442	6–12 yrs	67.0
		White children from Texas	435	6–12 yrs	79.0
Jamison[6]	1963	Tecumseh, Michigan (deciduous teeth only)	159	5–14 yrs	99.4
McHugh et al.[19]	1964	Dundee, Scotland, boys and girls	2905	13 yrs	99.4
Dutta[4]	1965	Calcutta, India, boys and girls	1424	6–12 yrs	89.8
Wade[29]	1966	Iraq	200	13–15 yrs	97.0
		London	222	13–15 yrs	
Sheiham[26]	1968	Nigeria	1620	10 yrs and older	99+
Sheiham[27]	1969	Surrey	756	11–17 yrs	99.7
Murray[21]	1969	West Hartlepool, 1.5–2.0 ppm fluoride			
		Boys	211	15 yrs	94.8
		Girls	175	15 yrs	86.3
		York, 0.2 ppm fluoride			
		Boys	202	15 yrs	95.5
		Girls	179	15 yrs	85.5
Downer[3]	1970	Secondary school children in London, England	373	11–14 yrs	79.0
Murray[22]	1972	West Hartlepool, 1.5–2.0 ppm fluoride			
		Boys	141	15–19 yrs	90.1
		Girls	449	15–19 yrs	88.4
		York, 0.2 ppm fluoride			
		Boys	61	15–19 yrs	86.9
		Girls	102	15–19 yrs	84.3
Jorkjend and Birkeland[7]	1973	Primary school children in Porsgrunn, Norway	154	11–13 yrs	99.0
Bowden et al.[1]	1973	Cheshire, England	622	15 yrs	81.2
Murray[23]	1974	West Hartlepool, 1.5–2.0 ppm fluoride			
		Boys	1470	8–18 yrs	92.9
		Girls	1406	8–18 yrs	91.1

17. Massler, M., Schour, I., and Chopra, B.: Occurrence of gingivitis in suburban Chicago school children. J. Periodontol., 21:146, 1950.
18. McCall, J. O.: The periodontist looks at children's dentistry. J. Am. Dent. Assoc., 20:1518, 1933.
19. McHugh, W. D., McEven, J. D., and Hitchin, A. D.: Dental disease and related factors in 13-year-old children in Dundee. Br. Dent. J., 117:246, 1964.
20. Messner, C. T., Gafaver, W. M., Cady, F. C., and Dean, H. T.: Dental Survey of School Children Ages 6 to 14 Years Made in 1933–1934 in 26 States. Public Health Bulletin 226. Washington, D.C., U.S. Government Printing Office, 1938.
21. Murray, J. J.: Gingivitis in 15-year-old children from high fluoride and low fluoride areas. Arch. Oral Biol., 14:951, 1969.
22. Murray, J. J.: Gingivitis and gingival recession in adults from high-fluoride and low-fluoride areas. Arch. Oral Biol., 17:1269, 1972.
23. Murray, J. J.: The prevalence of gingivitis in children continuously resident in a high fluoride area. J. Dent. Child., 41:133, 1974.
24. Russell, A. L.: Some epidemiological characteristics of periodontal disease in a series of urban populations. J. Periodontol., 28:286, 1957.
25. Schour, I., and Massler, M.: Gingival disease in post-war Italy (1945). I. Prevalence of gingivitis in various age groups. J. Am. Dent. Assoc., 35:475, 1947.
26. Sheiham, A.: The epidemiology of chronic periodontal disease in western Nigerian children. J. Periodont. Res., 3:257, 1968.
27. Sheiham, A.: The prevalence and severity of periodontal disease in Surrey school children. Dent. Pract., 19: 232, 1969.
28. Stahl, D. G., and Goldman, H. M.: Incidence of gingivitis among a sample of Massachusetts school children. Oral Surg., 6:707, 1953.
29. Wade, A. B.: Validity of anterior segment gingival scores in epidemiologic studies. J. Periodontol., 37:55, 1966.
30. Zimmerman, E. R., and Baker, W. A.: Effect of geographic location and race on gingival disease in children. J. Am. Dent. Assoc., 61:542, 1960.

TABLE 18–6. AVERAGE PERIODONTAL INDEX SCORES IN CIVILIANS (BOTH SEXES), AGED 40–49 YEARS, SURVEYED BY EXAMINERS OF THE NATIONAL INSTITUTE OF DENTAL RESEARCH, UNITED STATES*

Population Group	Average Periodontal Index Score
Baltimore, Maryland (white)	1.03
Colorado Springs, Colorado	1.04†
Alaska; primitive Eskimos	1.17‡
Ecuador	1.85
Ethiopia	1.86
Baltimore, Maryland (black)	1.99
Vietnam; Vietnamese	2.18
Colombia	2.21
Alaska; urban Eskimos	2.31‡
Uganda	2.50§
Chile	2.74
Lebanon; Lebanese	2.98
Thailand	3.30
Lebanon; Palestinian refugees	3.52
Burma	3.58
Jordan; Jordanian civilians	3.96
Vietnam; hill tribesmen	3.97
Trinidad	4.21
Jordan; Palestinian refugees	4.41

*Modified from Russell, A. L.: J. Periodontol., 38:585, 1967.
  †Ages 40–44 only
  ‡Males only
  §Age over 40

years, and 30 per cent at 50 years. Both data sets[32, 83] show a dramatic ninefold increase in the prevalence of destructive disease with pockets between 20 and 70 years of age. This pattern of disease with pockets closely parallels that of the reduction in bone height

that occurs with increasing age.[48] Although destructive periodontal disease is primarily a disease of adults, its onset during puberty has been reported with greater frequency in countries[80] other than the United States.[87]

Indicated by mean Periodontal Index scores, *the severity of periodontal disease increases with age* (Fig. 18–5). Between 35 and 40 years of age, the average adult enters the beginning phases of destructive disease. It takes approximately 20 years before the average adult, at ages 55 to 60, enters the advanced phases of destructive periodontal disease.[34]

Sex

In general, males consistently have a higher prevalence and severity of periodontal disease than females (Fig. 18–6). Before 20 years of age the difference between males and females is slight.[33, 87] At age 20, males have only a 30 per cent higher PI score (0.14 PI unit) than females.[31, 34] Between ages 18 and 74, males have almost 45 per cent more severe periodontal disease. Males enter the beginning phases of destructive periodontal disease at approximately 35 years of age, and females later at approximately 45 years of age. The advanced stages of periodontal disease begin at approximately 55 years of age for males and 75 years of age for females. However, some data suggest that women enter the advanced stages at closer to 65 rather than 75 years of age.[32]

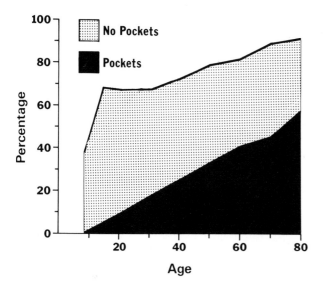

Figure 18–4. Prevalence of periodontal disease by age. Data are from the National Health Survey and cover the following periods: 1963 to 1965 (children, aged 6 to 11 years), 1966 to 1970 (youths, aged 12 to 17 years), and 1960 to 1962 (adults, aged 18 to 79 years). The percent distribution is by mild to moderate gingivitis (no pockets) and periodontal disease with one or more pockets; it is based on Periodontal Index (PI) scores. Data for males and females were combined. (Adapted from Kelly, J. E., and Sanchez, M. J.: Periodontal Disease and Oral Hygiene Among Children, United States. Washington, D.C., U.S. Department of Health, Education, and Welfare, 1972; Sanchez, M. J.: Periodontal Disease Among Youths 12–17 Years, United States. Washington, D.C., U.S. Department of Health, Education, and Welfare, 1974; and Kelly, J. E., and Van Kirk, L. E.: Periodontal Disease in Adults, United States 1960–1962. Washington, D.C., U.S. Department of Health, Education, and Welfare, 1966.)

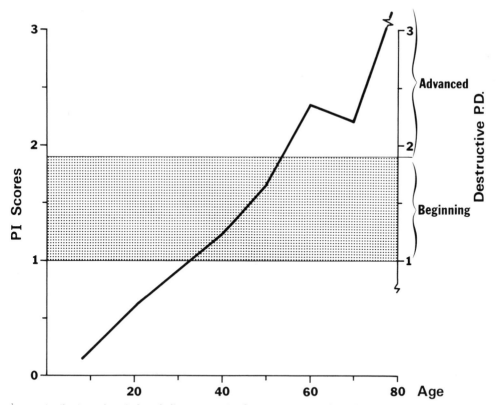

Figure 18–5. Distribution of periodontal disease severity by age. Data are from the National Health Survey and are combined for whites and blacks. Severity is indicated by mean Periodontal Index (PI) scores. The subdivisions of destructive periodontal disease approximate the group PI scores that correspond to the various clinical conditions (see Table 18–1). (Adapted from Kelly, J. E., and Sanchez, M. J.: Periodontal Disease and Oral Hygiene Among Children, United States. Washington, D.C., U.S. Department of Health, Education, and Welfare, 1972; Sanchez, M. J.: Periodontal Disease Among Youths 12–17 Years, United States. Washington, D.C., U.S. Department of Health, Education, and Welfare, 1974; and Kelly, J. E., and Van Kirk, L. E.: Periodontal Disease in Adults, United States 1960–1962. Washington, D.C., U.S. Department of Health, Education, and Welfare, 1966.)

Race

Figure 18–7 shows the severity of periodontal disease by racial-ethnic group from the NHS[33, 34, 87] and the Ten State Nutrition Survey (10SNS or National Nutrition Survey).[104] In the NHS data, blacks consistently appear to have more severe periodontal disease than whites.[34] Remarkably, after 20 years of age, blacks average 50 per cent more severe periodontal disease than whites.

Education

There are two important associations between periodontal disease and educational level (Fig. 18–8).[34] First, *periodontal disease is inversely related to increasing levels of educa-tion.*[30, 80] Whites have a 63 per cent or three fifths decrease in periodontal disease severity and blacks have a decrease of almost one half (47 per cent). Second, *the differences observed between whites and blacks with periodontal disease* (see Fig. 18–7) *can only be related to differences in education, because no significant differences exist between whites and blacks of similar education.* It is not surprising that occupation, which is so closely tied to education in the United States, shows a relationship to periodontal disease that is similar to that of education. For example, the prevalence and severity of periodontal disease are lower in office personnel than in factory workers, and are generally lower among persons in occupations that require more educational background.[4, 50]

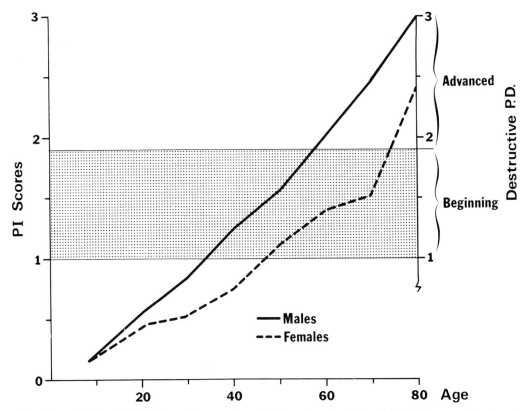

Figure 18–6. Severity of periodontal disease by sex and age. Data are from the National Health Survey and are for whites only. (Adapted from Kelly, J. E., and Sanchez, M. J.: Periodontal Disease and Oral Hygiene Among Children, United States. Washington, D.C., U.S. Department of Health, Education, and Welfare, 1972; Sanchez, M. J.: Periodontal Disease Among Youths 12–17 Years, United States. Washington, D.C., U.S. Department of Health, Education, and Welfare, 1974; Kelly, J. E., and Van Kirk, L. E.: Periodontal Disease in Adults, United States 1960–1962. Washington, D.C., U.S. Department of Health, Education, and Welfare, 1966.)

Income

Periodontal disease is inversely related to increasing levels of income. The association between periodontal disease and income is similar to that observed between periodontal disease and education. This decrease in the severity of periodontal disease that occurs with increasing income is 38 per cent for whites and 20 per cent for blacks,[34] but the observed differences (see Figure 18–7) were not influenced as strongly by income as by education. When the PI scores of whites and blacks are combined according to education

Figure 18–7. Severity of periodontal disease by racial-ethnic group and age. Data are from the National Health Survey and the Ten-State Survey (10–SNS) (1968 to 1970), high income ratio states. (Adapted from Kelly, J. E., and Sanchez, M. J.: Periodontal Disease and Oral Hygiene Among Children, United States. Washington, D.C., U.S. Department of Health, Education, and Welfare, 1972; Sanchez, M. J.: Periodontal Disease Among Youths 12–17 Years, United States. Washington, D.C., U.S. Department of Health, Education, and Welfare, 1974; Kelly, J. E., and Van Kirk, L. E.: Periodontal Disease in Adults, United States 1960–1962. Washington, D. C., U.S. Department of Health, Education, and Welfare, 1966; and Ten-State Nutrition Survey 1968–1970. Atlanta, Centers for Disease Control, 1972.)

Figure 18–8. Comparison of periodontal disease severity by education and racial-ethnic group. Data are from the National Health Survey and are for adults according to the number of years or the highest grade of elementary or high school completed. (Adapted from Kelly, J. E., and Van Kirk, L. E.: Periodontal Disease in Adults, United States 1960–1962. Washington, D.C., U.S. Department of Health, Education, and Welfare, 1966.)

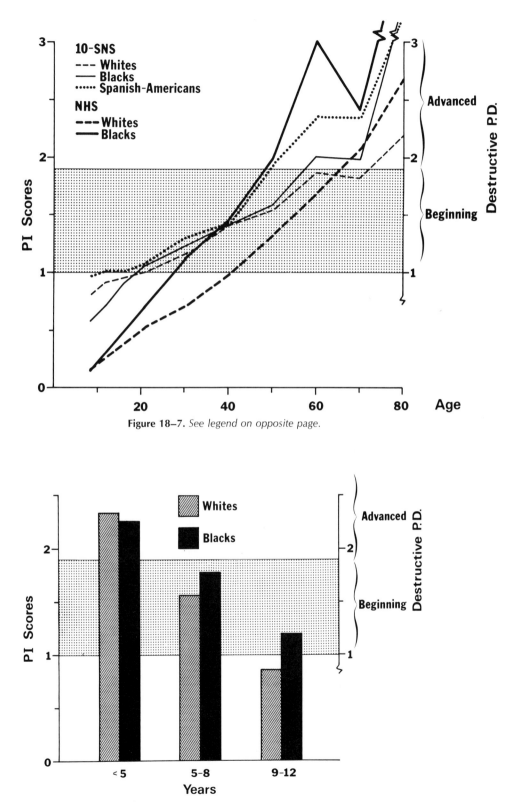

Figure 18–7. *See legend on opposite page.*

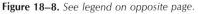

Figure 18–8. *See legend on opposite page.*

and income, the decrease associated with education is 55 per cent, whereas the decrease associated with income is only 28 per cent.

Residence

In general, the prevalence and severity of periodontal disease are slightly higher in rural areas than in urban areas.[6, 34]

Geographic Area

Within the United States, some investigators have shown geographic differences in the prevalence and severity of periodontal disease,[51, 110] others have shown none[32, 34] or only slightly higher periodontal index scores[33, 87] for children and youths living in the South.

Etiologic Factors

Plaque

Many researchers have reported strong positive relationships between poor oral hygiene and periodontal disease.[25, 26, 29, 35, 44, 97, 102] A vivid example of the relative importance of plaque and oral hygiene is a multiple correlation analysis of the combined effects of age, sex, and oral hygiene (OHI-S scores) on Periodontal Index (PI) scores of 752 South Vietnamese over 15 years of age.[86] It was demonstrated that 67 per cent of the variance was attributable to oral hygiene and approximately 31 per cent to age. The NHS also showed that oral hygiene correlated best with the prevalence and severity of periodontal disease.[87, 88] Therefore, *statistically as well as clinically, plaque is a primary etiologic factor in periodontal disease.*

Nutrition

The evidence of an association of nutritional deficiencies with human periodontal disease has been less than convincing.[96] In a series of nutrition surveys conducted by the Interdepartmental Committee on Nutrition for National Defense (ICNND),[82] no consistent correlation was found between nutrient levels and disease.

Therefore, *nutrition appears to be a secondary factor in the etiology of periodontal disease.*

Professional Dental Care

The incidence and severity of periodontal disorders are lower in individuals receiving regular dental care.[12, 45, 85, 102, 108] The prevalence and severity of disease increases with neglect.

DISTRIBUTION OF DISEASE IN DIFFERENT AREAS OF THE MOUTH

Löe and coworkers have shown that the interproximal area is most severely affected by gingivitis, followed by the buccal and lingual surfaces (Table 18–7). Evaluating the upper and lower arches has revealed that gingivitis is more severe on the interproximal and buccal areas of maxillary teeth, and the lingual areas of mandibular teeth.[42] Suomi and Barbano[100] detailed the same general pattern (listed in descending order): for facial surfaces, the most severely affected areas were the upper first and second molars, lower anteriors, upper anteriors, upper premolars, lower first and second molars, and lower premolars; for lingual surfaces, they were the lower first and second molars, lower premolars, lower anteriors, upper first and second molars, upper premolars, and upper anteriors. Other investigators[7, 100] have observed a slightly higher tendency for gingivitis on the right half of the mouth than on the left half. This may occur because right-handed people tend to have difficulty in brushing the right side.

The intraoral pattern of supra- and subgingival calculus is shown in Figure 18–9.[94] The upper first molars have the most supragingival calculus, followed by the lower centrals and laterals. The upper anteriors have the least supragingival calculus. The lower central and lateral incisors have the most subgingival calculus, followed by the upper first

TABLE 18–7. SEVERITY OF GINGIVITIS FOR THREE DIFFERENT AREAS BY ARCH*

Area	Arch	Mean Gingival Index Score
Interproximal	Upper > lower	1.44 > 1.20
Buccal	Upper > lower	1.23 > 1.13
Lingual	Lower > upper	0.89 > 0.46

*Adapted from Löe, H., Theilade, E., and Jensen, S. B.: J. Periodontol., 36:177, 1965.

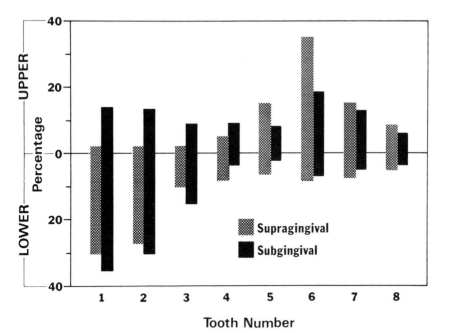

Figure 18–9. Intraoral prevalence of calculus by individual teeth. The percentage of supra- and subgingival calculus is presented by tooth and arch. Tooth numbers are defined as follows: 1 = central incisor, 2 = lateral incisor, 3 = canine, 4 = first premolar, 5 = second premolar, 6 = first molar, 7 = second molar, and 8 = third molar. (Adapted from Schroeder, H. E.: Formation and Inhibition of Dental Calculus, Vienna, H. Huber Publishers, 1969.)

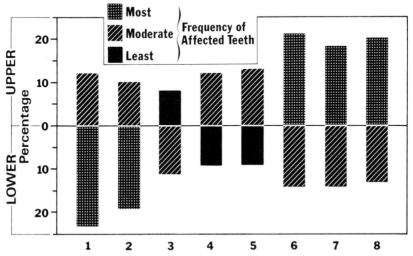

Figure 18–10. Intraoral prevalence of periodontal disease by individual teeth. The percentage of teeth affected by periodontal disease are classified as most, moderate, and least. Data are for industrial workers 40 to 44 years of age, with males and females combined. Tooth numbers are defined in legend for Figure 18–9. (Adapted from Bossert, W. A., and Marks, H. H.: J. Am. Dent. Assoc., *52*:429, 1956. Copyright by the American Dental Association. Reprinted by permission.)

molars; the upper anteriors and upper second molars have intermediate amounts of subgingival calculus; and the lower first and second premolars and the lower third molars have the least subgingival calculus. Combining both types of calculus, the lower centrals and laterals and the upper first molars have the most calculus; the upper second premolars and the upper second molars have less; and the lower second premolars and the lower third molars have the least calculus.[66, 94]

In general, the severity of bone loss follows the intraoral patterns of subgingival calculus and combined subgingival and supragingival calculus. The incisor and molar areas tend to be more severely involved than the canine and premolar areas,[22, 48, 55, 91, 103] and the least bone loss occurs in the lower canine and premolar region. Bone loss in the maxilla is generally more severe than that in the mandible,[5] with the situation reversed in the upper anterior region.[48, 108] Not surprisingly, the severity of bone loss is greater interproximally than it is on facial and lingual surfaces.

The upper and lower limits of the various patterns of plaque, gingivitis, calculus, and bone loss produce the intraoral pattern of periodontal disease shown in Figure 18–10.[11] *The teeth that are most severely affected by periodontal disease are the lower centrals, laterals, and all upper molars. The teeth that are moderately affected by periodontal disease are all the lower molars; the upper centrals, laterals, and premolars; and the lower canines. The teeth that are least affected by periodontal disease are the lower premolars and the upper canines.*

THE RELATIONSHIP BETWEEN PERIODONTAL DISEASE AND DENTAL CARIES

No clear-cut relationship has been established between the occurrence of periodontal disease and dental caries.[36] Some investigators consider these antagonistic processes, with the presence of one precluding the occurrence of the other.[13, 36] Several statistical studies have suggested a positive correlation between caries and gingival disease,[10] but this has not been a uniform finding[108] even though both have dental plaque as the chief etiologic factor.[54, 108]

Comparing the percentage of teeth extracted owing to caries with that caused by periodontal disease provides a common denominator for describing the relationship between the two processes (Fig. 18–11). The ravages of caries start shortly after the teeth erupt in the mouth, reach their greatest prevalence at approximately 20 years of age, and gradually decrease in a skewed pattern.[68] The greatest incidence of tooth extraction due to periodontal disease occurs between 20 and 50 years of age, and after 35 years of age more teeth are lost owing to periodontal disease than to dental caries.[2, 3] Even when there has been an absence of dental caries early in life, the need for tooth extraction is

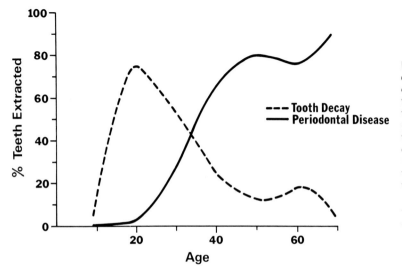

Figure 18–11. Tooth extractions due to dental caries and periodontal disease. A companion of the percentage of teeth indicated for extraction due to caries and periodontal disease by age was determined from almost 225,000 dental records of the U.S. Public Health Service facilities from 1948 through 1952. (Adapted from Pelton, W. J., Pennell, E. H., and Druzina, A.: J. Am. Dent. Assoc., 49:439, 1954. Copyright by the American Dental Association. Reprinted by permission.)

high before 40 years of age in those with moderate to advanced periodontal disease.[43]

It has been shown that periodontal disease is responsible for approximately 50 per cent of the total tooth loss after age 15, and caries for approximately 38 per cent. The remainder of the teeth are lost due to other causes such as accidents and impactions or are removed for orthodontic or prosthetic reasons.[68]

References

1. Ainamo, J., and Bay, I.: Problems and proposals for recording gingivitis and plaque. Int. Dent. J., 25:229, 1975.
2. Allen, E. F.: Statistical study of the primary causes of extraction. J. Dent. Res., 23:453, 1944.
3. Andrews, G., and Krogh, H. W.: Permanent tooth mortality. Dent. Prog., 1:30, 1961.
4. Arno, A., Waerhaug, J., Lovdal, A., and Schei, O.: Incidence of gingivitis as related to sex, occupation, tobacco consumption, toothbrushing and age. Oral Surg., 11:587, 1958.
5. Beagrie, G. S., and James, G. A.: The association of posterior tooth irregularity and periodontal disease. Br. Dent. J., 113:239, 1962.
5a. Bellini, H. T.: A System to Determine the Periodontal Therapeutic Needs of a Population. Oslo, Universitetsforlagets Trykningssentral, 1973.
6. Benjamin, E. M., Russell, A. L., and Smiley, R. D.: Periodontal disease in rural children of 25 Indian counties. J. Periodontol., 28:294, 1957.
7. Beube, F. E., Schwartz, M., and Thompson, R. H.: A comparison of effectiveness in plaque removal of an electric toothbrush and a conventional hand toothbrush. Periodontics, 2:71, 1964.
8. Bjorn, H., and Holmberg, K.: Radiographic determination of periodontal bone destruction in epidemiological research. Odontol. Revy, 17:232, 1966.
9. Bjorn, H., Halling, A., and Thyberg, H.: Radiographic assessment of marginal bone loss. Odontol. Revy, 20:165, 1969.
10. Black, G. V.: Something of the etiology and early pathology of the diseases of the periodontal membrane with suggestions as to treatment. Dent. Cosmos, 55:1219, 1913.
11. Bossert, W. A., and Marks, H. H.: Prevalence and characteristics of periodontal disease of 12,800 persons under periodic dental observation. J. Am. Dent. Assoc., 52:429, 1956.
12. Brandtzaeg, P., and Jamison, H. C.: The effect of controlled cleansing of the teeth on periodontal health and oral hygiene in Norwegian army recruits. J. Periodontol., 35:308, 1964.
13. Broderick, F. W.: Antagonism between dental caries and pyorrhea. Am. Dent. Surg., 49:103, 1929.
14. Carter, H. G., and Barnes, G. P.: The Gingival Bleeding Index. J. Periodontol., 45:801, 1974.
15. Chilton, N. W. (ed.): International Conference on Clinical Trials of Agents Used in the Prevention/Treatment of Periodontal Diseases. J. Periodont. Res., 9:(Suppl. 14):7–211, 1974.
16. Clemmer, B. A., and Barbano, J. P.: Reproducibility of periodontal score in clinical trials. J. Periodont. Res., 9(Suppl. 14):118, 1974.
17. Cohen, D. W., and Ship, I. I. (eds.): Clinical Methods in Periodontal Diseases Based on a Conference Held on May 20–23, 1967. J. Periodontol., 38:580–795, 1967.
18. Conroy, C. W., and Sturzenberger, O. P.: The rate of calculus formation in adults. J. Peridontol., 39:142, 1968.
19. Emslie, R. D.: Formal discussion. In Ramfjord, S. P.: Design of studies or clinical trials to evaluate the effectiveness of agents or procedures for the prevention, or treatment, of loss of the periodontium. J. Periodont. Res., 9:(Suppl. 14):78, 1974.
20. Ennever, J., Sturzenberger, O. P., and Radike, A. W.: Calculus Surface Index for scoring clinical calculus studies. J. Periodontol., 32:54, 1961.
21. Everett, F. G., and Fixott, H. C.: Use of an incorporated grid in the diagnosis of oral roentgenograms. Oral Surg., 16:1061, 1963.
22. Fleming, W. C.: Localization of pyorrhea involvement. Dent. Cosmos, 54:538, 1926.
23. Gjermo, P.: Formal discussion. In Hazen, S. P.: Indices for the measurement of gingival inflammation in clinical studies of oral hygiene and periodontal disease. J. Periodont. Res., 9(Suppl. 14):61, 1974.
24. Glass, R. L.: Hand and electric toothbrushing. J. Periodontol., 36:323, 1965.
25. Greene, J. C.: Periodontal disease in India: report of an epidemiological study. J. Dent. Res., 39:302, 1960.
26. Greene, J. C.: Oral hygiene and periodontal disease. Am. J. Public Health, 53:913, 1963.
27. Greene, J. C.: The Oral Hygiene Index—development and uses. J. Periodontol., 38:625, 1967.
28. Greene, J. C., and Vermillion, J. R.: Oral Hygiene Index: a method for classifying oral hygiene status. J. Am. Dent. Assoc., 61:172, 1960.
29. Greene, J. C., and Vermillion, J. R.: The Simplified Oral Hygiene Index. J. Am. Dent. Assoc., 68:7, 1964.
30. Harvey, C., and Kelly, J. E.: Decayed, Missing, and Filled Teeth Among Persons 1–74 Years, United States. Hyattsville, Md., U.S.P.H.S., U.S. Department of Health and Human Services, National Center for Health Statistics, DHHS Publication No. (PHS) 81–1673, Series 11, No. 223, 1981.
31. Johnson, E. S., Kelly, J. E., and Van Kirk, L. E.: Selected Dental Findings in Adults by Age, Race and Sex, United States 1960–1962. Washington, D.C., U.S. Department of Health, Education, and Welfare, National Center for Health Statistics, Publication No. 1000, Series 11, No. 7, 1965.
32. Kelly, J. E., and Harvey, C. R.: Basic Dental Examination Findings of Persons 1–74 Years, United States 1971–1974. Hyattsville, Md., U.S.P.H.S., U.S. Department of Health, Education, and Welfare, National Center for Health Statistics, DHEW Publication No. (PHS) 79-1662, Series 11, No. 214, 1979.
33. Kelly, J. E., and Sanchez, M. J.: Periodontal Disease and Oral Hygiene Among Children, United States. Washington, D.C., U.S.P.H.S., U.S. Department of Health, Education, and Welfare, National Center

for Health Statistics, Publication No. (HSM) 72-1060, Series 11, No. 117, 1972.

34. Kelly, J. E., and Van Kirk, L. E.: Periodontal Disease in Adults, United States 1960–1962. Washington, D.C., U.S.P.H.S., U.S. Department of Health, Education, and Welfare, National Center for Health Statistics, Publication No. 1000, Series 11, No. 12, 1966.

35. Kelly, J. E., Van Kirk, L. E., and Garst, C. C.: Oral Hygiene in Adults, United States 1960–1962. Washington, D.C., U.S.P.H.S., U.S. Department of Health, Education, and Welfare, National Center for Health Statistics, Publication No. 1000, Series 11, No. 16, 1966.

36. Kesel, R. G.: Are dental caries and periodontal disease incompatible? J. Periodontol., *21*:30, 1950.

37. Körber, K. H.: Periodontal pulsation. J. Periodontol., *41*:382, 1970.

38. Körber, K. H., and Körber, E.: Untersuchungen zur Biophysik des Parodontiums. Dtsch. Zahnärztl. Z., *17*:1585, 1962.

39. Lenox, J. A., and Kopczyk, R. A.: A clinical system for scoring a patient's oral hygiene performance. J. Am. Dent. Assoc., *86*:849, 1973.

40. Lobene, R. R.: The effect of an automatic toothbrush on gingival health. J. Periodontol., *35*:137, 1964.

41. Löe, H., and Silness, J.: Periodontal disease in pregnancy. Acta Odontol. Scand., *21*:533, 1963.

42. Löe, H., Theilade, E., and Jensen, S. B.: Experimental gingivitis in man. J. Periodontol., *36*:177, 1965.

43. Löe, H., Anerud, A., Boysen, H., and Smith, M.: The natural history of periodontal disease in man—study design and baseline data. J. Periodont. Res., *13*:550, 1978.

44. Lovdal, A., Arno, A., and Waerhaug, J.: Incidence of clinical manifestations of periodontal disease in light of oral hygiene and calculus formation. J. Am. Dent. Assoc., *56*:21, 1958.

45. Lovdal, A., Arno, A., Schei, O., and Waehaug, J.: Combined effect of subgingival scaling and controlled oral hygiene on the incidence of gingivitis. Acta Odontol. Scand., *19*:537, 1961.

46. Mandel, I. D.: Indices for measurement of soft accumulations in clinical studies of oral hygiene and periodontal disease. J. Periodont. Res., *9*(Suppl. 14):7, 1974.

47. Marshall-Day, C. D.: Chronic endemic fluorosis in Northern India. Br. Dent. J., *68*:409, 1940.

48. Marshall-Day, C. D., and Shourie, K. L.: A roentgenographic study of periodontal disease in India. J. Am. Dent. Assoc., *39*:572, 1949.

49. Massler, M.: The PMA Index for the assessment of gingivitis. J. Periodontol., *38*:592, 1967.

50. Massler, M., and Schour, I.: The PMA Index of Gingivitis. J. Dent. Res., *28*:634, 1949 (abstract).

51. Massler, M., Cohen, A., and Schour, I.: Epidemiology of gingivitis in children. J. Am. Dent. Assoc., *45*:319, 1952.

52. Massler, M., Schour, I., and Chopra, B.: Occurrence of gingivitis in suburban Chicago school children. J. Periodontol., *21*:146, 1950.

53. Miller, S. C.: Textbook of Periodontia, 3rd ed. Philadelphia, Blakiston, 1950.

54. Miller, S. C., and Seidler, B. B.: A correlation between periodontal disease and caries. J. Dent. Res., *19*:549, 1940.

55. Miller, S. C., and Seidler, B. B.: Relative alveoloclastic experience of the various teeth. J. Dent. Res., *21*:365, 1942.

56. Mühlemann, H. R.: Periodontometry, a method for measuring tooth mobility. Oral Surg., *4*:1220, 1951.

57. Mühlemann, H. R.: Tooth mobility. I. The measuring method--initial and secondary tooth mobility. J. Periodontol., *25*:125, 1954.

58. Mühlemann, H. R.: Ten years of tooth-mobility measurements. J. Periodontol., *31*:110, 1960.

59. Mühlemann, H. R., and Mazor, Z. S.: Gingivitis in Zurich school children. Helv. Odontol. Acta, *2*:3, 1958.

60. Mühlemann, H. R., and Son, S.: Gingival sulcus bleeding—leading symptom in initial gingivitis. Helv. Odontol. Acta, *15*:107, 1971.

61. Mühlemann, H. R., and Villa, P.: The Marginal Line Calculus Index. Helv. Odontol. Acta, *11*:175, 1967.

62. O'Leary, T. J.: Indices for measurement of tooth mobility in clinical studies. J. Periodont. Res., *9*(Suppl. 14):94, 1974.

63. O'Leary, T. J., and Rudd, K. D.: An instrument for measuring horizontal tooth mobility. Periodontics, *1*:249, 1963.

64. O'Leary, T. J., Drake, R. B., and Naylor, J. E.: The plaque control record. J. Periodontol., *43*:38, 1972.

65. Parfitt, G. J.: Development of an instrument to measure tooth mobility. J. Dent. Res., *37*:64, 1958 (abstract).

66. Parfitt, G. J.: A survey of the oral health of Navajo Indian children. Arch. Oral Biol., *1*:193, 1959.

67. Parfitt, G. J.: Measurement of the physiological mobility of individual teeth in an axial direction. J. Dent. Res., *39*:608, 1960.

68. Pelton, W. J., Pennell, E. H., and Druzina, A.: Tooth morbidity experience of adults. J. Am. Dent. Assoc., *49*:439, 1954.

69. Picton, D. C. A.: A method of measuring physiological tooth movements in man. J. Dent. Res., *36*:814, 1957.

70. Picton, D. C. A.: A study of normal tooth mobility and the changes with periodontal disease. Dent. Practit., *12*:167, 1962.

71. Podshadley, A. G., and Haley, J. V.: A method for evaluating patient hygiene performance by observation of selected tooth surfaces. Public Health Rep., *83*:259, 1968.

72. Proceedings of the Workshop on Quantitative Evaluation of Periodontal Diseases by Physical Measurement Techniques. J. Dent. Res., *58*:547, 1979.

73. Quigley, G., and Hein, J.: Comparative cleansing efficiency of manual and power brushing. J. Am. Dent. Assoc., *65*:26, 1962.

74. Ramfjord, S. P.: Indices for prevalence and incidence of periodontal disease. J. Periodontol., *30*:51, 1959.

75. Ramfjord, S. P.: The Periodontal Index (PDI). J. Periodontol., *38*:602, 1967.

76. Ramfjord, S. P.: Design of studies or clinical trials to evaluate the effectiveness of agents or procedures for the prevention, or treatment, of loss of

the periodontium. J. Periodont. Res., 9(Suppl. 14):78, 1974.

77. Ruffer, M. A.: Studies in the Palaeopathology of Ancient Egypt. Chicago, University of Chicago Press, 1921.

78. Rugg-Gunn, A. J., and Holloway, P. J.: Methods of measuring the reliability of caries prevalence and incremental data. Community Dent. Oral Epidemiol., 2:287, 1974.

79. Russell, A. L.: A system of classification and scoring for prevalence surveys of periodontal disease. J. Dent. Res., 35:350, 1956.

80. Russell, A. L.: A social factor associated with the severity of periodontal disease. J. Dent. Res., 36:922, 1957.

81. Russell, A. L.: The Geographical Distribution and Epidemiology of Periodontal Disease. World Health Organization Expert Committee on Dental Health (Periodontal Disease). WHO/DH/34. Geneva, 1960.

82. Russell, A. L.: International nutrition surveys: a summary of preliminary dental findings. J. Dent. Res., 42:233, 1963.

83. Russell, A. L.: Epidemiology of periodontal disease. Int. Dent. J., 17:282, 1967.

84. Russell, A. L.: Epidemiology and the rational bases of dental public health and dental practice. In Young, W. O., and Striffler, D. F. (eds.): The Dentist, His Practice, and His Community, 2nd ed. Philadelphia, W. B. Saunders Co., 1969, pp. 35–57.

85. Russell, A. L., and Ayers, P.: Periodontal disease and socioeconomic status in Birmingham, Ala. Am. J. Public Health., 50:206, 1960.

86. Russell, A. L., Leatherwood, E. C., Consolazio, C. F., and Van Reen, R.: Periodontal disease and nutrition in South Vietnam. J. Dent. Res., 44:775, 1965.

87. Sanchez, M. J.: Periodontal Disease Among Youth 12-17 Years, United States. Washington, D. C., U.S.P.H.S., U.S. Department of Health, Education, and Welfare, National Center for Health Statistics, Publication No. (HRA) 74-1623, Series 11, No. 141, 1974.

88. Sanchez, M. J.: Oral Hygiene Among Youths 12–17 Years, United States. Washington, D.C., U.S.P.H.S., U.S. Department of Health, Education, and Welfare, National Center for Health Statistics, Publication No. (HRA) 76-1633, Series 11, No. 151, 1975.

89. Sartwell, P. E. (ed.): Maxcy-Rosenau Preventive Medicine and Public Health, 10th ed. New York, Appleton-Century-Crofts, 1973, pp. 1–58.

90. Saxen, L.: Juvenile periodontics. J. Clin. Periodontol., 7:1, 1980.

91. Schei, O., Waerhaug, J., Lovdal, A., and Arno, A.: Alveolar bone loss as related to oral hygiene and age. J. Periodontol., 30:7, 1959.

92. Schour, I., and Massler, M.: Gingival disease in postwar Italy (1945). I. Prevalence of gingivitis in various age groups. J. Am. Dent. Assoc., 35:475, 1947.

93. Schour, I., and Massler, M.: Survey of gingival disease using the PMA Index. J. Dent. Res., 27:733, 1948.

94. Schroeder, H. E.: Formation and Inhibition of Den-

95. Shapiro, S., Pollack, B. R., and Gallant, D.: A special population available for periodontal research. Part II. A correlation and association analysis between oral hygiene and periodontal disease. J. Periodontol., 42:161, 1971.

96. Shaw, J. H., and Sweeney, E. A.: Nutrition in relation to dental medicine. In Goodhart, R. S., and Shils, M. E. (eds.): Modern Nutrition in Health and Disease. Philadelphia, Lea & Febiger, 1973, p. 756.

97. Sheiham, A.: The prevalence and severity of periodontal disease in Surrey school children. Dent. Practit., 19:232, 1969.

98. Shick, R. A., and Ash, M. M.: Evaluation of the vertical method of toothbrushing. J. Periodontol., 32:346, 1961.

99. Silness, P., and Löe, H.: Periodontal disease in pregnancy. Acta Odontol. Scand., 22:121, 1964.

100. Suomi, J. D., and Barbano, J. P.: Patterns of gingivitis. J. Periodontol., 39:71, 1968.

101. Suomi, J. D., Plumbo, J., and Barbano, J. P.: A comparative study of radiographs and pocket measurements in periodontal disease evaluation. J. Periodontol., 39:311, 1968.

102. Suomi, J. D., Greene, J. C., Vermillion, J. R., Doyle, J., Chang, J. J., and Leatherwood, E. C.: The effect of controlled oral hygiene procedures on the progression of periodontal disease in adults: results after third and final year. J. Periodontol., 42:152, 1971.

103. Tenenbaum, B., Karshan, M., Ziskin, D., and Nahoun, K. I.: Clinical and microscopic study of the gingivae in periodontosis. J. Am. Dent. Assoc., 40:302, 1950.

104. Ten-State Nutrition Survey 1968-1970, by Health Services and Mental Health Administration, U. S. Department of Health, Education, and Welfare. Atlanta Center for Disease Control. Atlanta, Publication No. (HSM) 72-8131, 1972, Vol. 3, pp. 111, 126–131.

105. Turesky, S., Gilmore, N. D., and Glickman, I.: Reduced plaque formation by the chloromethyl analogue of victamine. C. J. Periodontol., 41:41, 1970.

106. Volpe, A. R.: Indices for the measurement of hard deposits in clinical studies of oral hygiene and periodontal disease. J. Periodont. Res., 9(Suppl. 14):31, 1974.

107. Volpe, A. R., Manhold, J. H., and Hazen, S. P.: In vivo calculus assessment: a method and its reproducibility. J. Periodontol., 36:292, 1965.

108. White, C. L., and Russell, A. L.: Some relations between dental caries experience and active periodontal disease in two thousand adults. N.Y. J. Dent., 32:211, 1962.

109. Wilkinson, F. C., Adamson, K. T., and Knight, F.: A study of the incidence of dental disease in the aborigines, from the examination of 65 in the collection found in the Melbourne University. Aust. J. Dent., 33:109, 1929.

110. Zimmerman, E. R., and Baker, W. A.: Effect of geographic location and race on gingival disease in children. J. Am. Dent. Assoc., 61:542, 1960.

tal Calculus. Berne, Stuttgart, Vienna, H. Huber Publishers, 1969, pp. 66–68.

Glossary

Abrasion, dental: Loss of substance induced by mechanical wear other than that of mastication.

Abscess, gingival: Localized purulent inflammation of the gingiva.

Abscess, periapical: Localized purulent inflammation of the periapical tissue.

Abscess, periodontal: Localized purulent inflammation of the periodontal tissue.

Acute herpetic gingivostomatitis: Infection of the oral cavity caused by herpes simplex virus.

Acute necrotizing ulcerative gingivitis (ANUG): Inflammatory destructive disease of the gingiva, probably caused by a complex of bacterial organisms (fusiform bacilli, spirochetes, and others) and underlying tissue changes that facilitate the pathogenic activity of the bacteria.

Alveolar bone: The bone that forms the tooth sockets and supports the teeth.

Antibody: Proteins, primarily derived from mature plasma cells, that are effectors of humoral immunity.

Ascorbic acid: Vitamin C.

Atrophy, gingival: Recession of the gingiva without overt inflammation.

Attached gingiva: Gingival tissue that is tightly bound to the underlying periosteum of the alveolar bone.

Attrition, dental: Wear and tear of the tooth caused by opposing teeth.

Bacteremia: Presence of bacteria in the blood.

Bacterial endocarditis: Disease in which infective microorganisms colonize the damaged endocardium or heart valve.

Bacterial plaque: Complex, organized mass of bacterial colonies attached to the tooth surface or to calculus.

Bass method of toothbrushing: The bristles of a soft brush are placed at a 45-degree angle to the long axis of the teeth, vibrating pressure is exerted on the long axis of the bristles, and attempts are made to force the bristle ends into the gingival sulci.

Bleeding Points Index: Assessment of the presence or absence of bleeding in the interproximal, facial, and lingual surfaces of the teeth, made by drawing a periodontal probe along the sulci and examining for bleeding after 30 seconds.

Bone graft: A surgical procedure using any of a variety of materials in an effort to actively induce bone formation, deposit new bone, or act as a scaffolding for bone formation in periodontal defects.

Bone Loss: Reduction in the height of alveolar bone as a consequence of periodontal disease.

Bruxism: The clenching or grinding of the teeth when the individual is not chewing or swallowing.

Calculus, subgingival: Mineralized bacterial plaque below the crest of the marginal gingiva.

Calculus, supragingival: Mineralized bacterial plaque above the crest of the marginal gingiva.

Carcinoma: Malignant epithelial tumor.

Caries: Demineralization and cavitation of the mineralized tooth structures.

Cementum: Calcified mesenchymal tissue forming the outer covering of the roots of teeth; may be acellular *(primary)* or cellular *(secondary)*.

Centric occlusion: The position of the teeth when the mandible is in the retruded position.

Charters method of toothbrushing: A medium or hard brush is used with the bristles at a 45-degree angle to the occlusal plane and activated with short back-and-forth strokes.

Chlorhexidine: A diguanidohexane with pronounced antiseptic properties, used to inhibit plaque formation.

Chronic desquamative gingivitis: Intense redness and desquamation of the epithelial surfaces of the oral mucosa from unknown causes.

Clefts: Indentations extending from and into the gingival margin for varying distances.

Col: The valley-like depression of the interdental gingiva between two teeth, under the contact, formed where buccal and lingual papillae are connected.

Connective tissue: The lamina propria, consisting of densely collagenous tissue with few elastic fibers.

Crevicular epithelium: The epithelial lining of the sulcus or periodontal pocket.

Crown, anatomic: The portion of the tooth covered by enamel.

Crown, clinical: The portion of the tooth denuded of epithelium and projecting into the oral cavity.

Curettage: Scraping of the gingival wall of a periodontal pocket to separate and remove diseased soft tissue.

Defense mechanisms: Resistance to bacterial and mechanical aggressions, provided by saliva, epithelial surface, and inflammatory response.

Dehiscence: Facial root surface denuded of bone, including the surrounding marginal bone.

Diabetes: Disease characterized by hypofunction of the beta cells of the islets of Langerhans in the pancreas, leading to high blood glucose levels and excretion of sugar in the urine.

Diet: The total intake of food, water, and nutrients.

Down's syndrome (mongolism, trisomy 21): Congenital disease caused by a chromosomal abnormality, resulting in mental deficiency and growth retardation.

Epidemiology: The study of the pattern (distribution) and dynamics of dental diseases in a human population.

Epithelial attachment: The mechanism of union of the epithelial cells with the tooth surface.

Epithelial migration: The apical displacement of the epithelial cells along the root surface as a result of periodontal disease.

Epithelial rests: Strands of epithelial cells in the periodontal ligament.

Epulis: Generic term used to describe benign localized growths of the gingiva.

Exfoliative cytology: A diagnostic procedure consisting of the microscopic examination of cells obtained by scraping the surface of the suspected area or by rinsing the oral cavity.

Fenestrations: Isolated areas in which the root is denuded of bone, with persistence of the marginal bone.

Festoons: Lifesaver-shaped enlargements of the marginal gingiva, occurring most frequently in the canine and premolar regions on the facial surfaces.

Flap: A section of gingiva and/or mucosa surgically separated from the underlying tissues to provide visibility of and access to the bone and root surfaces. The flap also allows the gingiva to be positioned in a different location in patients with mucogingival problems.

Frenectomy: An operation for complete removal of the frenum including its attachment to the underlying bone.

Frenotomy: Incision of the frenum.

Furcation involvement: A commonly occurring condition in which the bifurcation or trifurcation of multirooted teeth is denuded by periodontal disease.

Gingiva: The part of the oral mucosa that covers the alveolar processes of the jaws and surrounds the necks of the teeth.

Gingival curettage: The removal of the inflamed soft tissue lateral to the pocket wall.

Gingival enlargement: An increase in the size of the gingiva.

Gingival fluid: The material that seeps into the gingival sulcus from the gingival connective tissue, containing plasma proteins that enhance adhesion and have antimicrobial properties.

Gingival Index (GI): Measuring system to assess the severity of gingivitis and its location.

Gingival inflammation: The most common form of gingival disease, characterized by redness, swelling, and the tendency of the gingiva to bleed.

Gingival pocket: A pocket formed by gingival enlargement without destruction of the underlying periodontal tissues.

Gingival recession (atrophy): Exposure of the tooth by apical migration of the epithelial attachment.

Gingival sulcus: The shallow crevice or space around the tooth, bounded by the surface of the tooth on one side and by the epithelium lining the free margin of the gingiva on the other.

Gingivectomy: Excision of the gingiva to provide visibility of and access to the root surface.

Gingivitis: Inflammation of the gingiva.

Gingivoplasty: Artificial reshaping of the gingiva to create physiologic gingival contours.

Gracey curette: A specially designed, area-specific curette that is used for subgingival scaling and root planing.

Halitosis: Foul or offensive odor emanating from the mouth.

History: Past occurrence of some condition.

Hormones: Organic substances produced by the endocrine glands.

Host response: The ability of the individual body to mediate the insult of destructive forces such as microorganisms or trauma.

Hypertension: High blood pressure.

Inadvertent curettage: Partial removal of the inflamed soft tissue lateral to the pocket wall, performed unintentionally during scaling and root planning.

Incision: The cut produced with a sharp instrument to open the field in a surgical operation.

Indices: Graduated scales to measure clinical conditions.

Infrabony pockets (subcrestal or intra-alveolar): A periodontal pocket that extends apical to the level of the adjacent alveolar bone.

Instruments: Periodontal tools designed for specific purposes such as calculus detection, calculus removal, and measurement of probing depth.

Interdental bone: Alveolar bone situated between two adjacent teeth.

Interdental cleansing aids: Devices used to remove plaque between teeth, such as dental floss or interproximal brushes.

Interdental gingiva: Gingiva situated between two adjacent teeth, usually made up of two papillae (facial and lingual) and the col.

Interdental papillae: Elevated portions of the interdental gingiva connected by the col under the contact point.

Interdental septum: See *Interdental bone.*

Junctional epithelium: Gingival epithelium united to the tooth surface by epithelial attachment.

Juvenile periodontitis: Advanced destructive periodontal lesions in children and adolescents; may be localized or generalized.

Keratin: Fibrous protein found in the epidermis, hair, and nails, which is produced by keratinocytes.

Keratinization: The biochemical and morphologic process by which superficial epithelial cells become impregnated with keratin. The surface cells form scales and lose their nuclei, and keratohyalin granules appear in the cells of the subsurface layer.

Leukocytes: White blood cells.

Lichen planus: Inflammatory disease of skin and mucous membranes characterized by the eruption of papules; relatively common in the mouth.

Mastication: The process of chewing.

Microorganisms: Microscopic living organisms including bacteria, viruses, fungi, and others.

Mobility: Movement of the tooth within the socket in response to various forces; may be physiologic or pathologic.

Mouth breathing: Inspiration and expiration of air through the oral cavity due to habit and/or nasal obstruction, which may result in gingival pathology.

Mucogingival defects: Abnormalities that appear in the gingivo–mucous membrane relationship. They consist of pockets extending to or beyond the mucogingival junction, absence of attached gingiva with no pocket formation, isolated gingival recession, and high frenum insertions.

Mucogingival junction: The line separating the attached gingiva from the alveolar mucosa; also called the *mucogingival line.*

Mucogingival line: See *Mucogingival junction.*

Mucogingival surgery: Plastic surgical procedures for the correction of abnormal gingivo–mucous membrane relationships.

Mucous Membrane: See *Oral mucosa.*

Nutrition: The complex relationship between the individual's total health status and the intake, digestion, and utilization of nutrients.

Occlusion: The contact relationship of the teeth.

Oral mucosa: The tissue that lines the oral cavity, including the gingiva; also called *mucous membrane.*

Orthodontic therapy: Correction of malpositions of teeth.

Osseous defects: Alterations in the morphology of the alveolar bone due to periodontal disease. These include vertical and angular defects, osseous craters, bulbous bone contours, and inconsistent margins and ledges.

Osseous surgery: The procedure by which changes in the alveolar bone are accomplished to rid it of deformities caused by periodontal disease or other, related factors. It can be additive (attempts to restore the alveolar bone to its original level) or subtractive (recontouring of the existing bone to a more normal shape).

Pack: Dressings used for the protection of periodontal surgical wounds.

Parakeratinization: The process of keratinization in which the superficial layers of the epithelium retain their nuclei, albeit pyknotic, but show some signs of being keratinized. (See also *Keratinization*.)

Pemphigus: Chronic vesiculobullous lesion involving the skin and mucous membranes and invariably affecting the oral mucosa; currently considered to have autoimmune etiology.

Pericoronitis: Inflammation of the gingiva in relation to the crown of an incompletely erupted tooth.

Periodontal disease: Pathologic processes involving the tooth-supporting structures.

Periodontal Disease Index (PDI): Epidemiologic index developed by Ramfjord that estimates periodontal disease in six preselected teeth for each individual.

Periodontal emergencies: Conditions requiring immediate treatment, such as periodontal abscesses and ANUG.

Periodontal flap: See *Flap*.

Periodontal health: Condition of the periodontal tissues in the absence of disease.

Periodontal Index (PI): Epidemiologic index developed by Russell that measures the presence or absence of gingival inflammation and its severity; pocket formation; and masticatory function.

Periodontal ligament: The connective tissue structure that surrounds the tooth root and connects it to the bone.

Periodontal pocket: A pathologically deepened gingival sulcus.

Periodontal surgery: Treatment procedures that involve intentional severing or incising of gingival tissue for the purpose of controlling, eliminating, and preventing periodontal disease.

Periodontal therapy: Procedures performed for the control and correction of periodontal disease and its effects on the tissues.

Periodontitis: The most common type of periodontal disease, resulting from the extension of the inflammatory process initiated in the gingiva to the supporting periodontal tissues.

Plaque: See *Bacterial plaque*.

Pregnancy gingivitis: Accentuation of the gingival inflammatory response to local irritants, induced by the hormone changes associated with pregnancy.

Puberty gingivitis: Accentuation of the gingival inflammatory response to local irritants, induced by the hormone changes associated with puberty.

Radiographic examination: Adjunct to clinical examination, consisting of the analysis of intraoral roentgenograms.

Restorative dentistry: The phase of clinical dentistry concerned with the restoration of teeth.

Root: The portion of the tooth embedded in alveolar bone (*clinical root*) or that portion of the tooth covered with cementum (*anatomic root*).

Root planing: The removal of plaque, embedded calculus, and altered cementum from root surfaces, using periodontal curettes and scalers.

Scaling: The removal of plaque and calculus from the crown and root surfaces of the teeth, using curettes and scalers.

Stomatitis: Any inflammatory disease of the oral mucosa.

Subgingival curettage: The removal of the inflamed soft tissue lateral and apical to the pocket wall and extending to the osseous crest.

Subgingival scaling: The removal of subgingival calculus.

Sulcular fluid: See *Gingival fluid*.

Suprabony pocket (supracrestal or supra-alveolar): A periodontal pocket that extends coronal to the level of the adjacent alveolar bone.

Suture: Material and technique used in closing a surgical wound.

Systemic disease: Disease pertaining to or affecting the body as a whole.

Temporomandibular joint (TMJ): Articulation of the temporal bone with the mandible.

Tooth: Hard, calcified structure located in the alveolar processes of the mandible or maxilla.

Vitamin deficiency: Disease occurring from lack of needed amounts of one or more organic compounds required in trace amounts and not synthesized by the body.

Index

Note: Page numbers in italic refer to illustrations; page numbers followed by (t) indicate tables; page numbers followed by (g) indicate Glossary entries.

Tooth (teeth) (*Continued*)
  attrition of, 119, *119*
  bone loss around, in juvenile periodontitis, 74, *75*
  calculus on, distribution of, 272, *273, 274*
  clinical examination of, 128–133
  deciduous, carious, 70
    loose, 70
    malposed, 70
    periodontium of, 69–70
    shedding of, and periodontium, 72
  developmental grooves in, and prognosis of individual teeth, 153
  eruption of, and gingivitis, 70
    gingival changes and, 69
    partial, and pericoronitis, 41–42, *42*
  examination of, 128–133
  extraction of, due to caries, *274, 274*–275
    due to periodontal disease, *274, 274*–275
  individual, prognosis of, 151–153
  irregular, and gingival enlargement, *33*
  loosening of, radiation therapy and, 113
  loss of, maintenance therapy and, 249–251, *250*
    periodontal disease and, *274, 274*–275
    radiation therapy and, 113
  malposition of, and gingival recession, 30, *32*
  migration of, distolabial, in juvenile periodontitis, 74
    mesial, 17
    pathologic, 132, *132*
      causes of, 132–133
    physiologic, 17
    with diastema formation, in juvenile periodontitis, 74, *75*
  mobility of, 282(g)
    and prognosis of individual teeth, 151
    assessment of, techniques for, 259
    clinical examination of, *131*, 131–132
    in juvenile periodontitis, 74, *75*
    pathologic, causes of, 132
    postoperative, 217
  morphology of, and prognosis of individual teeth, 151–152
  occlusal wear of, *119*, 119–120, *120*
    and aging, 17, *18*
  proximal wear of, 17
  roots of. See *Root(s).*
  rotational axis of, *11*
  sensitivity of, patient education about, 218–219
  stains on, 129–131
  tilted, *108*, 109
  unreplaced missing, and pathologic migration, 133
    complications from, *108*, 109
  wasting disease of, 128–129
Toothache, periodontal pocket and, 47
Toothbrushes, 195–196
  bristle types in, 196
  electrically powered,196, 201
Toothbrushing, aggressive, and abrasion, 129, *129*
  frequency of, and plaque control, 206
  methods of, 197–201. See also names of specific methods, e.g., *Bass method; Charters method.*

Toothbrushing (*Continued*)
  postoperative, contraindications for, 217
  resumption of, postoperative, 218
  trauma from, 111–113, *112*, 196
Toothpicks, improper use of, and gingival inflammation, 112
Toothsetting, in bruxism, 120
Torques, and bone formation and resorption, 121
Trabecula(ae), cancellous, 14, *15*
Transseptal fibers, 5
  of periodontal ligament, 9, *11*
Trauma, from occlusion, acute, 121–122
  and marginal periodontitis, 123, *123*, 125
  and pathologic migration, 133
  and periodontitis, 47
  and reattachment process, 150
  and tooth mobility, 132
  causes of, 122
  changes produced by, 123
  chronic, 122
  faulty dental restorations and, 105
  occlusal forces and, 121
  periodontal findings in, 138–139
  primary, 122
  radiographic signs of, *124*, 125
  secondary, 122
  stages of, 122–123
  from toothbrushing, 111–113, *112*
Trifurcation, See also *Furcation involvement.*
  and prognosis of individual teeth, 153, *153.*
  angular bone loss and, radiographic appearance of, *142*
  denudation of, in periodontal disease, 64
Trisomy 21. See *Down's syndrome.*
Tuberculosis, periodontal manifestations of, 80
Tumors, and gingival enlargement, 32, 34, *34*
  gingival, 22
    benign, 37
    giant cell, 37
    malignant, 37
  jaw, and tooth mobility, 132
  periodontal manifestations of, 80
Turesky-Gilmore-Glickman modification, of Quigley-Hein Plaque Index, 261, 261(t)

Ulceration, and bone loss, in periodontal disease, 58
  gingival, chemicals and, 113
    radiation therapy and, 113
  in periodontal pocket wall, 52, *52*

Valium, for sedation, in periodontal surgery, 212
Vancomycin, in bacterial endocarditis prophylaxis, 166(t)
Veillonella, and plaque mineralization, 100
Vertical bone defects, in juvenile periodontitis, 62
  in periodontal disease, 62, *62*
Vitamin C deficiency, and periodontal disease, 157–158